# EFFECTS OF DISEASES ON LABORATORY TESTS

# *Jerome J. Berner,* M.D.

Associate Pathologist
Lutheran Medical Center
and
Assistant Clinical Professor of Pathology
Case Western Reserve University School of Medicine
Cleveland, Ohio

# EFFECTS OF DISEASES ON LABORATORY TESTS

*J.B. Lippincott Company*

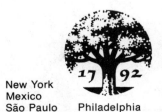

New York                   London
Mexico                     St. Louis
São Paulo    Philadelphia    Sydney

*Acquisitions Editor:*   Lisa A. Biello
*Sponsoring Editor:*   Richard Winters
*Manuscript Editor:*   Barbara Farabaugh
*Indexer:*   Julia B. Schwager
*Art Director:*   Maria S. Karkucinski
*Designer:*   Ronald Dorfman
*Production Supervisor:*   J. Corey Gray
*Production Assistant:*   Edward Scirrotto
*Compositor:*   Bi-Comp, Inc.
*Printer/Binder:*   R.R. Donnelley & Sons Company

The author and publisher have exerted every effort to ensure that drug selection and dosage set forth in this text are in accord with current recommendations and practice at the time of publication. However, in view of ongoing research, changes in government regulations, and the constant flow of information relating to drug therapy and drug reactions, the reader is urged to check the package insert for each drug for any change in indications and dosage and for added warnings and precautions. This is particularly important when the recommended agent is a new or infrequently employed drug.

1        3        5        6        4        2

**Library of Congress Cataloging in Publication Data**

Berner, Jerome J.
    Effects of diseases on laboratory tests.
    Bibliography: p.
    Includes index.
    1. Diagnosis, Laboratory.  I. Title.
[DNLM:  1. Diagnosis, Laboratory.  QY 4 B525d]
RB37.B47   1984        616.07′5        82-23936
ISBN 0-397-50580-9

# *PREFACE*

*T*his unique book is for medical technologists, nurses, medical students, physicians, and anyone else who would like a clearer understanding of diseases and the effects of each disease on laboratory tests. Through my years of teaching medical technologists I have been aware of the need for a book like *Effects of Diseases on Laboratory Tests*. The text is designed to help bridge the gap between clinical medicine and laboratory medicine. I feel that a better understanding of the interrelationship of diseases and laboratory tests will benefit everyone who orders, performs, or interprets such tests.

The chapters are arranged according to body systems rather than laboratory disciplines. The text includes only the most common medical disorders and only those that affect laboratory tests. Diseases that are diagnosed solely by history and physical examination or biopsy or that are exclusively monitored by electrocardiograms, pulmonary-function tests, or radiologic techniques are not included. A distinctive feature of this text is the emphasis on explanations and descriptions of the causes and fundamental mechanisms of each disease. There is only limited discussion of the clinical features of the diseases. Discussions of differential diagnoses, epidemiologies, therapies, and prognoses are intentionally omitted. The text attempts to be selective rather than all-inclusive and elucidating rather than confusing.

The Laboratory Findings sections in each chapter include the most commonly performed and affected laboratory tests. The major, but not sole, reference source for this information is the third edition of *Interpretation of Diagnostic Tests* by J. Wallach (Boston, Little, Brown, 1978). Laboratory methods and normal ranges are excluded, as are nonlaboratory diagnostic modalities.

I have used illustrations from many different sources in an attempt to clarify concepts or disease processes with which readers might be unfamiliar.

Each chapter was reviewed by a panel of medical technologists, pathologists, and physicians whose specialty was appropriate to that chapter. I could not have written this book without the many valuable comments and suggestions offered by these experts.

Jerome J. Berner, M.D.

# ACKNOWLEDGMENTS

*I* could not have written this book without the critical and helpful comments provided by the many medical technologists, physicians, and nurses who reviewed various chapters. I thank you all most appreciatively. If this text has reached its goal, it will have been only with your help.

*Review panel, Chapters 1–11:* C. Finegan, MT(ASCP); A. Mozil, MT(ASCP);
    K. Ott, MT(ASCP); I. Pillay, M.D.; J. Wingenfeld, MT(ASCP);
    B. Wolpert, MT(ASCP)
*Chapter 1:* P. Maroo, M.D.; M. Mellino, M.D.; A. Robertson, Jr., M.D. Ph.D.;
    W. Sinclair, M.D.; T. Tuthill, M.D.
*Chapter 2:* P. Kondapalli, M.D.; W. Sinclair, M.D.; T. Tuthill, M.D.
*Chapter 3:* P. Greenwalt, M.D.; M. Henoch, M.D.; M. Petrelli, M.D.;
    T. Tuthill, M.D.
*Chapter 4:* P. Greenwalt, M.D.; M. Henoch, M.D.; M. Petrelli, M.D.
*Chapter 5:* P. Hall, M.D.; M. C. Park, M.D.; E. Ricanati, M.D.
*Chapter 6:* W. Jeffries, M.D.; S. Johnson, I(ASCP); H. Taylor, M.D.
*Chapter 7:* B. Banker, M.D.; C. Barusch, M.D.; J. Morris, M.D.
*Chapter 8:* T. Bidari, M.D.; J. Hogan, M.D.; D. Maslar, MT(ASCP);
    G. McLaren, M.D.; A. Snyder, MT(ASCP)S.H.; R. Weisman, M.D.
*Chapter 9:* J. Aponte, M.D.; I. Kushner, M.D.; N. Zein, M.D.
*Chapter 10:* E. Hirsch, M.D.; I. Kushner, M.D.; I. Schafer, M.D.;
    A. Walker, M.D.
*Chapter 11:* T. Gavan, M.D.; K. V. Gopalakrishna, M.D.;
    K. Jarmuziewicz, MT(ASCP); D. Kiraly, R.N.; L. Sykes, MT(ASCP)

I also want to thank my secretaries, Barbara Foreman and Marilyn Longmore, for their patience, persistence, and skills in interpreting my writing and notations, for their rendering of my many revisions, and for their production of a fine-looking manuscript.

I want to thank the librarians at Lutheran Medical Center, Rosary Martin and Irene Szentkiralyi, who helped me track down and obtain all of the references I needed. The staff at the Cleveland Medical Library was also of great assistance.

The original illustrations were skillfully drawn by Barbara Hawekotte.

Photographers Gerry Daley, Willie Hernandez, and Joe Tyrpak of the Visual Aids Department of Lutheran Medical Center photographed all of the borrowed illustrations in preparation for publication. I am deeply grateful to them for their excellent contribution toward the production of this book.

I appreciate the generous permissions granted by many publishers and authors to use their illustrations.

I appreciate the encouragement, support, and guidance of Lisa Biello and Richard Winters of J.B. Lippincott Company.

# CONTENTS

## *3* GASTROINTESTINAL DISEASES     72

## 6   ENDOCRINE DISEASES                                   158

## 7   NEUROLOGIC DISEASES                                  192

# 8  HEMATOLOGIC DISEASES

## 9 MUSCULOSKELETAL AND CONNECTIVE-TISSUE DISEASES

# *10* NUTRITIONAL AND METABOLIC DISEASES     295

# EFFECTS OF DISEASES ON LABORATORY TESTS

# 1

# *CARDIOVASCULAR DISEASES*

Congenital Heart Disease
Acute Rheumatic Fever and Rheumatic
    Heart Disease
Hypertension
Coronary-Artery Disease and Myocardial
    Infarction
Cor Pulmonale (Pulmonary Heart
    Disease)
Pericarditis
Infective Endocarditis
Cardiomyopathies
Congestive Heart Failure

Atherosclerosis
Aneurysm
Syphilitic Cardiovascular Diseases
Raynaud's Phenomenon
Arterial Thrombosis and Embolism
Gangrene
Hypersensitivity Vasculitis
Polyarteritis Nodosa
Temporal Arteritis
Peripheral Venous Disease
Shock

## *CONGENITAL HEART DISEASE*

Approximately one baby in 100 is born with a congenital abnormality of the cardiovascular system. In only about 3% of these births can a cause be ascribed. One cause is maternal rubella (German measles) occurring during the first two months of pregnancy. Chromosomal abnormalities, such as Down's syndrome (mongolism), may also result in cardiac malformations. Most cardiovascular malformations result in either an obstruction of blood flow or an abnormal routing of blood flow through the heart. Rerouting indicates the presence of a shunt, which is an abnormal passage of blood from one side of the heart directly to the other. In a right-to-left shunt, some poorly oxygenated venous blood bypasses the lungs and appears in the left ventricle, in the aorta, and throughout the body. This poorly oxygenated circulating blood imparts a bluish tint, known as cyanosis, to the skin, lips, and nail beds. These infants are therefore termed *blue babies*. In a left-to-right shunt, fully oxygenated arterial blood passes abnormally to the right side of the heart. This oxygenated blood does not impart cyanosis. Malformations in which there are obstructions, but not rerouting, of blood flow do not result in cyanosis.

    Diagnosis of congenital heart disease is accomplished through use of medical history, physical examination, electrocardiogram, echocardiography, and chest x-ray examination. In cases in which further diagnostic confirmation is necessary or surgery is required, cardiac catheterization and angiocardiography are performed. The latter involves the instillation of a radiopaque solution into the heart and observation of the course of blood flow on x-ray film. An intracardiac catheter may also be used to obtain pressure readings and blood-oxygen saturation measurements from various sites in the heart.

## LABORATORY FINDINGS

### Right-to-Left Shunt

Decreased arterial $PO_2$

Increased red blood cell (RBC) count, hemoglobin, hematocrit; this secondary erythrocytosis results from arterial hypoxemia and tissue hypoxia, which stimulate renal erythropoietin formation and erythropoiesis

X-ray contrast material used in angiocardiography contains iodine, which causes alteration of some laboratory tests that evaluate thyroid status

### Laboratory Findings of Complications

Secondary hypertension

Myocardial infarction

Cor pulmonale (pulmonary heart disease)

Pericarditis

Infective endocarditis, with or without embolization

Congestive heart failure

## ACUTE RHEUMATIC FEVER AND RHEUMATIC HEART DISEASE

Group A streptococci may cause infection of the throat or tonsils. If untreated, this may produce an immunologic reaction to the streptococci in about 2 weeks to 3 weeks. This reaction is known as *acute rheumatic fever*. Migrating polyarthritis, an inflammation of the large joints of the body, occurs in about 85% of affected patients. Inflammation of the heart is seen in about 65% of cases. The myocardial lesions are probably the result of autoimmunity induced by streptococcal antigens that cross-react with heart muscle, but this has not yet been proved. During the acute phase of the disease, the valves of the heart may become inflamed and boggy with fluid. The heart muscle and covering of the heart may also be involved.

Rheumatic heart disease occurs years after the patient has had acute rheumatic fever. Rheumatic fever does not inevitably result in heart damage, but anyone who has had the illness is at increased risk of recurrent attacks of rheumatic fever. The heart disease affects the heart covering (pericardium), heart muscle (myocardium), and heart lining and valves (endocardium). Damage to the heart valves interferes with their normal opening or closing and may result in heart failure. Rheumatic valvulitis also increases the susceptibility of those valves to subsequent infective endocarditis. Thrombi may form on the injured endocardial lining of the valves, atrium, or atrial appendage. Thrombi may fragment and circulate as emboli, occluding arteries and causing brain, kidney, intestine, spleen, or limb infarction.

## LABORATORY FINDINGS

### Rheumatic Fever

There is no specific laboratory test for rheumatic fever. However, laboratory tests may be helpful in confirming the presence of inflammation and the recent occurrence of a streptococcal infection.

*Nonspecific Test Results Indicating Inflammation*

Increased sedimentation rate, increased C-reactive protein, leukocytosis; these are used to follow disease activity and response to therapy

Mild normocytic anemia, chronic disease type (hemoglobin 8 g/dl–12g/dl); occasionally microcytic

Increased fibrinogen, increased $\alpha_2$-globulin; these are acute phase reactants, which indicate acute inflammation

Decreased albumin (due to hemodilution)

*Test Indicating Present Infection*

Throat culture showing Group A streptococci

*Tests Indicating Prior Recent Streptococcal Infection*

Elevated serum anti–streptolysin O (ASO) titer—occurs in 80% of patients convalescing from streptococcal sore throat. This appears 2 weeks after infection, peaks at 4 weeks to 6 weeks after infection, and may remain elevated for months. The titer is not related to the severity of the disease, and its rate of fall is not related to the course of the disease.

Increased anti–deoxyribonuclease (DNase) B titer

Increased "Streptozyme" titer; this measures several streptococcal antibodies

### Rheumatic Heart Disease

*Laboratory Findings of Complications:*

Active rheumatic fever

Infective endocarditis

Congestive heart failure

Arterial embolism with infarction of brain, kidney, intestines

## *HYPERTENSION*

Hypertension in adults is the sustained elevation of arterial blood pressure above 140 mm Hg systolic pressure and 90 mm Hg diastolic pressure.

Maintenance of normal blood pressure is achieved through a complex interaction of many organs and systems (Fig. 1-1). The primary factors that control

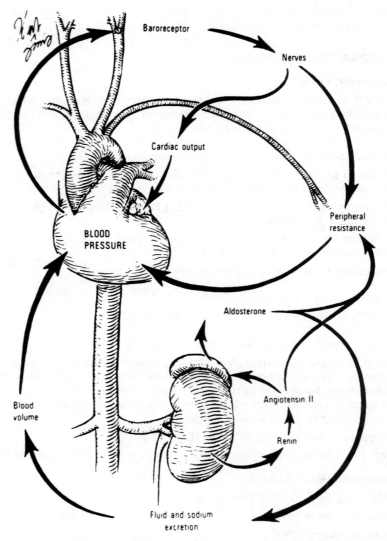

**Fig. 1-1.** The mechanism of blood-pressure regulation. (DeBakey M, Gotto A: The Living Heart, p 195. New York, Raven Press, 1977)

blood pressure are cardiac output, aortic elasticity, peripheral resistance of small blood vessels, and blood and extracellular fluid volumes. These are affected by the nervous system (pressure receptors, sympathetic nerves, emotional states, and mental stress), the kidneys (renin and salt regulation), and the adrenal glands (aldosterone, epinephrine, norepinephrine). When any of these factors is altered without normal compensation occurring, the result is hyper- or hypotension.[17]

The renal enzyme *renin* plays a key role in blood-pressure control. This enzyme is contained in the juxtaglomerular apparatus surrounding the afferent glomerular arterioles in the kidneys (Fig. 1-2). Its secretion is influenced by mean arteriolar pressure, sodium content of the tubular fluid, and the neural innervation of the juxtaglomerular cells. A fall in blood pressure, sodium, or fluid volume stimulates renin release. When released into the bloodstream, renin splits the substrate angiotensinogen to produce angiotensin I, which is further split to produce angiotensin II. The latter is the most potent blood-pressure substance known. It regulates the secretion of aldosterone from the adrenal cortex. Obstructive lesions of a renal artery result in decreased arterial pressure to the affected kidney. This stimulates the release of renin, which produces more angiotensin, resulting in renovascular hypertension.

The adrenal glands also play an important role in blood-pressure control. As stated above, angiotensin stimulates the secretion of aldosterone from the adrenal cortex. Aldosterone promotes renal sodium and water retention, potassium excretion and arteriolar constriction. The retained fluid and constricted vessels are major factors in producing hypertension. The adrenal medulla is the source of epinephrine and norepinephrine, which together are known as *catecholamines*. These maintain peripheral vascular resistance and cardiac output. A rare tumor of the adrenal medulla, pheochromocytoma, secretes increased amounts of catecholamines, resulting in hypertension.

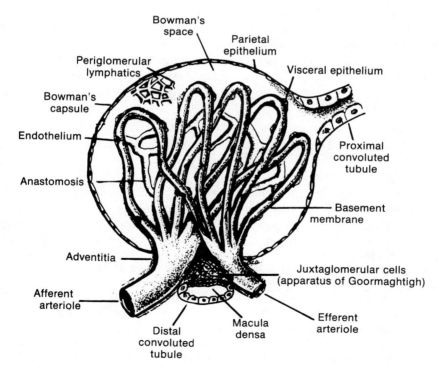

**Fig. 1-2.** A normal glomerulus. (Allen AC: The Kidney, 2nd ed, p 27. New York, Grune & Stratton, 1962, by permission)

The complications of hypertension include heart failure, renal failure, blindness, accelerated atherosclerosis, aneurysm formation, and cerebral hemorrhage.

About 85% to 95% of cases of hypertension are classified as primary, or *essential*. This indicates that the disorder is not secondary to any identifiable cause. It is diagnosed by the exclusion of the various disorders that are known to cause hypertension. Factors known to influence blood pressure or to be associated with primary hypertension include heredity, age, race, sex, body weight, sodium ingestion, alcohol consumption, heart rate, previous blood pressures, plasma glucose, and serum uric acid.

The major causes of *secondary* hypertension include renal parenchymal diseases, such as glomerulonephritis, pyelonephritis, and diabetic renal disease; renal vascular diseases, such as renal-artery narrowing due to arteriosclerosis or fibromuscular hyperplasia; adrenal cortical hyperactivity, such as Cushing's syndrome or primary aldosteronism; pheochromocytoma; coarctation or segmental narrowing of the aorta; and hyperthyroidism. The causes of secondary hypertension are shown in Figure 1-3. Laboratory studies are done to help detect the secondary causes of hypertension.[2]

## LABORATORY FINDINGS

### Renal Parenchymal Diseases

Mechanism—retention of salt and water, followed by small-vessel constriction (see Chronic Renal Failure, Chap. 5)

Urine—presence of protein, glucose, red blood cells (RBC), white blood cells (WBC), casts; decreases in volume, sodium, osmolality, and specific gravity

Serum—increased creatinine, blood urea nitrogen (BUN), uric acid; decreased albumin, total protein

Decreased creatinine clearance

Anemia, normocytic (see Anemia of Chronic Renal Insufficiency, Chap. 8)

### Renal Vascular Disease

Mechanism—production of increased renin by the kidney in response to decreased renal blood supply

This should be suspected in patients under 30 years or over 50 years of age who *suddenly* develop hypertension, who have no family history of hypertension, and whose laboratory screening tests indicate no renal parenchymal disease. Laboratory confirmation requires that both renal veins be catheterized, that plasma renin activity (PRA) be measured in both veins, and that the PRA on the affected side be at least one and one half times that on the contralateral side.

The use of peripheral venous PRA as a *screening* test for renal vascular hypertension is fraught with the likelihood of many false-positive and false-negative results. Gifford recently concluded, "There is no justification for including the renin–sodium profile in the routine diagnostic evaluation of hypertensive patients, because it is not helpful as a screen for secondary hypertension or as a guide to prognosis or selection of drugs."[6]

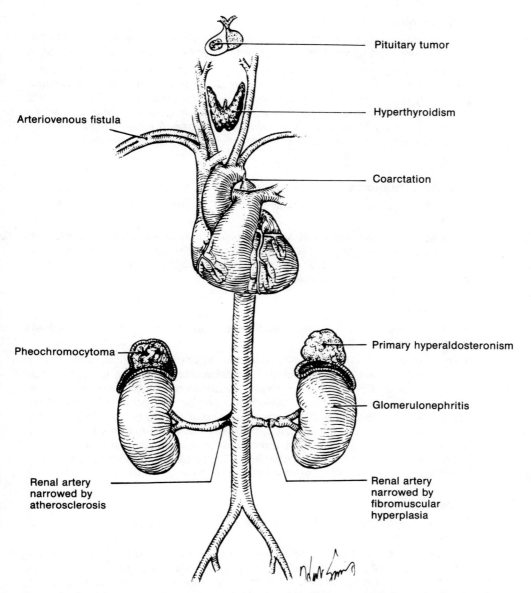

**Fig. 1-3.** Some causes of secondary hypertension. Other causes include Cushing's disease, birth control pills, anemia, and beriberi. (DeBakey M, Gotto A: The Living Heart, p 197. New York, Raven Press, 1977)

## Aldosteronism

Mechanism—production of increased aldosterone by an adrenal cortical tumor; this causes retention of salt and water and loss of serum potassium (see Chap. 6)

An excess of aldosterone is suggested by the presence of serum potassium below 3 mEq/l and urine potassium above 30 mEq/day. The loss of potassium frequently results in metabolic alkalosis, (*i.e.,* high $p$H and high $CO_2$ content). Aldosteronism is further suggested if PRA is below 1 ng/ml/hr and is usually confirmed by increased plasma or urine aldosterone. A recently described screening test uses an elevated aldosterone–PRA ratio following administration of diuretics and salt restriction.[8]

## Cushing's Syndrome

Mechanism—production of increased cortisol by the adrenal cortex (see Chap. 6)

Hyperactivity of the adrenal cortex results in a clinical syndrome that includes hypertension. The syndrome is diagnosed by the finding of increased levels of cortisol in the plasma and urine. The increased cortisol is not suppressible by giving the patient dexamethasone.

## Pheochromocytoma

Mechanism—production of increased catecholamines by a tumor of the adrenal medulla (see Chap. 6)

This adrenal medullary tumor is a very rare cause of hypertension (0.04% of all cases). If it is clinically suspected, the best laboratory screening test is a 24-hour urine test for metanephrines, which are metabolic products of epinephrine and norepinephrine. Because the disease is not prevalent, a positive test must be repeated for confirmation. If it is again positive, it should be reconfirmed using the less sensitive, but more specific, estimation of 24-hour urinary vanillylmandelic acid (VMA). The most accurate diagnostic test is the measurement of plasma catecholamines.[1] Elevated catecholamines are not suppressible after administration of clonidine hydrochloride.

## Hyperthyroidism

Mechanism—production of increased thyroxine by the thyroid gland (see Chap. 6)

Hyperactivity of the thyroid gland results in increased cardiac output, producing systolic or high-output hypertension. Hyperthyroidism is diagnosed by the finding of increased blood levels of triiodothyronine ($T_3$) or thyroxine ($T_4$).

## Miscellaneous

Other, less common, causes of secondary hypertension include the following:

Polycythemia, in which increased blood viscosity increases both resistance to blood flow and the work demand on the heart, resulting in hypertension.

Severe anemia, in which increased demand for cardiac output to supply oxygen to tissues results in systolic or high-output hypertension.

**Laboratory Findings of Complications**

Myocardial infarction

Congestive heart failure

Cerebral hemorrhage

Renal failure

## CORONARY-ARTERY DISEASE AND MYOCARDIAL INFARCTION

Despite the relatively small size of the heart, about 20% of the total cardiac output is needed to provide nourishment for the heart itself. The cardiac blood supply is carried by the *coronary arteries,* which are so named because they encircle the heart like a crown. Approximately 15 gallons of blood are pumped through these arteries each hour. The heart muscle extracts more oxygen from the blood than does any other tissue in the body. A cross-sectional reduction of 60% to 70% in the arterial lumen is usually required before clinical symptoms of reduced coronary blood flow appear.

The major underlying cause of coronary-artery obstruction is the development of atherosclerotic plaques. Recent studies have demonstrated that increased platelet aggregation and coronary-arterial spasm may contribute to the formation of thrombi or blood clots in the coronary arteries.[12] A thrombus may partially or completely occlude a coronary artery. When the vessel lumen is partially obstructed, inadequate amounts of blood and oxygen are available to support the needs of the heart muscle. This condition is known as *myocardial ischemia.* If the blood and oxygen supplies to a portion of heart muscle become severely or totally reduced, death of heart cells results. This is called a *myocardial infarction* or *heart attack* (Fig. 1-4). If collateral blood vessels have formed, as occurs when vessel narrowing is gradual, coronary-artery occlusion might not result in infarction. An infarct is diagnosed by clinical signs and symptoms, electrocardiogram (ECG), and the finding of an elevation of certain enzymes in the blood. In approximately 30% of patients with myocardial infarction, the ECG shows no evidence of an infarct. This is most frequently the case postoperatively, in diabetics, in hypertensives, in patients with electrical cardiac conduction defects, or in those with previous myocardial infarctions. In these situations, findings of elevated cardiac enzymes in the circulation are essential for establishing the diagnosis.

### LABORATORY FINDINGS

#### Cardiac Enzymes

When heart-muscle fibers die, their intracellular enzymes are released from the cells into the surrounding tissue and ultimately appear in the circulating bloodstream. Different enzymes reach peak blood levels at different times following a myocardial infarction (Fig. 1-5). The enzymes of greatest diagnostic value for myocardial infarction are creatine phosphokinase (CPK) and lactate dehydrogenase (LDH).[5]

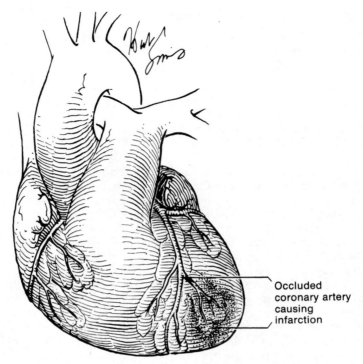

**Fig. 1-4.** Myocardial infarction caused by blockage of a branch of the anterior descending coronary artery. (DeBakey M, Gotto A: The Living Heart, p 123. New York, Raven Press, 1977)

CPK is found primarily in skeletal and myocardial muscle and also in the brain and intestines. There is little or no CPK activity in the lungs, liver, kidneys, pancreas, or RBC. CPK activity in the blood begins to rise about 4 hours to 8 hours after myocardial infarction, reaching levels of five times to ten times the upper limit of normal, depending on the size of the infarct. Peak activity usually occurs 18 hours to 24 hours after infarction, and CPK activity returns to normal by the fifth day. CPK activity provides a highly sensitive test, but its low specificity is a drawback to its usefulness as the sole diagnostic laboratory test for myocardial infarction.

LDH activity is found in almost all human tissues. The liver and skeletal muscle have the greatest concentrations, followed by the heart. LDH is also found in RBC, the kidneys, the lungs, the pancreas, and the brain. LDH activity in the blood starts to rise about 12 hours to 24 hours after myocardial infarction, often reaching levels of two to three times the upper limit of normal. Peak activity usually occurs on the third day following infarction, and activity may remain raised for as long as 10 days postinfarction. This is a sensitive test; however, its wide tissue distribution decreases its specificity.

The specificity of both CPK and LDH may be greatly increased by electrophoretically separating and quantitating their isoenzymes. An *isoenzyme*

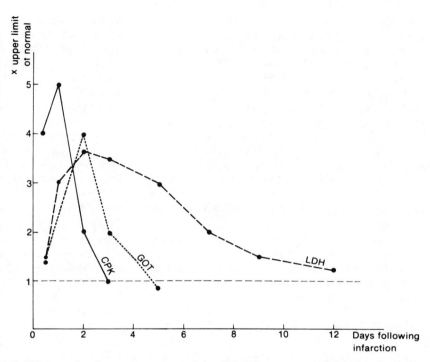

**Fig. 1-5.** Change in serum enzyme activity following myocardial infarction. (Raphael SS: Lynch's Medical Laboratory Technology, 3rd ed, p 281. Philadelphia, WB Saunders, 1976)

is a varied molecular form of an enzyme. All of the isoenzymes of a particular enzyme have similar catalytic effects on substrates but differ in their physical characteristics.

LDH may be electrophoretically separated into five isoenzymes; these are designated as $LDH_1$ (fastest migration), $LDH_2$, $LDH_3$, $LDH_4$, and $LDH_5$ (slowest migration) (Table 1-1).

Release of increased $LDH_1$ isoenzyme from the myocardium into the bloodstream following a myocardial infarction results in the preponderant isoenzyme changing from $LDH_2$ (in normal serum) to $LDH_1$. This reversal of isoenzyme predominance is referred to as a *"flipped-LDH"* pattern. This is seen

**Table 1-1.** Distribution of LDH Isoenzymes in Normal Tissues

| ISOENZYME | NORMAL SERUM (%) | HEART MUSCLE (%) | LIVER (%) | SKELETAL MUSCLE (%) |
|-----------|------------------|------------------|-----------|---------------------|
| $LDH_1$ | 25 | 40 | 0 | 0 |
| $LDH_2$ | 35 | 35 | 5 | 0 |
| $LDH_3$ | 20 | 20 | 10 | 10 |
| $LDH_4$ | 10 | 5 | 15 | 30 |
| $LDH_5$ | 10 | 0 | 70 | 60 |

following acute myocardial or renal infarction and in hemolysis associated with prosthetic heart valves, hemolytic anemia, or pernicious anemia. Elevation and predominance of $LDH_1$ show far greater specificity for infarction than does elevation of the total LDH enzyme. The flipped pattern occurs within 12 hours to 24 hours of the infarction; by 48 hours after infarction, 80% of patients show this pattern. Fewer than 50% of these patients still have flipped patterns after 7 days.

CPK may also be electrophoretically separated into isoenzymes: $CPK_1$ (BB), $CPK_2$ (MB), $CPK_3$ (MM) (Table 1-2). Each CPK isoenzyme is made up of a combination of B and/or M subunits. The B polypeptide chain is so called because it has been isolated from the brain, and the M chain is found in skeletal muscle. The isoenzyme found in the brain consists of two similar units, termed *BB*. The isoenzyme found in the skeletal muscle consists of two other identical subunits and is termed the *MM* isoenzyme. Heart tissue has a virtually specific isoenzyme, which is a hybrid of both subunits and is termed *MB*.

CPK-BB, occurring predominantly in brain tissue, is rarely seen in serum even after cerebral infarction because the enzyme does not usually cross the blood–brain barrier. CPK-BB has been found in serum in patients who have had neurosurgery, in patients with certain tumors, and in some patients with bowel infarction. CPK-MM, found predominantly in skeletal muscle, increases in the serum in cases of muscle trauma, in muscular dystrophy, following intramuscular injections, in shock, after major surgical procedures, and following acute myocardial infarction.

CPK-MB, found almost exclusively in heart muscle, is usually indicative of an acute myocardial infarction when it is found in serum. This is more specific for myocardial damage than is $LDH_1$. Following acute myocardial infarction, CPK-MB appears in 4 hours to 8 hours, reaches peak activity at 18 hours to 24 hours, and may last for another 2 days. CPK-MB always precedes the appearance of a flipped-LDH pattern. CPK-MM, which also occurs in heart muscle, remains elevated 4 days to 5 days following myocardial infarction. Myocardial injury other than infarction may also result in serum elevation of CPK-MB. Examples of conditions that injure heart muscle include myocarditis, heart trauma, open heart surgery, coronary angiography, cardiomyopathy, cardiac resuscitation, and electrical cardioversion. CPK-MB may also be present, usually in small amounts, in the following neuromuscular disorders: muscular dystrophies, polymyositis, dermatomyositis, viral myositis, malignant hyperpyrexia, severe skeletal-muscle trauma, and Reye's syndrome.

The highest sensitivity and specificity in diagnosing acute myocardial infarction are obtained by testing for both LDH and CPK enzymes and isoenzymes on admission, after 24 hours, and again at 48 hours after the onset of symptoms; some suggest testing at 12 hours and 24 hours. The presence of CPK-MB and

**Table 1-2.** Distribution of CPK Isoenzymes in Normal Tissues

| ISOENZYME | NORMAL SERUM (%) | SKELETAL MUSCLE (%) | HEART (%) | BRAIN (%) |
|---|---|---|---|---|
| $CPK_1$ (BB) | 0 | 0 | 0 | 90 |
| $CPK_2$ (MB) | 0 | 0 | 40 | 0 |
| $CPK_3$ (MM) | 100 | 100 | 60 | 10 |

flipped LDH within 48 hours of the onset of symptoms offers laboratory confirmation of acute myocardial infarction. The presence of CPK-MB *alone* is insufficient evidence for diagnosing acute myocardial infarction. If CPK-MB does not appear within 48 hours of the onset of chest pain, acute myocardial infarction may be ruled out. CPK-MB occurs in some cases of myocardial infarction in the absence of abnormally elevated total CPK activity.

**Other Laboratory Findings**

Leukocytosis—12,000/$\mu$l to 20,000/$\mu$l with 75% to 90% neutrophils

Increased sedimentation rate starts after 2 days, peaks after 4 days to 5 days, and persists for 2 months to 6 months. The degree of increase does not correlate with the severity of the infarction or with prognosis.

Increased serum glucose and urine glucose, attributed to adrenal cortical stimulation secondary to stress or to shock

Decreased arterial $PO_2$ and oxygen saturation—frequent occurrence, 2 days to 3 days following infarction; especially abnormal in the presence of shock, left ventricular failure, or pulmonary edema; this reflects impaired arterial oxygenation in the lungs

Metabolic acidosis (decreased $p$H, decreased $HCO_3^-$, increased lactic acid) due to impaired circulation and consequent tissue hypoxia

## COR PULMONALE (PULMONARY HEART DISEASE)

Cor pulmonale is heart disease that occurs secondary to lung disease. Cor pulmonale may be a consequence of any of the following long-standing pulmonary disorders: advanced emphysema, chronic bronchitis, pulmonary fibrosis, and cystic fibrosis. These disorders all cause a decreased cross-sectional area of the pulmonary vascular bed and hypoxemia, resulting in pulmonary arterial hypertension. Increased pulmonary vascular resistance causes the right ventricle of the heart to enlarge and fail, resulting in right-sided congestive heart failure.

Arterial hypoxemia and tissue hypoxia stimulate erythropoietin formation. This might result in secondary erythrocytosis and hypervolemia, which further aggravate congestive failure.

### LABORATORY FINDINGS

Decreased arterial $PO_2$ and oxygen saturation due to underlying lung disease

Increased RBC, hemoglobin, hematocrit, blood volume, and red cell mass, all reflecting erythrocytosis secondary to tissue hypoxia

**Laboratory Findings of Underlying Lung Disease***

Chronic bronchitis

Pulmonary emphysema

Pulmonary embolism and infarction

* See Chapter 2.

## PERICARDITIS

Inflammation of the pericardial sac around the heart is called *pericarditis*. Acute pericarditis is associated with the accumulation of fluid in the pericardial cavity (Fig. 1-6). When the fluid causes pressure on the heart, interfering with blood flow into the heart's chambers, this compression is called *cardiac tamponade*. If the inflammation persists, *chronic pericarditis* results; the formation of fibrous tissue in the pericardium is referred to as *constrictive pericarditis*.

Acute pericarditis is usually caused by infection with coxsackie B virus, echovirus, or influenza virus. Viruses are assumed to be bloodborne, but they may originate from viral myocarditis. Pyogenic bacteria usually invade the pericardium from an adjacent infected site such as the lung, pleura, or mediastinum. Pericarditis may also be due to rheumatic fever, bacterial infection, uremia, surgery, radiation, metastatic malignant tumors, or myocardial infarction.

Chronic pericarditis is usually due to tuberculosis, hypothyroidism, metastatic tumor, or lupus erythematosus. Chronic constrictive pericarditis, especially following tuberculosis, may result in congestive heart failure and marked hepatic congestion.

### LABORATORY FINDINGS

#### Acute Pericarditis

Pericardial fluid (Table 1-3)

WBC—elevated in bacterial pericarditis, normal or low in viral or tuberculous pericarditis

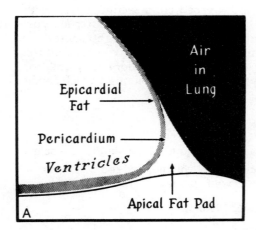
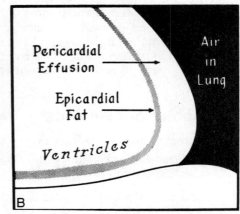

**Fig. 1-6.** Radiographic identification of the epicardial fat line in the diagnosis of pericardial effusion. (*A*) Postero-anterior (PA) view of the normal heart. (*B*) PA view of the heart showing pericardial effusion. (Jorgens J, Kundel R, Lieber A: The cinefluorographic approach to the diagnosis of pericardial effusion. Am J Roentgenol 87:911, 1962)

**Table 1-3.** Pericardial Fluid: Transudate *vs.* Exudate

| LAB FINDING | TRANSUDATE (*e.g.*, UREMIA, LUPUS, RHEUMATIC FEVER) | EXUDATE (*e.g.*, TUMOR, BACTERIAL INFECTION) |
|---|---|---|
| LDH | <60% of serum level | >60% of serum level |
| Protein | <50% of serum level | >50% of serum level |
| Clot | Absent | Present |
| Cells | Few lymphocytes or RBC | Many segmented neutrophils |
| Glucose | Same as serum | Decreased because of consumption by WBC or bacteria |

Positive pericardial culture for bacteria, mycobacteria, and viruses

Fourfold rise in viral antibody titers from acute to convalescent sera

**Constrictive Pericarditis**

Increased LDH (especially $LDH_5$) and decreased albumin, due to hepatic congestion

Laboratory findings of congestive heart failure

## INFECTIVE ENDOCARDITIS

Inflammation of the lining of the heart or heart valves is called *endocarditis*. This is most frequently caused by bacteria, but it may also result from fungal or rickettsial infection. Altered or abnormal endocardial surfaces are particularly susceptible to the deposition and aggregation of circulating bacteria. Altered endocardial surfaces occur on a valve that has been previously damaged by rheumatic fever or syphilis. These are less common today than heretofore. Certain congenital malformations of the heart, or the presence of an artificial heart valve or graft, also predispose a patient to the development of endocarditis.

Endocarditis usually involves the mitral and aortic valves, producing small, wartlike growths or vegetations (Fig. 1-7). The growths, which usually contain a mixture of bacteria, blood cells, and fibrin, may deform or even destroy heart valves. Vegetations may break off, seed the bloodstream with bacteria, and enter the circulation as emboli. Emboli block peripheral arteries, forming small abscesses and infected foci of tissue necrosis known as *septic infarcts*. These may occur in the brain, kidneys, spleen, or heart.

Acute bacterial endocarditis results from circulating virulent bacteria, such as *Staphylococcus aureus* and gram-negative cocci. These bacteria are deposited on intact heart valves and cause their destruction. The severe damage to heart valves usually results in heart failure. More frequently, the process of infection is slow and is referred to as *subacute bacterial endocarditis* (SBE). SBE is caused by organisms of low virulence that occur normally in the upper-respiratory and gastrointestinal tracts. Such transient bacteremia may occur following dental extraction, tonsillectomy, endoscopic examination, barium enema, or even vigorous chewing. *Streptococcus viridans* and group D streptococci are the most frequent causes of SBE. These bacteria are deposited on previously damaged heart valves and produce smaller vegetations than those occurring in acute

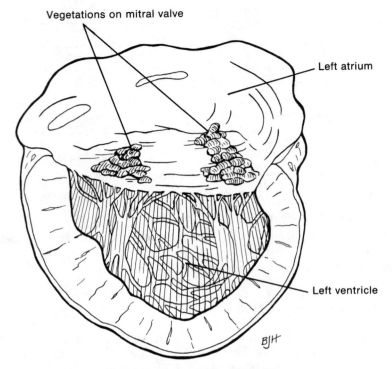

Vegetations on mitral valve

Left atrium

Left ventricle

BJH

**Fig. 1-7.** Bacterial endocarditis.

bacterial endocarditis. In SBE, the valves are not usually destroyed. Bacteria multiply and are discharged from endocardial vegetations into the circulation at a relatively constant rate. They are frequently sources of embolization, characteristically producing capillary thrombi and petechiae.

Hospital-acquired infections and septicemia in addicts using intravenous drugs have resulted in an increased incidence of infections with *Staphylococcus epidermidis,* gram-negative bacilli, *Candida,* and "opportunistic" microorganisms. The increased incidence of hospital-acquired infections is associated with greater use of intravascular prostheses, including prosthetic cardiac valves, and with the use of invasive mechanical life-support and monitoring systems.[19]

Death may occur as a result of congestive heart failure, neurologic involvement, or overwhelming infection.

### LABORATORY FINDINGS

Positive blood culture is essential to establishing the diagnosis and is positive in 80%–90% of patients. *Streptococcus viridans,* group D streptococci and *Staphylococcus aureus* cause more than 75% of cases of endocarditis. Other bacteria, fungi, or rickettsiae are responsible for the remaining cases. The diagnosis should be based on two or more cultures that are positive for the same organism. Three separate blood cultures should be collected as quickly as possible for severe, life-threatening septicemia. For suspected SBE, the three blood cultures should be taken within the first 24 hours, at intervals no shorter than 1 hour. In patients already on antibiotic therapy, four to six separate blood cultures should be collected within the first 48 hours. Positive blood cultures are difficult to obtain in patients already on antibiotics and in patients whose endocarditis is due to unusual or fastidious organisms.

Normocytic anemia—the degree of anemia is related to the duration of illness, rather than to the virulence of the organism

WBC—normal or elevated to 15,000/$\mu$l with 65%–85% neutrophils

Increased sedimentation rate indicates active inflammation

Increased $\gamma$-globulins reflect chronic inflammation

Albuminuria and hematuria—the former occurs even without renal involvement

## CARDIOMYOPATHIES

Disease of the heart muscle that is not due to impaired coronary circulation and ischemia is called *cardiomyopathy*.[3] This may be either primary or secondary to a specific disease, which often also involves other organs.

Factors that have been suggested as possible causes of *primary* cardiomyopathy include viral infections, hyperimmune responses, genetic abnormality of the heart muscle, nutritional deficiency, lack of oxygen, toxins, and drugs.

*Secondary* cardiomyopathy occurs associated with many disorders. A recent classification follows.[13]

**Infective Cardiomyopathies**
Viral—coxsackie B virus and echovirus are the most frequent causes of myocarditis
Rickettsial, fungal, parasitologic
**Metabolic Cardiomyopathies**
Endocrine—thyrotoxicosis, hypothyroidism, adrenal cortical insufficiency, pheochromocytoma, acromegaly
Familial storage disease—hemochromatosis, glycogen storage disease
Deficiency—potassium-metabolism disturbances, magnesium deficiency, and nutritional disorders
Amyloidosis
**General System Diseases**
Connective tissue disorders—systemic lupus erythematosus, polyarteritis nodosa, rheumatoid arthritis, scleroderma, dermatomyositis
Infiltrations and granulomas—sarcoidosis, leukemia
**Heredofamilial Cardiomyopathies**
Muscular dystrophies
Friedreich's ataxia
**Sensitivity and Toxic Reactions**
Sulfonamides
Penicillin
Alcohol

Two principal functional types of cardiomyopathy are described: *hypertrophic* and *dilated*. The former results in an increased muscle mass, usually of the left ventricle. This diminishes the volumes of the left ventricular chamber and the blood flowing through it. In dilated cardiomyopathy, the volumes of one or both ventricular chambers increase. This impairs normal cardiac pumping function. Dilated cardiomyopathy is also termed *congestive cardiomyopathy*, because the impaired circulation results in the vascular congestion of most organs.

## LABORATORY FINDINGS

Increased serum CPK, CPK-MB, LDH, and $LDH_1$ are the result of severe myocardial damage; levels do not approach those encountered in myocardial infarction

Increased blood eosinophils suggest trichinosis, polyarteritis, or allergic endomyocarditis.

Fourfold rise in coxsackie virus or echovirus antibody titer from acute-phase to convalescent-phase sera

### Laboratory Findings of Complications
Congestive heart failure

Systemic or pulmonary emboli

Pericardial effusion

### Laboratory Findings of Underlying Nonmyocardial Diseases

## *CONGESTIVE HEART FAILURE*

Congestive heart failure is a symptom complex that is a consequence of impaired cardiac pumping ability and fluid retention. Impaired cardiac pumping ability may be due to hypertension or to diseases of heart valves, heart muscle, or coronary arteries.

When there is a decrease in cardiac output, increased backward pressure on the venous circulation causes the volume of blood within the cardiovascular system to become abnormally expanded. This diminishes blood flow in all organs and tissues. There is also an excessive accumulation of fluid in the lungs, legs, and other body tissues. This fluid accumulation is known as *edema*. Renal retention of salt and water further increases edema.

In congestive heart failure, diminished blood flow and vascular engorgement result in impairment of function of the liver, kidneys, and lungs.

## LABORATORY FINDINGS

### Renal Functions
Urine specific gravity <1.020 as a result of diminished renal-concentrating ability

Decreased urine sodium and urine volume due to the effects of increased renin and aldosterone formation

**Table 1-4.** Characteristics of Transudates

| LABORATORY TEST | RESULT |
|---|---|
| Specific gravity | <1.016 |
| Protein | <50% of serum level |
| LDH | <60% of serum level |
| WBC | <1000/$\mu$l |
| Differential WBC | Mononuclear cells predominate |
| Glucose | Same as serum |
| $p$H | Same as blood |

Slight albuminuria (<1 g/day)

Occasional urine RBC, WBC, casts

Decreased creatinine clearance and increased serum BUN (usually <60 mg/dl); this occurs in severe heart failure

Decreased serum sodium, chloride, protein, and albumin due to dilution by increased blood volume and edema fluid; the increased blood volume is due to increased renin and aldosterone formation

Metabolic acidosis (decreased $p$H and decreased $HCO_3^-$) due to superimposed chronic renal failure.

**Liver Functions**

Increased serum bilirubin (1 mg/dl–5 mg/dl), urine bilirubin, and urobilinogen; reflects severity of the heart failure and hepatic congestion

Decreased erythrocyte sedimentation rate due to decreased fibrinogen synthesis by the liver

Increased LDH, especially $LDH_5$, due to severe heart failure and congestive hepatocellular necrosis

Mild to moderate increase in alkaline phosphatase due to hepatic congestion and impaired enzyme excretion by the liver

Slight increase in prothrombin time due to decreased fibrinogen synthesis by the liver

**Pulmonary Functions**

Decreased arterial $PO_2$ due to impaired gas exchange in congested lungs

Respiratory alkalosis (increased $p$H and decreased $PCO_2$) due to hyperventilation in response to hypoxemia

Respiratory acidosis (decreased $p$H and increased $PCO_2$); acute pulmonary edema impairs ventilation and blood flow resulting in $CO_2$ retention.

Table 1-4 shows the characteristics of pleural and peritoneal effusions that occur in congestive heart failure.

## ATHEROSCLEROSIS

*Arteriosclerosis* refers to the process of thickening and loss of elasticity of the arterial wall in any artery. *Atherosclerosis* is the most common type of arteriosclerosis and is characterized by complex degenerative changes involving predominantly the inner, or intimal, layer of medium to large arteries. Atherosclerosis is regarded as a pathologic response of the vessel wall to chronic multifactorial injury. Endothelial damage, platelet aggregation, and smooth-muscle proliferation are important early events in the development of an atherosclerotic lesion.[18] Platelets contribute to the development of atherosclerosis in at least two different ways: by the release from activated platelets of chemical mediators that damage the vessel wall or alter its metabolism and by repeated microthrombus and microembolus formation, which augment occlusion of already damaged arteries.

The evolution of an atherosclerotic lesion from childhood includes the following stages:[15] (Fig. 1-8)

1. Damage to the endothelial lining
2. Focal accumulation of intimal lipids (fatty streak)
3. Proliferation of smooth-muscle cells (fibrous plaque)
4. Cell death and injury
5. Formation of a necrotic, lipid-rich, complicated lesion

It is generally accepted that the cholesterol of the atheromatous plaque is derived chiefly from plasma cholesterol. When an atheromatous plaque develops, it interferes with the normal oxygenation and nourishment of the arterial wall, producing further damage. Bleeding may occur into a plaque, or the plaque surface may ulcerate. These events stimulate formation of an overlying blood clot or thrombus, which results in partial or complete obstruction of the arterial lumen, bringing about impairment or complete interruption of circulation. The latter causes death of tissue, known as *infarction* or *gangrene*.

The consequences of impaired blood flow depend on which organ or tissue is affected and on the rapidity of the process. Gradual vascular occlusion results in the formation of many new small collateral vessels, which can maintain tissue viability with diminished function. Involvement of the aorta or coronary, cerebral, or peripheral vessels is quite variable, and many patients may have more than one area affected. Coronary arteries tend to be involved earlier than are cerebral or peripheral arteries.

Atherosclerosis may not produce occlusive disease but, in some patients, it leads to a "ballooning out" of the arterial wall; this is called an *aneurysm*. The consequences of atherosclerotic occlusion of different vessels include the following:

Coronary artery—myocardial infarct (heart attack)
Cerebral artery—cerebral infarct (stroke)
Peripheral artery—gangrene
Renal artery—renal infarct
Mesenteric artery—gangrene of the intestines

Most people who die or are disabled from atherosclerosis exhibit one or more identifiable characteristics called *risk factors*.[7] These risk factors are considered to be present more frequently in people who develop atherosclerosis than in the general population. Estimates of the occurrence of major risk factors in persons with atherosclerosis vary from 50% to 80%. The risk-factor hypothesis is as follows: If a person has a risk factor, he is more likely to develop clinical

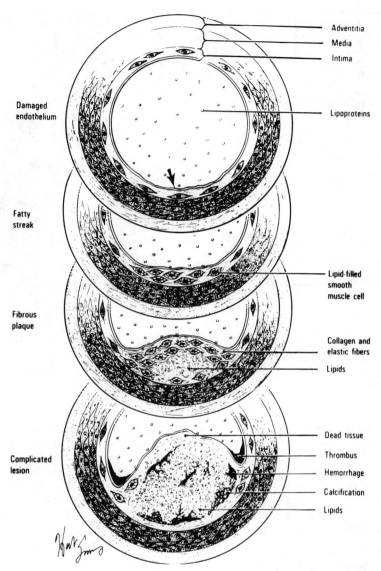

**Fig. 1-8.** Types of atherosclerotic lesions. (DeBakey M, Gotto A: The Living Heart, p 111. New York, Raven Press, 1977)

manifestations of atherosclerosis, and he is likely to do so earlier than is a person with no risk factors. Three modifiable primary risk factors that have been identified for premature coronary-artery disease are hypercholesterolemia, hypertension, and smoking. The additive effects of these factors are shown in Figure 1-9. Elevated serum cholesterol is considered to be the single most important

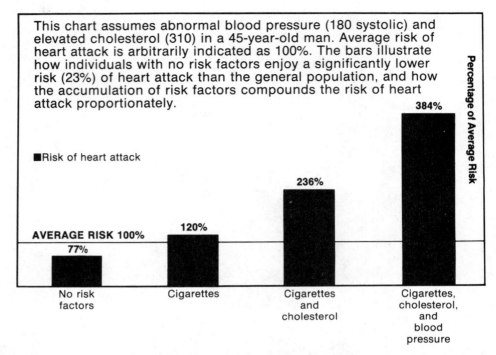

This chart assumes abnormal blood pressure (180 systolic) and elevated cholesterol (310) in a 45-year-old man. Average risk of heart attack is arbitrarily indicated as 100%. The bars illustrate how individuals with no risk factors enjoy a significantly lower risk (23%) of heart attack than the general population, and how the accumulation of risk factors compounds the risk of heart attack proportionately.

Percentage of Average Risk

■Risk of heart attack

384%

236%

AVERAGE RISK 100%     120%

77%

No risk factors — Cigarettes — Cigarettes and cholesterol — Cigarettes, cholesterol, and blood pressure

**Fig. 1-9.** Risk factors for heart attack. (Source: The Framingham, MA Heart Study) (Stein EA: Coronary Heart Disease: You Can Live Without It, p 9. Medfield, MA, Corning Medical, 1979)

factor in the pathogenesis of atherosclerosis and coronary heart disease.[10] Hypertension accelerates atherosclerosis in persons with hypercholesterolemia.

*Hyperlipidemia* is an elevation of plasma cholesterol or triglyceride. Water-insoluble cholesterol and other plasma lipids are carried in the bloodstream by emulsified water-soluble compounds called *lipoproteins*. Plasma lipoproteins may be separated and classified by means of ultracentrifugation and electrophoresis. Through ultracentrifugation, several types of lipoproteins have been identified based on their different densities:

1. Chylomicrons
2. Very low-density lipoproteins (VLDL)
3. Low-density lipoproteins (LDL)
4. High-density lipoproteins (HDL).

Through electrophoresis, the lipoproteins are classified on the basis of their migration:

1. Chylomicrons do not leave their points of origin.
2. VLDL (prebetalipoproteins) migrate near the $\beta$-globulins.
3. LDL ($\beta$-lipoproteins) migrate with the $\beta$-globulins.
4. HDL ($\alpha$-lipoproteins) migrate with the $\alpha$-globulins.

Using electrophoresis of the plasma lipoproteins, measurement of plasma cholesterol and triglyceride, and observation of plasma clarity or opacity, Fredrickson, Levy, and Lees of the National Heart Institute proposed a system for classifying the hyperlipoproteinemias into several types (see Chap. 10).[4] It has been observed that patients with Type II hyperlipoproteinemia, which has the highest $\beta$ fraction (LDL), have the greatest incidence of coronary heart disease. LDL is found to be associated with cholesterol in atherosclerotic plaques; LDL thus appears to be the most atherogenic of all lipoproteins.

## LABORATORY FINDINGS

Until recently, the major laboratory test used to classify the risk of developing coronary heart disease (CHD) has been a total cholesterol assay. However, only when the serum cholesterol is above 350 mg/dl (which occurs in less than 1% of the population) is there a significantly increased risk of CHD. Most patients have cholesterol values between 150 mg/dl and 300 mg/dl, whether or not they have CHD. The Framingham Heart Institute Study has shown that if the HDL cholesterol value is less than 45 mg/dl, the rate of CHD is very high.[7,10] On the other hand, when the HDL cholesterol exceeds 55 mg/dl, the rate of CHD is very low. HDL appears to have a salutary effect on CHD. It functions to remove cholesterol from atherosclerotic vessels and from other tissues and returns the cholesterol to the liver for excretion in bile. The higher the levels of HDL, the greater the degree of lipid excretion.

A statistical analysis of the roles of various lipids in predicting the risk of CHD showed a significant inverse relationship between HDL cholesterol and myocardial infarction.[11] HDL cholesterol was shown to be the most sensitive single predictor of a patient's risk of developing CHD by the age of 50; the HDL measurement is eight times more sensitive than measurement of the total cholesterol level. Various combinations of lipid measurements as ratios further increased the predictability of CHD. Probably the best predictor is the LDL–HDL ratio; the tests for this ratio require that the patient be fasting. The total cholesterol–HDL cholesterol ratio is almost as good a predictor.[20] The tests for this ratio may be done in a nonfasting patient. HDL cholesterol is determined by first separating HDL from the other plasma lipids, through precipitation or electrophoresis, and then measuring the cholesterol content of the separated HDL.

The total cholesterol–HDL cholesterol ratio in various populations is shown in Table 1-5.

## *ANEURYSM*

The word *aneurysm* is from the Greek, meaning *a widening*. An aneurysm is a localized abnormal dilatation or ballooning of an artery. It is the result of weakening of the wall of an artery, which is usually secondary to atherosclerosis; it may also be caused by syphilis or aging. Due to the combined effects of the pulsatile nature of blood flow and its pressure, the affected artery tends to become progressively larger and frequently ruptures (Fig. 1-10). An aneurysm

**Table 1-5.** Total Cholesterol–HDL Cholesterol Ratios in Populations in Order of Increased CHD Risk

| POPULATION | RATIO |
|---|---|
| Vegetarians | 2.8 |
| Eskimos | 3.2 |
| Those with ½ average risk of CHD | 3.4 |
| Marathon runner | 3.4 |
| Female, normal | 4.5 |
| Male, normal | 5.0 |
| Those with CHD | 5.3–5.7 |
| Those with 2× average risk of CHD | 7–10 |
| Those with 3× average risk of CHD | 11–23 |

either dilates throughout its entire circumference, giving a fusiform appearance, or balloons out like a large bubble at only one area on the artery wall. The latter is known as a *sacciform* or *saccular* aneurysm (Fig. 1-11). Although an aneurysm may develop in any artery, the abdominal aorta below the origin of the renal arteries is the most common site.

A dissecting aneurysm occurs when a tear in the inner lining of the artery wall allows blood to enter the middle layer, creating a new channel within the arterial wall and blocking the arterial branches from the aorta. The tear is usually located in the ascending aorta. The cause of spontaneous aortic dissection is usually unknown, and intrinsic abnormality in the wall of the aorta is usually not identified. About 70% of patients with aortic dissection have, or have had, systemic hypertension. The most frequent mechanism of death is rupture of the aorta. Diagnosis is usually based on the clinical signs and symptoms that occur when the aneurysm ruptures or occludes various aortic branches.

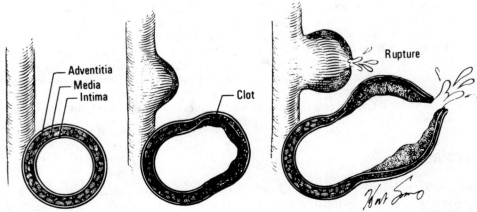

**Fig. 1-10.** A normal artery (*left*) is weakened by arteriosclerosis or atherosclerosis and gradually balloons out, forming an aneurysm, which may be partially lined with a blood clot (*center*). Eventually, the aneurysm may rupture (*right*). (DeBakey M, Gotto A: The Living Heart, p 166. New York, Raven Press, 1977)

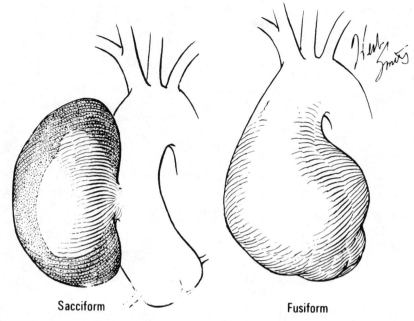

Sacciform                    Fusiform

**Fig. 1-11.** Types of aneurysm. (DeBakey M, Gotto A: The Living Heart, p 166. New York, Raven Press, 1977)

### LABORATORY FINDINGS

#### Rupture of Aneurysm

Leukocytosis

Increased sedimentation rate

Findings associated with shock

#### Interference With Blood Supply to the Following

Heart (see Myocardial Infarction and Congestive Heart Failure)

Brain (see Cerebral Infarction, Chap. 7)

Kidney (see Renal Infarction, Chap. 5)

Intestines (see Mesenteric Infarction, Chap. 3)

## SYPHILITIC CARDIOVASCULAR DISEASES*

Syphilis is a generalized infection caused by the spirochete *Treponema pallidum.* Syphilis is acquired through sexual contact. Multiple serious effects on the cardiovascular system appear many years after a patient contracts the original

* See also Chapters 7 and 11.

infection. There is damage to the aortic valve ring, resulting in dilatation and backward leakage of blood from the aorta, through the dilated aortic valve, into the left ventricle during each diastole. This backward leakage through the aortic valve is known as *insufficiency*. The additional workload placed on the left ventricle causes enlargement of the heart and often results in congestive heart failure.

Another late cardiovascular complication of syphilis is damage to the medial layer of the ascending or thoracic aorta. This results in an aneurysm, which may cause pressure on adjacent thoracic structures and nerves.

### LABORATORY FINDINGS

Positive serum FTA-ABS test (95% of patients) and VDRL (77% of patients)

Laboratory findings of congestive heart failure due to aortic-valve insufficiency

Laboratory findings of myocardial infarction due to narrowing of coronary-artery openings

Laboratory findings of aneurysm

## RAYNAUD'S PHENOMENON

Raynaud's phenomenon is a condition in which the smallest arteries supplying the fingers or toes go into spasm on exposure to cold or as a result of emotional stresses. Because the small veins remain open, the blood drains out of the capillaries and the fingers or toes become pale, cold, and numb. This may result in ulcers, or even gangrene, of the affected tissues. The condition may be primary or secondary to another disease. The secondary form of Raynaud's phenomenon is associated with one of the connective-tissue diseases, such as scleroderma, rheumatoid arthritis, or systemic lupus erythematosus.

### LABORATORY FINDINGS

Cold agglutinins are occasionally present.

Cryoglobulins may be present in multiple myeloma or leukemia.

Laboratory findings of scleroderma, systemic lupus erythematosus, rheumatoid arthritis (see Chap. 9)

## ARTERIAL THROMBOSIS AND EMBOLISM

In arterial thrombosis, the initiating features are vascular injury and platelet aggregation. In contrast to its primary occurrence in venous thrombosis, activation of the clotting mechanism is a secondary occurrence in arterial thrombosis. Sudden occlusion of an artery may occur if a thrombus forms at the site of an atherosclerotic plaque or if a thrombus that has formed in the heart or aorta is carried by the bloodstream as an embolus to a peripheral artery. When an artery is blocked suddenly, time is not allowed for collateral circulation to develop. Tissues supplied by the occluded vessel consequently have diminished blood supplies. Such diminished blood supply is known as *ischemia*. Other arteries in the affected region undergo secondary spasm, further reducing the blood supply. This may result in tissue death, known as *ischemic necrosis*, or gangrene. Gangrene is ischemic necrosis plus suppurative inflammation. A segmental zone of necrosis involving only the region supplied by the occluded vessel is called an *infarct*. An infarct secondary to thrombotic or embolic arterial occlusion may involve the extremities, heart muscle, kidney, brain, or intestines.

Arterial emboli may originate from thrombi in the left heart chambers, from the lining of an atherosclerotic artery, or from an aneurysm of the aorta or any of its branches. Cardiac thrombi may form in the left atrium or its appendage in patients with rheumatic heart disease, with narrowing (stenosis) of the mitral valve, or with an irregular heart rhythm, such as atrial fibrillation. A thrombus may also form on the endothelial lining of the heart following a myocardial infarction. This type is known as a *mural thrombus*. Large emboli may block large arteries, whereas small emboli usually occlude small arteries.

In bacterial or infective endocarditis, emboli consisting of bacteria, fibrin, and blood cells from involved heart valves are usually disseminated throughout the systemic circulation, causing petechiae, small abscesses, and septic infarcts.

## LABORATORY FINDINGS

### Laboratory Findings of Underlying Disorders
Infective endocarditis

Rheumatic heart disease

Myocardial infarction with mural thrombus

### Laboratory Findings of Embolic Occlusion and Infarction
Heart (see Coronary Artery Disease and Myocardial Infarction)

Kidney (see Renal Infarction, Chap. 5)

Brain (see Cerebral Infarction, Chap. 7)

Intestine (see Mesenteric Infarction, Chap. 3)

Extremity (see Gangrene)

## *GANGRENE*

The most frequent cause of arterial occlusion is atherosclerosis. As occlusion progresses and the blood supply diminishes, the organ or tissue supplied by that artery becomes ischemic, infarcted, and then (possibly) gangrenous. *Gangrene* is ischemic necrosis, or death of tissue, with superimposed infection. This most frequently affects the extremities or the intestines when the arterial blood flow is interrupted. When venous occlusion also occurs this is referred to as "wet" gangrene because fluid is retained in the tissues.

### LABORATORY FINDINGS

Increased C-reactive protein and sedimentation rate; the former usually precedes the latter

Leukocytosis

If there is extensive tissue necrosis, there will be increased LDH (especially $LDH_1$), CPK (especially CPK-MM), and serum glutamic-oxaloacetic transaminase (SGOT).

## HYPERSENSITIVITY VASCULITIS

The necrotizing vasculitides are a group of inflammatory diseases of the blood vessels in which there is destruction of the vessel wall. The most common form of necrotizing vasculitis is allergic, or hypersensitivity, vasculitis.[16] This involves small blood vessels, is manifested by palpable small hemorrhages (purpura) of the skin, and appears to be due to immune-complex deposition in the involved vessels.

In addition to cutaneous involvement, there may also be involvement of small vessels of the kidneys, joints, gastrointestinal tract, lungs, or central nervous system.

The most common causes include streptococcal infection and drug ingestion. Other causes include hepatitis antigen, foreign proteins, and exposure to insecticides or petroleum products.

Immunofluorescent studies of biopsy specimens from active lesions demonstrate immunoglobulins and complement distributed in a granular pattern within the vessel walls. This finding is presumptive evidence that the disease is due to immune complexes. An *immune complex* is a substance composed of antigen (*i.e.*, streptococcal protein or hepatitis B surface antigen [$HB_sAg$]) that is combined with an antibody. If relatively small, this complex remains soluble within the circulation and causes no problems. If large, it is usually cleared by phagocytes. In some patients, however, this complex may deposit within vessel walls, bind and activate complement, and attract leukocytes. Neutrophils release enzymes that damage vessel walls, allowing red cells to leak into the surrounding tissue. This results in the formation of palpable purpura.

### LABORATORY FINDINGS

Skin biopsy showing characteristic necrotizing vasculitis; lesions less than 24 hours to 36 hours old may show immunofluorescent deposits of immunoglobulins and complement

Presence of circulating immune complexes

Decreased serum complement

Detection of specific infectious agents, such as streptococci or $HB_sAg$

Positive ASO test indicating prior streptococcal infection

Findings of connective-tissue disease, indicated by presence of rheumatoid factor, antinuclear antibody, anti-DNA.

Findings of renal involvement, such as proteinuria or decreased creatinine clearance

Presence of occult blood in stool, indicating gastrointestinal involvement

# POLYARTERITIS NODOSA

Polyarteritis nodosa is an inflammatory disease of the medium-sized muscular arteries. It is thought to be due to an immunologic mechanism. The sites of inflammation and necrosis are segmental and are usually at points of vascular branching. Formation of microaneurysms results in the development of small nodules on the vessels; these nodules give us the term *nodosa*. When this process involves the inner, or intimal, layer of the artery, thrombosis and occlusion occur; this may result in infarction. The most frequent sites involved are the kidneys, liver, heart, and gastrointestinal tract. (See Chap. 5.)

## LABORATORY FINDINGS

### Indicators of Inflammation

Increased leukocytes and neutrophils; eosinophilia suggests pulmonary involvement

Marked increase in sedimentation rate

Increased complement

Increased $\alpha_2$-globulin and $\gamma$-globulin

### Indicators of Renal Involvement

Increased urine protein, RBC, and granular casts

Decreased serum albumin is the result of marked proteinuria, which occurs in nephrosis

Microcytic anemia due to blood loss and renal failure

### Other Findings

Increased platelets

# TEMPORAL ARTERITIS

Temporal arteritis is a chronic, generalized inflammatory disease of unknown cause. It principally involves the temporal and occipital arteries of patients over the age of 50.[9] The histologic reaction is characterized by localized foci of inflammation, called *granulomas,* which contain many giant cells. This disease is often called *giant cell arteritis* or *granulomatous arteritis.* The inflammatory reaction causes a marked thickening of the inner layer of the artery with narrowing and occlusion of the lumen.

Headache and scalp tenderness are common symptoms and are probably due to inflammation of the cranial arteries. Visual manifestations are generally caused by ischemia of the optic nerve or involvement of the ophthalmic artery.

Severe pain in the jaw muscles results from narrowing or occlusion of the temporal or maxillary arteries. Polymyalgia rheumatica occurs in about 50% of patients (see Chap. 9).

### LABORATORY FINDINGS

Marked increase in sedimentation rate (50mm/hr–132 mm/hr, Westergren method) is a characteristic finding.

Moderate normocytic anemia (mean hemoglobin = 11.4 g/dl)

Slight increase in WBC (up to 20,000/$\mu$l)

Increased fibrinogen and $\alpha_2$-globulin parallel the sedimentation rate. These are indicators of inflammation.

Biopsy of the temporal artery is required for definitive diagnosis.

## PERIPHERAL VENOUS DISEASE

*Peripheral venous disease* refers to any interference with venous return of deoxygenated blood from the tissues to the heart and lungs. Veins that carry blood from regions of the body below the heart must work in opposition to the force of gravity. The direction of flow is aided by skeletal-muscle contractions and by venous valves, which prevent blood from flowing backward (Fig. 1-12).

The most common problem affecting the venous system is that of varicosity; this dilatation occurs most often in the superficial veins of the legs. The actual cause is uncertain, although heredity may play a role. Varicosities may develop because the valves fail to function properly. This results in backward blood flow, increased venous resistance, venous stagnation, pooling, venous dilatation, and possibly thrombus formation. A thrombus or clot in a vein may partly or completely stop the flow of blood.

In the presence of diminished blood flow, the fluidity of blood is maintained by an intact endothelium, abundant plasma coagulation inhibitors, and vigorous fibrinolysis. When the last two mechanisms fail, a thrombus may be formed, even over an intact endothelium. Activation of the coagulation system is primarily responsible for the formation of venous thrombi. Platelet aggregation, vascular stasis, and endothelial damage play secondary roles. This process is in contrast to that in arterial thrombosis, in which vascular injury and platelet aggregation are of primary importance.

Venous thrombosis is a serious medical disorder because of its possible complication: pulmonary embolism. If a portion of a venous thrombus breaks off, it is called an *embolus*. Major emboli are more likely to come from thrombi proximal to the knee, which usually have extended from the calf. An embolus is carried in the venous circulation into the right side of the heart and, through the pulmonary arteries, into the lungs. This results in decreased circulation to the affected portion of the lung and may cause localized death of tissue or infarction (see Chap. 2).

Venous thromboembolism may occur in an apparently healthy person, but it is more likely to strike the elderly, those who are immobilized for a long time (*e.g.*, stroke and arthritis victims and patients in plaster casts), those who have

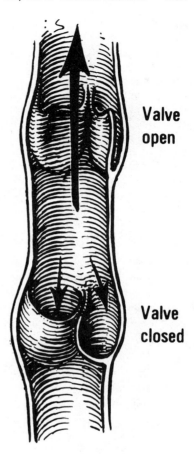

**Valve open**

**Valve closed**

**Fig. 1-12.** One-way valves in the veins prevent blood from flowing backward. (DeBakey M, Gotto A: The Living Heart, p 63. New York, Raven Press 1977)

stasis of blood due to varicosities, and those who have recently undergone surgery, childbirth, heart failure, or shock. It may also occur after certain infections and malignant tumors or with the use of oral contraceptives. It is one of the most common causes of death following major orthopedic surgery and is a contributing factor in deaths among patients with chronic cardiac and pulmonary diseases.

### LABORATORY FINDINGS*

Laboratory findings of underlying disease (*e.g.,* carcinoma of the pancreas, polycythemia)

Leukocytosis with increased bands and positive blood culture often occurs in septic phlebitis.

Laboratory findings of pulmonary infarction

* If a patient is maintained on anticoagulant therapy, the effect of Coumadin or heparin should be monitored in the laboratory.

## *SHOCK*

Shock is the state of circulatory collapse that is frequently associated with insufficient return of blood to the heart and manifested by persisting deficiency of blood flow to peripheral tissues. Any condition that causes deficient blood volume, peripheral vasodilatation, cardiac insufficiency, or combinations of these factors may initiate a series of functional alterations and compensatory responses that constitute the clinical syndrome of shock. Shock may follow severe trauma, major surgery, massive hemorrhage, dehydration, myocardial infarction, overwhelming infection, poisoning, or a drug reaction.[14]

Circulatory collapse is manifested by a fall in cardiac output, a decrease in blood volume, a fall in blood pressure, and a rapid pulse rate. The diagnosis is based primarily on the patient's history and clinical findings. The laboratory findings are secondary.

### LABORATORY FINDINGS

WBC: Increased with hemorrhage; decreased when shock is severe, as in gram-negative septicemia; increased neutrophils, decreased lymphocytes and eosinophils

Increased hematocrit, hemoglobin, BUN, and albumin due to hemoconcentration, which occurs in dehydration and burns

Decreased hematocrit and hemoglobin due to hemodilution, which occurs in hemorrhage, crush injury, and skeletal trauma

Early increase in blood glucose due to increased epinephrine formation in response to stress

Metabolic acidosis (low $pH$, low $CO_2$ content, increased lactic acid) due to tissue hypoxia when shock is severe

Decreased urine volume, low urine specific gravity, proteinuria; increased serum creatinine, BUN, and potassium; all due to decreased renal circulation

Increased LDH, proportionate in all five isoenzymes; if shock is due to myocardial infarction or cardiogenic shock, $LDH_1$ will be predominant; if there is severe hepatic congestion and necrosis, $LDH_5$ will be increased

## *REFERENCES*

1. Bravo EL, Tarazi RC, Gifford RW, Stewart BH: Circulating and urinary catecholamines in pheochromocytoma. N Engl J Med 301:682–686, 1979
2. Burke MD: Hypertension: Test strategies for diagnosis and management. Diagn Med 2:72–84, 1979
3. Fowler NO: Differential diagnosis of cardiomyopathies. Prog Cardiovasc Dis 14:113–128, 1971
4. Frederickson DS, Levy RI, Lees RS: Fat transport and lipoproteins: An integrated approach to mechanisms and disorders. N Engl J Med 276:34–44, 94–103, 148–156, 215–225, 273–281, 1967
5. Galen RS: Isoenzymes and myocardial infarction. Diagn Med 1:40–52, 1978
6. Gifford R: Is the renin–sodium profile helpful in evaluating hypertension? JAMA 244:35–37, 1980
7. Gotto AM: Diagnosis and management of risk factors for atherosclerosis. Atherosclerosis: A Scope Publication. Kalamazoo, Upjohn, 1977

8. Hiramatsu K, Yamada T, Yukimura Y et al: A screening test to identify aldosterone-producing adenoma by measuring plasma renin activity. Arch Intern Med 141:1589–1593, 1981
9. Hunder GG, Allen GL: Giant cell arteritis: A review. Bull Rheum Dis 29:980–987, 1978–1979
10. Inkeles S, Eisenberg D: Hyperlipidemia and coronary atherosclerosis: A review. Medicine 60:110–123, 1981
11. Kannel WB, Castelli WB, Gordon T: Cholesterol in the prediction of atherosclerotic disease. Ann Intern Med 90:85–91, 1979
12. Oliva PB: Pathophysiology of acute myocardial infarction. Ann Intern Med 94:236–250, 1981
13. Report of the WHO/ISFC task force on the definition and classification of cardiomyopathies. Br Heart J 44:672–673, 1980
14. Riede U, Sandritter W, Mittermayer C: Circulatory shock: A review. Pathology 13:299–311, 1981
15. Robertson AL: The pathogenesis of human atherosclerosis. Atherosclerosis: A Scope Publication. Kalamazoo, Upjohn, 1977
16. Sams WM: Allergic vasculitis. Postgrad Med 70:193–200, 1981
17. Sheps SG, Kirkpatrick RA: Hypertension. Mayo Clin Proc 50:709–720, 1975
18. Steinberg D: Underlying mechanisms in atherosclerosis. J Pathol 133:75–87, 1981
19. Washington JA: The role of the microbiology laboratory in the diagnosis and antimicrobial treatment of infective endocarditis. Mayo Clin Proc 57:22–32, 1982
20. Zampogna A, Luria MH, Manubens SJ et al: Relationship between lipids and occlusive coronary artery disease. Arch Intern Med 140:1067–1069, 1980

## BIBLIOGRAPHY

**American Heart Association:** American Heart Association Heartbook. New York, Elsevier-Dutton, 1980
**DeBakey M, Gotto A:** The Living Heart. New York, Raven Press, 1977
**Stein EA:** Coronary Heart Disease: You Can Live Without It. Medfield, MA, Corning Medical, 1979

# 2
# *RESPIRATORY DISEASES*

Croup
Bronchiolitis
Whooping Cough
Viral Pneumonias
Bacterial Pneumonias
Mycoplasmal Pneumonia
Legionnaires' Disease
Tuberculosis
Mycobacterial Diseases Other Than
       Tuberculosis
Actinomycosis and Nocardiosis
Histoplasmosis
Coccidioidomycosis
Blastomycosis
Cryptococcosis
Aspergillosis
Chronic Bronchitis
Pulmonary Emphysema
Asthma
Bronchiectasis
Pneumoconiosis
Sarcoidosis
Pleural Effusion
  Circulatory Disorders
    Congestive Heart Failure

Pulmonary Embolism or Infarction
  Hypoalbuminemia
Pulmonary Infectious Diseases
Neoplasms
Collagen Diseases
Trauma
Intra-abdominal Disorders
  Abscess
  Pancreatitis
  Cirrhosis of the Liver
  Meigs' Syndrome
Miscellaneous
  Uremia
  Myxedema
Lung Abscess
Allergic Pulmonary Parenchymal
      Diseases
  Hypersensitivity Pneumonitis
  Eosinophilic Pneumonias
Pulmonary Edema
Pulmonary Embolism and Infarction
Fat Embolism
Respiratory Distress Syndrome
Respiratory Failure
Bronchogenic Carcinoma

## CROUP

Croup is a clinical syndrome in children. It is characterized by an inspiratory, high-pitched "crowing" sound and a barking cough. This is due to acute inflammation of the epiglottis, larynx, trachea, and bronchi. Inflammation and edema of the larynx produce the characteristic clinical manifestations. Croup occurs most commonly in children between two and six years of age. Epiglottitis is most frequently caused by *Hemophilus influenzae* type B. Acute laryngotracheobronchitis is most often associated with parainfluenza viruses. Involvement of the trachea and bronchi, with accumulation of dried secretions, may further obstruct the airway.

### LABORATORY FINDINGS

Leukocytosis with increased granulocytes

Nasopharyngeal cultures usually show *H. influenzae* type B.

Positive blood cultures for *H. influenzae* (in up to 50% of cases)

Isolation of parainfluenza viruses from nasopharyngeal secretions

## BRONCHIOLITIS

Bronchiolitis is an acute viral respiratory infection of infants under one year old that is characterized by obstruction of the terminal branches of the bronchial tree. Thick secretions and bronchiolar edema produce the obstruction. This results in the trapping of air and hyperinflation of the lungs. The virus that is most frequently implicated is the respiratory syncytial virus. Bronchiolitis results from the spread of an upper respiratory infection.

### LABORATORY FINDINGS

Isolation of respiratory syncytial and parainfluenza viruses

Rise in titer of viral antibodies during convalescence

## WHOOPING COUGH

Whooping cough is an acute infectious disease of the tracheobronchial tree; it may also involve the lungs. It is caused by *Bordetella pertussis*. The organism is not invasive but it attaches to the surfaces of respiratory epithelial cells. An exotoxin causes necrosis of the cells. Necrotic cellular debris and mucus accumulate, irritate the mucosa, and initiate coughing. Secondary pneumonia is common and obstruction of the bronchi by mucus may cause anoxia.

### LABORATORY FINDINGS*

Fluorescent antibody staining of organisms in nasopharyngeal smears provides a rapid, specific diagnosis.

Leukocytosis (<100,000/$\mu$l) with marked lymphocytosis (<90%), especially in patients over six months of age

Negative blood cultures

---

* Serologic tests are of little diagnostic value because antibodies appear late.

## VIRAL PNEUMONIAS

Viruses are generally considered to be common etiologic agents in early childhood pneumonias.[9] Respiratory syncytial virus is now recognized as the major cause of serious lower respiratory tract disease in young children, especially in those less than six months of age. Parainfluenza virus infections are very common and usually occur in a slightly older age group. Influenza virus causes lung disease in children, but it is milder in children than in adults. Adenoviruses are also common respiratory pathogens in children.

The most common viral agent causing pneumonia in adults is the influenza virus. The frequency of pneumonia resulting from influenza infection tends to increase with underlying cardiopulmonary disease and with increasing age. Influenza is transmitted through inhalation of the virus. Influenza virus contains an enzyme that enables it to penetrate respiratory mucus. The organism infects most of the surface epithelial cells of the entire respiratory tract. Infected cells show characteristic intracellular viral inclusions and a change from respiratory epithelium to squamous epithelium. The respiratory epithelial cells of the large and medium-sized airways die and are sloughed off, down to the basement membrane. Systemic symptoms are probably due to the absorption of breakdown products of dying cells into the bloodstream. Viremia is not a common occurrence.

Alveolar walls swell with dilated vessels, edema fluid, and monocytic exudate. Red blood cells (RBC), mononuclear cells, and fibrin leak into the air spaces. Fibrin may adhere to the walls of the alveoli, forming "hyaline" membranes. All of these pathologic changes interfere with the exchange of oxygen and carbon dioxide and may alter pulmonary function.

The influenza virus hampers migration and phagocytosis by granulocytes and macrophages and probably also depresses cell-mediated immunity. Secondary bacterial tracheobronchitis or bacterial pneumonia occurs in about 10% of patients. The most frequent accompanying bacterial organism is *Streptococcus pneumoniae*. Secondary bacterial pneumonia is the major cause of death.

Viral pneumonia may also occur as part of systemic viral diseases, such as measles and chickenpox. In immunocompromised hosts, the most important virus associated with pulmonary infection is cytomegalovirus.

### LABORATORY FINDINGS

Isolation of influenza, parainfluenza, or respiratory syncytial virus from nasopharyngeal or throat swab or from throat washings

Complement-fixing antibodies; these appear 8 days to 9 days after the onset of illness; antibody titer against the specific causative virus shows a fourfold rise in serum specimens taken two to three weeks apart

Fluorescent staining of viral antigens in nasopharyngeal or bronchial epithelial cells establishes the diagnosis while the patient is acutely ill

Sputum—no bacteria; polymorphonuclear, mononuclear, and bronchial epithelial cells; the latter are those sloughed from the infected air passages

White blood cell (WBC) count may be normal or decreased with relative lymphocytosis. Leukocytosis above 15,000/$\mu$l usually indicates the presence of a secondary bacterial infection.

## BACTERIAL PNEUMONIAS

Pneumonia is an acute infection of the alveolar air spaces of the lung. It may involve an entire lobe of the lung (lobar), a portion of a lobe adjacent to a bronchus (bronchial), or the alveolar septa (interstitial); it may also result in the destruction of lung tissue (necrotizing). These forms of pneumonia are shown in Figure 2-1.

Streptococcus pneumoniae is the most common cause of bacterial pneumonia.[14] It is usually transmitted by healthy carriers, especially in crowded environments. Pneumococcal pneumonia develops most often during the course of viral infection of the upper respiratory tract. At that time, abundant mucous secretions from the nose and pharynx carry pneumococci through the air passages into the lungs. Edematous lungs are more susceptible to pneumococcal infection than are normal lungs. Edema fluid provides a suitable culture medium for pneumococci and interferes with phagocytosis. Conditions producing pulmonary edema and enhancing pneumococcal pneumonia include inhalation of irritating anesthetics, chest trauma, heart failure, and influenzal pneumonia. Bacteremia occurs in approximately 30% of patients with pneumococcal pneumonia.

Staphylococcal pneumonia is often a complication of influenza, measles, or cystic fibrosis; it may also occur in debilitated hospitalized patients. Pneumonia due to group A streptococci is uncommon except as a complication of measles, influenza, streptococcal sore throat, or scarlet fever. Klebsiella pneumoniae is frequently acquired in a hospital and usually causes necrotizing pneumonia in elderly debilitated patients and in alcoholics. Thick gelatinous secretions interfere with phagocytosis and antibiotic penetration. Hemophilus influenzae pneumonia is most common in children less than two years of age, but it has

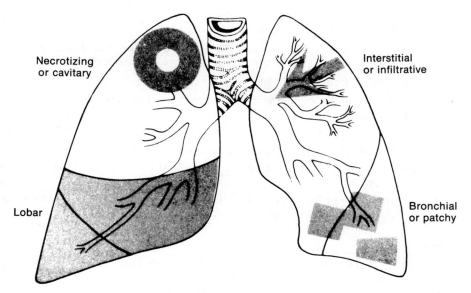

**Fig. 2-1.** Forms of pneumonia. (Geschickter CF: The Lung in Health and Disease, p 115. Philadelphia, JB Lippincott, 1973)

been found with increasing frequency in elderly patients with preexisting chronic lung disease.

Pulmonary infection usually occurs whenever foreign bodies, gastric contents, or lipids are aspirated into the lungs. This is often secondary to loss of consciousness, seizures, or alcoholic intoxication.

Pneumonia is usually caused by organisms that are normally present in the mouth and throat. Whether a lung infection occurs is determined primarily by the virulence of the bacteria and the cellular defenses of the host. Normal host defenses may be decreased by alcohol, diabetes, acidosis, uremia, blood diseases, and various medical and surgical therapies. Disorders that predispose individuals to bacterial pneumonias include chronic obstructive pulmonary diseases, lung disease due to inhaled dust, congestive heart failure, bronchial obstruction, viral pneumonia, and cystic fibrosis.

Proliferating bacteria damage lung capillaries, allowing edema fluid, leukocytes, and erythrocytes to fill the alveoli. The fluid and cells interfere with the exchange of oxygen and carbon dioxide. Bacteria are removed initially by polymorphonuclear leukocytes and later by alveolar macrophages. Phagocytosis is impaired by bacterial capsules, which are present on *Streptococcus pneumoniae, Hemophilus influenzae,* and *Klebsiella pneumoniae.* The healing process usually takes 2 weeks to 3 weeks and leaves the lungs undamaged. Complications include spread of the infection into the pleural space producing empyema (pus in the pleural cavity), abscess formation, and destruction of lung tissue. Organisms may enter the bloodstream and cause meningitis, endocarditis, or arthritis.

Interference with gas exchange results in decreased arterial oxygen and stimulates ventilation, which in turn decreases arterial carbon dioxide. Severe hypoxemia may result in reduced consciousness, cardiac arrhythmias, or death.

## LABORATORY FINDINGS

Leukocytosis—usually 15,000/$\mu$l with 70%–90% granulocytes; in overwhelming infections or in aged patients, WBC may be normal or even decreased.

Blood culture is frequently positive.

Increased sedimentation rate and C-reactive protein are nonspecific indicators of acute infection.

Decreased albumin and increased $\alpha_2$-globulin result from chronic inflammation.

Decreased arterial $PO_2$ due to impaired oxygenation in lung

Decreased arterial $PCO_2$ and increased $pH$ (respiratory alkalosis) are the result of stimulated ventilation.

Urine—commonly proteinuria, WBC, and casts; ketones may occur with severe infections; glucose may be found, indicating underlying diabetes

### Sputum

Specimen should show fewer than 10 squamous epithelial cells and more than 25 WBC/low-power field ($\times$ 100) to be acceptable for culture.

Gram's stains show a predominant bacterial species.

Culture on appropriate media shows the causative organisms.

Counterimmunoelectrophoresis can be used to detect the pneumococcal antigen.

## MYCOPLASMAL PNEUMONIA

This very common disease was formerly known as *primary atypical pneumonia.*[7] It is caused by *Mycoplasma pneumoniae* (Eaton agent). Mycoplasmas are the smallest organisms that are free living (*i.e.,* they do not require cells for growth, as do viruses). The organisms are intermediate in size between bacteria and rickettsiae. Mycoplasmas differ from other bacteria in that they are unable to synthesize rigid cell walls and their growth is inhibited by specific antibodies.

The organism does not enter host cells nor does it penetrate beneath the epithelial surface. It impairs ciliary activity and destroys bronchiolar epithelium by releasing hydrogen peroxide into cells. Infection results in acute pharyngitis, bronchitis, and bronchiolitis with formation of a tenacious exudate. Lungs are only mildly involved, and the infection resolves without permanent damage. Most infections are subclinical and bacterial superinfection is rare. Antibodies do not confer immunity and reinfection does occur.

### LABORATORY FINDINGS

Complement-fixing antibody—fourfold rise in titer is diagnostic in serum drawn 3–4 weeks after onset. This is present in 80%–90% of patients. If only convalescent serum is available, a titer $>1:64$ is suggestive of prior infection. Titers may remain elevated for one or more years after infection. IgM antibody first appears 7–9 days after infection, peaks at 4–6 weeks, and does not start to decline until 4–6 months later.

Cold hemagglutinins—fourfold rise in titer during illness is suggestive but not diagnostic. This is positive at the seventh day, peak level is at four weeks, and it is negative by four months. Only 25%–50% of patients develop cold agglutinins; therefore, a negative test does not exclude the disease. Many other conditions show elevated cold agglutinin titers. These include infectious mononucleosis, rubella, mumps, influenza, adenovirus, dysproteinemias, hemolytic anemia, paroxysmal hemoglobinuria, Raynaud's disease, and scleroderma.

Indirect fluorescent antibodies—rise in titer may be demonstrated by this sensitive and specific test

Isolation of organism from sputum, throat washing, or upper-respiratory-tract secretions

Sputum—leukocytes and monocytes; normal bacterial flora on smear and culture

WBC—normal to 20,000/$\mu$l (average 10,000/$\mu$l–12,000/$\mu$l); predominant granulocytes.

Increased sedimentation rate

## *LEGIONNAIRES' DISEASE*

*Legionella pneumophila* is a recently described, unique soil organism that, when inhaled in sufficient quantity, may cause either mild or severe disease. There is no evidence of person-to-person transmission.

The disease's effects may range from headache and sore muscles to overwhelming pneumonia and death. Fatalities may have been at least partly due to host factors such as middle age, alcohol intake, cigarette smoking, and underlying respiratory disease.

### LABORATORY FINDINGS

Elevated antibody titer in serum, using immunofluorescent techniques

Identification of organism in sputum using immunofluorescent techniques

Isolation and culture of the organism require special media.

No leukocytosis

## *TUBERCULOSIS*

Tuberculosis is a disease caused by *Mycobacterium tuberculosis.*[11] It is acquired by inhaling viable tubercle bacilli into the lungs. Though primarily a disease of the lungs, it might involve any organ in the body. The host response following an initial infection is different from that following a reinfection. On first exposure, the bacilli in the lungs are slowly engulfed by phagocytes, but they may remain viable and multiply. They form a focus of tuberculous pneumonia, usually in the lower lung fields, and then spread to the regional draining lymph nodes. The bacilli may be killed or may remain viable, encased in scar tissue or within macrophages. In most cases this host-defense process controls further spread of the infection and the host–parasite relationship settles into a state of equilibrium. Some organisms are slowly destroyed as lesions heal, but significant numbers of bacilli retain their viability in a dormant condition. Dissemination by the bloodstream throughout the body may occur. Limited foci of infection then develop in the upper lungs, kidneys, bones, and cerebral cortex. Two weeks to four weeks after the primary infection, the patient develops acquired cell-mediated immunity, which limits further multiplication of the bacilli and results in healing of the lesions. Once a person has developed acquired immunity to tubercle bacilli, it is uncommon for him to develop a new airborne infection.

This immunologic response to the bacilli and their products is clinically evident by the appearance of a positive tuberculin skin test and pathologically evident by the formation of tubercles (Fig. 2-2). Tubercles are localized foci of chronic infection called *granulomas,* which are comprised of macrophages containing tubercle bacilli, sensitized lymphocytes, giant cells, and central zones of necrosis. The necrotic central zone is cheeselike; it is therefore called *caseous.* The infection is usually arrested at this stage and the lung and lymph nodes become fibrotic and, often, calcified. In a small number of patients the infection is not brought under control and the primary lesions become progressively

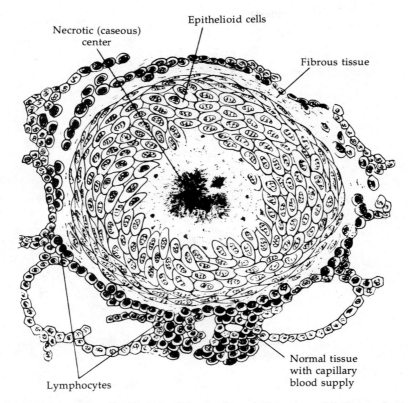

Necrotic (caseous) center

Epithelioid cells

Fibrous tissue

Lymphocytes

Normal tissue with capillary blood supply

**Fig. 2-2.** Caseous tubercle. (American Lung Association: Introduction to Lung Diseases, 5th ed, p 39. New York, American Lung Association, 1973)

larger, coalesce, and liquefy. When this necrotic material is released, a cavity is formed in the lung. This process allows the infection to spread through the bronchi to other regions of the lung. Fibrous scar tissue also forms, which limits the spread of infection. Most patients show both progressive and healing areas.

Tubercle bacilli at different sites throughout the body remain dormant but viable following the primary infection. They may become activated years or decades later to produce a secondary reinfection. Foci of infection may be reactivated at any time, especially if cellular immunity wanes owing to chronic illness, use of steroid or immunosuppressive drugs, or old age. Diseases that increase the likelihood of reactivation include alcoholism, uncontrolled diabetes mellitus, silicosis, leukemia, and Hodgkin's disease. Reactivated tuberculosis usually involves the upper lung zones, possibly because of the higher oxygen content there. There may be cavity formation and extension of infection through the bronchi to other areas of the lungs (Fig. 2-3). Infection also extends into the pleural space or throughout the body through the lymphatics or bloodstream. When it extends into the bloodstream, it is known as *miliary tuberculosis*. The most commonly involved sites of extrapulmonary infection include the meninges, bones and joints, genitourinary system, lymph nodes, pleura, and

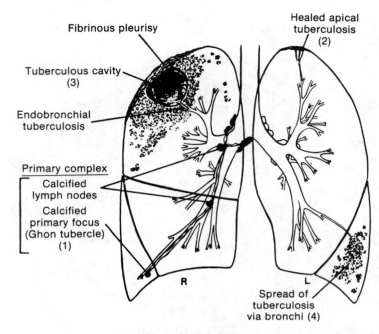

**Fig. 2-3.** Lungs showing progressive stages (1–4) of pulmonary tuberculosis. (American Lung Association: Introduction to Lung Diseses, 5th ed, p 35. New York, American Lung Association, 1973)

peritoneum. Extrapulmonary disease commonly develops as a result of reactivation of dormant lesions seeded during the primary infection.

### LABORATORY FINDINGS

Presence of characteristic organisms seen on carbol-fuchsin or auramine–rhodamine-stained smears of suspected secretions or tissue

Characteristic cultures from involved sites of concentrates of suspected material: sputum, bronchial washings, gastric fluid, pleural fluid, urine, cerebrospinal fluid, pus, bone marrow, endometrial scrapings, tissue biopsy

WBC—usually normal, except for lymphocytosis or monocytosis; leukemoid reaction or leukopenia may occur in miliary disease; pancytopenia is suggestive of bone-marrow involvement

Moderate normocytic, normochromic anemia in advanced disease

Increased sedimentation rate in disseminated disease; this is not an index of disease activity

Decreased serum albumin reflects severe chronic infection

Laboratory findings of extrapulmonary tuberculosis (*e.g.,* meningitis, renal disease, pleural or pericardial effusion, arthritis, liver disease)

## MYCOBACTERIAL DISEASES OTHER THAN TUBERCULOSIS

There are at least a dozen species of nontuberculous mycobacteria. This group of organisms has been called atypical, anonymous, and opportunistic. Organisms in the environment are the usual source of infection. There is no evidence of person-to-person transmission. Some of these organisms may be harbored as saprophytes in the mouth and pharynx of a healthy person and may occasionally be grown from the bronchial secretions of patients with chronic bronchitis, emphysema, or bronchiectasis. These mycobacteria are less pathogenic than are tubercle bacilli.[13] When disease does occur, it is often related to some reduction in host defense, as in the case of malignancy or chemotherapy. The most common conditions that predispose the patient to these infections are silicosis, chronic obstructive pulmonary diseases, and healed tuberculosis. Diseases produced by the nontuberculous mycobacteria are clinically, radiologically, and histologically similar to tuberculosis.

Within the lung, the inflammatory reaction and the resulting necrosis reflect the cellular immune response of the host. Extrapulmonary spread through lymphatic channels and bloodstream is uncommon.

The nontuberculous mycobacteria were initially categorized into the following groups, based primarily on pigment production:

Photochromogens—produce pigment only in the light
Scotochromogens—produce pigment in the dark as well as in the light
Nonphotochromogens—do not produce pigment
Rapid growers—grow in 3–5 days, in contrast to the 4–8 weeks required by most other mycobacteria

For specific species identification, many additional microbiologic and biochemical tests are required.

Wolinsky has formulated a clinically useful classification of mycobacteria based on human pathogenicity.[16] The most common pathogenic species and the diseases they cause are listed below:

Chronic pulmonary disease in adults
  *Mycobacterium avium-intracellulare*
  *M. kansasii*
Local lymphadenitis in children
  *M. scrofulaceum*
  *M. avium-intracellulare*
Bone and joint infection
  *M. kansasii*
  *M. avium-intracellulare*
Disseminated disease
  *M. avium-intracellulare*
  *M. kansasii*
Cutaneous and subcutaneous diseases
  Swimming-pool granuloma—*M. marinum*
  Sporotrichoid lesions—*M. marinum*

Local abscess—*M. fortuitum complex*
Buruli ulcer—*M. ulcerans*
Skin and soft-tissue infections—*M. kansasii*

## LABORATORY FINDINGS

A definite diagnosis requires either repeated isolation and identification of multiple colonies of the same strain of nontuberculous mycobacteria or isolation under sterile conditions of the organism from a closed lesion. These criteria are necessary to differentiate pathogenic organisms from saprophytic organisms.

# ACTINOMYCOSIS AND NOCARDIOSIS

*Actinomyces* and *Nocardia* are bacteria that are microbiologically similar to *Mycobacteria* and produce similar clinical and pathologic manifestations. The organisms are not fungi.

*Actinomyces israelii* is normally found as a saprophyte in such sites as the tonsillar crypts, gums, teeth, and gastrointestinal tract. Disease occurs when organisms penetrate damaged mucosal surfaces, gain access to dead or devitalized tissues, or spread in association with viral or bacterial infections. This causes a chronic infection, which tends to form destructive abscesses with burrowing sinus tracts to the skin surface and fistulous tracts between organs. When these organisms are aspirated into the lungs, diffuse chronic necrotizing pneumonia may occur. This is often followed by infection of the pleural cavity and chest wall with sinus-tract formation. Approximately 15% of actinomycotic infections involve the lungs.

In contrast to *Actinomyces, Nocardia asteroides* does not occur in healthy persons. The organism grows as a saprophyte in soil. When organisms in soil are inhaled, they cause scattered areas of pneumonia, lung abscesses, empyema, or (occasionally) draining chest-wall sinus tracts. *Nocardia* often gain access to the bloodstream and spread throughout the body, especially to the brain and meninges. This disease is particularly pathogenic in patients whose normal defenses are depressed.

## LABORATORY FINDINGS

### Actinomycosis

Organism is seen on Gram's stain or material from infected sinus tracts, abscess cavities, or empyema fluid. The organism may be found normally in sputum and the tonsils and pharynx.

Presence of yellowish particles (sulfur granules) within pus or infected sputum; the granules comprise *Actinomyces* colonies embedded in a matrix of calcium phosphate

Growth of organism on culture of pus or biopsy tissue

Increased sedimentation rate

Normocytic, normochromic anemia reflects chronic infection

**Nocardiosis**

Organism shows gram-positive filaments and is weakly acid-fast.

Growth of organism on Sabouraud's medium without antibiotics and on blood agar; it usually grows very slowly, is often mixed with other organisms and some strains may be killed by mycobacterial concentration techniques; occasional strains may grow rapidly on blood agar

## *HISTOPLASMOSIS*

Infections with the fungus *Histoplasma capsulatum* are endemic to certain areas, particularly to the Mississippi and Ohio River valleys.[6] The spores thrive in soil contaminated by excreta of birds and bats.

Inhaled spores cause a mild localized pneumonia. A few days later, the inhaled spores are transformed into the parasitic yeast form of the fungus. Yeasts are phagocytosed by macrophages, and localized foci of infection called *granulomas* are formed in the lungs and lymph nodes of the chest. The initial infection may pass unnoticed or appear as a self-limited respiratory infection. In many infected patients, there is bloodstream invasion with systemic dissemination. There is usually involvement of the liver and spleen. Within 4 to 8 months caseating granulomas, similar to those of tuberculosis, are found. These usually heal by calcification and contain nonviable organisms.

Rather than becoming inactive and calcifying, sometimes the primary lung lesions remain active and develop into a chronic pulmonary disease with formation of cavities. This tends to occur in persons with underlying chronic obstructive pulmonary disease, such as emphysema. Disseminated histoplasmosis may occur in infants, children, or immunosuppressed or older adults.

### LABORATORY FINDINGS

Culture of *H. capsulatum* from skin or mucosal ulcers, sputum, blood, spinal fluid, bone marrow, or tissues is required for definitive diagnosis.

Tissue biopsy of bone marrow, mucosal ulcers, liver, lymph nodes, lung with identification of *H. capsulatum*

Polyvalent fluorescent antibody reagent for the detection and identification of *H. capsulatum*

Complement fixing antibody titers—positive in 80% of chronic cases, but in only 50% of acute cases; appear in 3rd to 6th week; may persist for months or years if the disease remains active. When paired acute and convalescent sera are available, a fourfold or greater rise in titer is highly suggestive of recent infection. Titer above 1:32 is strong presumptive evidence of active infection. Because of cross-reactivity, titers may be positive in blastomycosis, aspergillosis, and coccidioidomycosis. The test thus has low specificity. False-positive and false-negative results may occur with chronic cavitary and disseminated disease. This test is more sensitive than the immunodiffusion test in patients with subclinical infection.

Latex agglutination test—this is often positive in acute disease because it detects IgM antibody. It is not dependable in chronic infections because it becomes negative in 5 to 8 months, even with persistent active disease.

Immunodiffusion and counterimmunoelectrophoresis tests are useful screening procedures. Precipitin bands of diagnostic value are designated *h* and *m*. The *m* band has been considered presumptive evidence of infection with *H. capsulatum*. If the patient has not had a recent histoplasmin skin test, detection of an *m* band may serve as an indicator of early disease, because this band appears before the *h* band and disappears more slowly.

It is important to note that levels of complement-fixing, precipitating, and agglutinating antibodies to *H. capsulatum* may be significantly increased in histoplasmin-sensitized persons after a single histoplasmin skin test.

## COCCIDIOIDOMYCOSIS

*Coccidioides immitis* is a fungus commonly found in the soil of the southwestern United States. Inhaled spores reach the alveoli, where they are transformed into spherules; these multiply and rupture, releasing more spores, which form more spherules until this process is arrested by the host's defenses. Granulomas form and the disease usually remains limited to the lungs.[2] About 60% of infections are mild, unrecognized, and detected only serologically. About 40% of patients develop acute pneumonia. Some patients ultimately develop chronic pulmonary cavitary disease, resembling tuberculosis. Although rare, widespread systemic dissemination may occur and be fatal.

### LABORATORY FINDINGS

Identification of organism by direct or phase-contrast microscopy of tissue or body secretions

Isolation of organism by culture of sputum, gastric contents, cerebrospinal fluid, exudate, synovial fluid, tissue

Precipitin antibodies are IgM, appear early, and are detectable by the 3rd week of illness in approximately 90% of symptomatic patients; they are uncommon after the 5th month. The latex agglutination test also detects IgM antibodies of early primary infection. This test is more sensitive than the precipitin test but is less specific. Neither of these tests provides information about disease severity or prognosis.

Complement-fixing antibodies are IgG, and they appear later and persist longer than do precipitin antibodies. They appear 4 to 5 weeks after exposure and decrease after 4 to 8 months, but they may remain positive for years. The antibody titer correlates with disease severity and response to therapy. These antibodies are positive in approximately 50% of nondisseminated primary infections and in 96% to 100% of disseminated infections. Antibodies in spinal fluid indicate involvement of meninges.

The immunodiffusion test, with antibody to the complement-fixing antigen, is negative in early primary infection but is a good screening test for other stages.

# BLASTOMYCOSIS

Blastomycosis is caused by the fungus *Blastomyces dermatitidis*. It begins in the lung after the spores have been inhaled from soil and converted into parasitic budding yeasts.[6] There is usually a mild, self-limited pulmonary infection starting as bronchopneumonia, which then forms tuberculoid granulomas. This is usually followed by dissemination to the skin, bones, viscera, and meninges. Healing occurs by fibrosis, usually without calcification.

## LABORATORY FINDINGS

Identification of organism by direct or phase-contrast microscopy of sputum, pus, or tissue

Isolation of organism by culture of sputum, pus, or tissue is required for definitive diagnosis.

Complement-fixing antibodies may be positive or negative with systemic infection. Cross-reaction with *H. capsulatum* further detracts from the diagnostic usefulness of this test.

The immunodiffusion test for blastomycosis is specific and has a sensitivity of approximately 80%. Negative tests, therefore, do not exclude the diagnosis.

Leukocytosis and increased sedimentation rate occur in active disease.

# CRYPTOCOCCOSIS

*Cryptococcus neoformans* is a fungus that is inhaled and initially infects the lungs. Pigeon excreta are an important source of infection. In contrast to infections from other bacteria and fungi, only a minimal inflammatory reaction is evoked. It is likely that silent infections of the lung are common and that only a very small proportion of these becomes disseminated. Patients with sarcoidosis, those with hematologic malignancies, and those with drug immunosuppression are at increased risk for disseminated infection with this fungus. Bloodstream invasion usually carries the organism to the brain (see Cryptococcal Meningitis, Chap. 7).

## LABORATORY FINDINGS

Identification of organism in sputum or spinal fluid using India ink or Nigrosin preparation

Isolation of organism by culture of cerebrospinal fluid, blood, pus, urine, stool, sputum, bone marrow, or tissue

Spinal fluid—lymphocytosis, increased protein, decreased glucose

Latex slide agglutination on serum and spinal fluid specifically detects cryptococcal antigen. This is a screening test. The titer is usually proportional to the extent of infection. This is more sensitive in diagnosing cryptococcal meningitis than is the India ink test.

Tests for cryptococcal antibody—indirect fluorescent antibody test and tube agglutination test; the latter is more specific; a positive antibody test may occur early in the course of the disease and in localized infections; the antibody test may have prognostic value; these tests usually become positive after the latex agglutination test becomes negative.

# ASPERGILLOSIS

*Aspergillus fumigatus* is a fungus that grows well in compost and in organic debris. The spores are commonly inhaled but only invade tissue when the host's defenses are diminished. Aspergillosis is a common problem in asthmatics and in patients with suppressed immunity. In immunosuppressed patients the fungus might invade the lungs, producing pulmonary disease, which may spread throughout the body. *Aspergillus* species are responsible for several forms of allergic pulmonary diseases.[8] These fungi also tend to inhabit preexisting cystic lung lesions or residual cavities in patients with healed tuberculosis, sarcoidosis or bronchiectasis. Fungus aggregates within lung cavities are termed *fungus balls*.

## LABORATORY FINDINGS

Identification of organism on smear; culture of organism from sputum or lung tissue; because the organisms are usually saprophytes, their isolation is not diagnostic but must be correlated with clinical information. Diagnosis requires demonstrating the fungus *in tissues*.

Immunodiffusion test for antibody, when used with reference sera, is 100% specific. Conversion of the immunodiffusion antibody test from negative to positive is diagnostic of infection. Demonstration of one or more precipitating antibodies indicates infection, fungus ball formation, or allergy due to an *Aspergillus* species.

Laboratory findings of an underlying disease, such as tuberculosis, asthma, bronchiectasis, or bronchogenic carcinoma

# CHRONIC BRONCHITIS

Chronic bronchitis is defined clinically by the presence of a chronic cough productive of excessive sputum. Symptoms are generally present on most days for at least three months of the year and for at least two successive years. Bronchitis is usually associated with cigarette smoking and usually coexists with pulmonary emphysema. The term *chronic obstructive lung disease* or *pulmonary disease* is often used to include a syndrome of chronic bronchitis, pulmonary emphysema, and (often) asthma. Bronchitis frequently is complicated by viral and bacterial infections of the tracheobronchial tree. This results in an excess of viscid-mucus secretions, which obstruct the air passages and make breathing difficult. Impaired gas exchange in the lungs results in severe hypoxemia, which might be manifested as cyanosis. Hypoxemia may also be responsible for secondary polycythemia. Another complication is heart failure with hepatic congestion and peripheral edema.

The most consistent pathologic abnormality in chronic bronchitis is an increase in size and number of bronchial mucus-secreting glands.[1] The glandular layer of the bronchi is thicker than normal. The characteristic chronic productive cough is the consequence of an increased volume of bronchial mucus. Obstruction to air flow is probably the result of narrowing of peripheral airways.[12] Inflammation is not a characteristic finding in patients with chronic bronchitis. Excessive mucus production and stasis of bronchial secretions provide a favorable environment for bacterial multiplication.

## LABORATORY FINDINGS

Leukocytosis occasionally occurs when acute infection is present.

Increased eosinophil count indicates an allergic component to the disease.

Increased sedimentation rate indicates acute infection.

Polycythemia is secondary to hypoxemia of long duration.

Sputum is clear and mucoid. When there is secondary infection, cultures frequently yield *Streptococcus pneumoniae* and *Hemophilus influenzae*.

Decreased arterial $PO_2$ due to impaired oxygen exchange

Decreased $PCO_2$ and increased $p$H (respiratory alkalosis) due to compensatory increased ventilation

Increased $PCO_2$ and decreased $p$H (respiratory acidosis) due to severely impaired and decreased ventilation

Polyclonal gammopathy indicates chronic infection.

Laboratory findings of associated disorders, such as emphysema and bronchiectasis

## *PULMONARY EMPHYSEMA*

Pulmonary emphysema is a disease of the lungs that is characterized by enlargement of the alveoli accompanied by destruction of alveolar walls.[1] Although emphysema is a disorder of air-flow obstruction, the site of obstruction is not readily demonstrable. It is generally felt that the obstructive phenomenon is at the level of the respiratory bronchioles.[12] Several factors combine to produce bronchiolar obstruction: excess mucus, spasm of smooth muscles, mucosal edema and proliferation, collapse of weakened bronchiolar walls, and even obliteration of bronchiolar lumina.[5] Up to 30% of lung tissue may be destroyed by emphysema without a result of demonstrable air-flow obstruction. Normally bronchiolar walls are supported by the attached alveolar septa, which exert forces of radial traction. With the loss of alveolar septa in emphysema there is a decrease in bronchiolar traction, rendering the bronchioles more collapsible. As a result, during expiration, when the pressure in adjoining alveoli exceeds the luminal pressure in the bronchioles, the bronchioles become compressed and collapse (Fig. 2-4). There is also loss of the elastic recoil of the bronchioles and

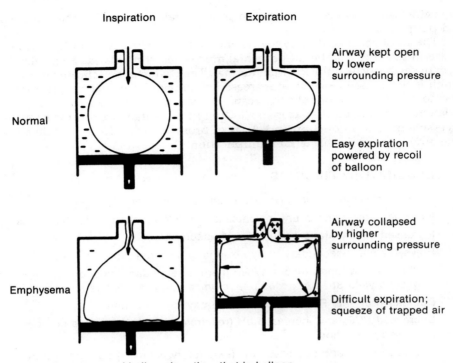

Inspiration          Expiration

Normal

Emphysema

Airway kept open
by lower
surrounding pressure

Easy expiration
powered by recoil
of balloon

Airway collapsed
by higher
surrounding pressure

Difficult expiration;
squeeze of trapped air

− = pressure around balloon less than that in balloon
+ = pressure around balloon greater than that in balloon

**Fig. 2-4.** The balloon-and-piston analogy illustrates the mechanism of expiratory bronchiolar collapse with emphysema. (American Lung Association: Chronic Obstructive Pulmonary Disease, 5th ed, p 34. New York, American Lung Association, 1977)

lung tissues. Bronchiolar obstruction due to loss of alveolar structure is irreversible and poorly responsive to bronchodilator drug therapy.

Involvement of the central portions of lung acini is referred to as *centriacinar emphysema,* whereas diffuse involvement is called *panacinar emphysema* (Fig. 2-5). The two types may coexist. The former is thought to represent a complication of chronic bronchitis, whereas the latter is considered to be a primary disorder of lung tissue. Centriacinar emphysema has a predilection for the upper parts of the lungs, where the mechanical stresses acting to expand alveoli are the greatest. This is the characteristic form found in long-term cigarette smokers.

Panacinar emphysema is frequently associated with an inherited deficiency of the antiproteolytic substance $\alpha_1$-antitrypsin. This suggests that emphysema might result from autodigestion of lung tissue by the unopposed action of trypsin and other proteases released from leukocytes and alveolar macrophages. These cells are found in increased numbers in smokers, in whom emphysema is of greater frequency and severity. Increased numbers of WBC release large amounts of trypsin, which could overcome pulmonary antiproteases, even when blood levels of $\alpha_1$-antitrypsin are normal. Furthermore, cigarette smoke may cause a major reduction in the protease-inhibitor activity of $\alpha_1$-antitrypsin. Thus, smoking has multiple adverse effects on the balance between proteases and their inhibitors.

Impaired ventilation and impaired gas exchange initially result in hypoxemia, but later progress to increased $CO_2$ retention, respiratory acidosis, and finally respiratory failure. Chronic hypoxemia may be a stimulus for secondary erythrocytosis. Pulmonary vascular obstruction and pulmonary hypertension may result in pulmonary heart disease.

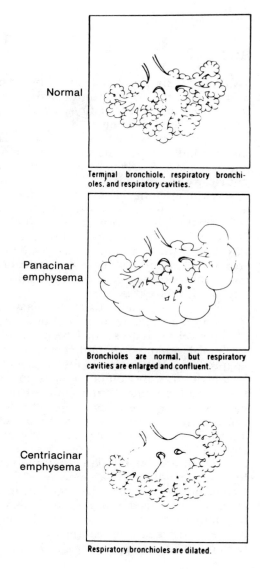

Normal

Terminal bronchiole, respiratory bronchioles. and respiratory cavities.

Panacinar emphysema

Bronchioles are normal, but respiratory cavities are enlarged and confluent.

Centriacinar emphysema

Respiratory bronchioles are dilated.

**Fig. 2-5.** Normal lung and lung showing two types of emphysema. (American Lung Association: Chronic Obstructive Pulmonary Disease, 5th ed, p 14. New York, American Lung Association, 1977)

## LABORATORY FINDINGS

Normal arterial $PO_2$, decreased $PCO_2$, and increased $pH$ (respiratory alkalosis) due to compensatory increased ventilation in response to hypoxemia

Increased $PCO_2$ and decreased $pH$ (respiratory acidosis) due to impaired and decreased ventilation

Decreased serum $\alpha_1$-antitrypsin may exist in persons with positive family histories of emphysema.

Laboratory findings of pulmonary heart disease

## *ASTHMA*

Asthma is a disease characterized by an increased responsiveness of the trachea and bronchi to various stimuli. This disorder is manifested by extensive reversible narrowing of the airways, which changes in severity either spontaneously or as a result of treatment.

*Extrinsic asthma* is that form of the disease in which episodes of asthma may be attributed to an immunologic response of the patient to exposure to an allergen. *Intrinsic asthma* is that form of the disease in which an inciting cause is not clearly identifiable.

Asthmatic attacks are characterized by narrowing of the large and small airways because of bronchial smooth-muscle spasm, edema, and eosinophilic inflammation in the bronchial mucosal wall. There is also production of tenacious mucus; this results in bronchiolar plugging and decreased ventilation (Fig. 2-6). These abnormalities lead to hyperinflation of the lungs, with an increase in residual volume and functional residual capacity, increased pulmonary arterial pressure, and a ventilation–perfusion imbalance with a variable degree of hypoxemia.

The major pathogenic mechanism in allergic asthma is sensitization of respiratory mast cells with IgE antibody and subsequent antigen-induced release of chemical mediators from the mast cells. The several chemical mediators include histamine, eosinophil chemotactic factor, and slow-reacting substance of anaphylaxis. In addition to the exaggerated mast-cell response, there appears to be a major dysfunction of the parasympathetic nervous system, contributing to the respiratory smooth-muscle constriction and mucous-gland secretion. According to the direct theory of pathogenesis, the chemical mediators directly cause airway smooth-muscle stimulation. According to the indirect theory, mast-cell secretions stimulate the vagus nerves to produce bronchial constriction.

Continued blood flow to underventilated areas of the lung results in hypoxemia with little change in $pH$ or $PCO_2$. The patient responds to the hypoxemia by hyperventilating. This results in decreased $PCO_2$ and respiratory alkalosis. With further progression of an asthmatic attack, the patient's capacity to compensate by increased ventilation of unobstructed areas of the lung is further impaired by more extensive airway narrowing. Arterial hypoxemia worsens and $PCO_2$ begins to rise, leading to respiratory acidosis.

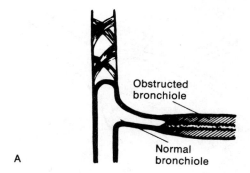

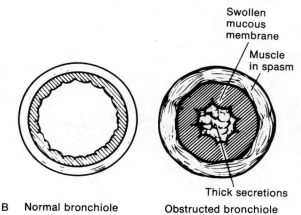

**Fig. 2-6.** Two views of an obstructed bronchiole show how it may be completely blocked by muscle spasm, swelling of mucosa, and thick secretions during an attack of asthma. (*A*) Longitudinal section of bronchiolar obstruction. (*B*) Enlarged cross section. (Brecher R, Brecher E: Breathing . . . What You Need To Know, p 61. New York, American Lung Association, 1973)

## LABORATORY FINDINGS

Sputum—usually yellow or white and mucoid; it may contain eosinophils, crystals, and mucous casts; neutrophils and bacteria indicate superimposed infection

Increased blood and nasal eosinophils

Early decrease in arterial $PO_2$; there is a greater decrease as the condition becomes more severe

Early decrease in $PCO_2$ as a result of compensatory hyperventilation

$PCO_2$ increases toward normal as compensation fails.

$p$H—increases early (respiratory alkalosis); decreases as condition worsens (respiratory acidosis)

Theophylline blood levels are useful in monitoring therapy.

## *BRONCHIECTASIS*

Bronchiectasis is a chronic disease characterized by weakened bronchial walls and resulting in an abnormal irreversible dilatation of the bronchi. Bronchial

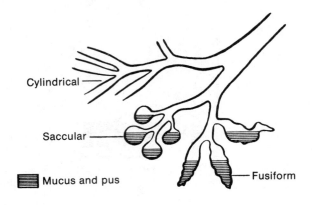

Cylindrical

Saccular

Mucus and pus

Fusiform

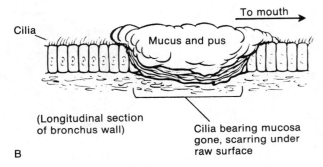

To mouth →

Cilia

Mucus and pus

(Longitudinal section of bronchus wall)

Cilia bearing mucosa gone, scarring under raw surface

B

**Fig. 2-7.** Bronchiectasis. (*A*) Three types of bronchial dilatation. (*B*) A permanently damaged bronchial wall with loss of ciliary action in clearing out mucus. (American Lung Association: Introduction to Lung Diseases, 5th ed, p 21. New York, American Lung Association, 1973)

infections are nearly always evident at one time or another, owing to impaired clearance of mucus and bacteria from the involved airways. Infections are the chief cause of intercurrent complications and progression of the process. Infection destroys the supporting elastic and muscular components of the bronchial wall, resulting in characteristic bronchial dilatation. Dilated bronchi are the site of accumulated mucus and pus (Fig. 2-7). The adjacent lung tissue shows extensive scarring. This disease is commonly seen in association with cystic fibrosis. Respiratory insufficiency is common and resembles that occurring in chronic bronchitis and emphysema.

## LABORATORY FINDINGS

Sputum—abundant and mucopurulent during acute infections; cultures yield multiple aerobic and anaerobic organisms

Mild normocytic anemia—chronic-disease type

Leukocytosis and increased sedimentation rate during acute infections

Mild to moderate arterial hypoxemia due to venous admixture with arterial blood

Polyclonal gammopathy reflects chronic infection.

Laboratory findings of immunodeficiency disease (Chap. 8) or cystic fibrosis (Chap. 10)

Laboratory findings of complications such as pneumonia, brain abscess, aspergillosis, sepsis, cor pulmonale, pulmonary hemorrhage

## PNEUMOCONIOSIS

*Pneumoconiosis* refers to a group of lung diseases that result from the inhalation of various types of dust. The most common disorders are silicosis, asbestosis, and coal-workers' pneumoconiosis (CWP). Clinical disease requires three essential factors: exposure to a specific substance capable of causing disease, exposure to particles that are of the appropriate size to be retained in the lungs, and exposure for a sufficient length of time to retain enough particulate matter to be capable of causing detectable disease.

Disease results from one of the following mechanisms:

1. Retention of particles that may produce damage in the form of inflammation and scarring; the disease may progress after exposure has ceased
2. Direct chemical or physical injury to the mucosal lining of the tracheobronchial tree or lung tissue; because the material is not retained in the lung, no further damage occurs when exposure ceases
3. Immunologic damage, such as allergy or hypersensitivity, which is usually self-limited, but which might persist when the allergen is permanently retained in the lung
4. The development of cancer, which requires many years of exposure to the foreign substance; the number of agents definitely known to be carcinogenic is small

Most inhaled dusts are entirely harmless. The coal smoke or soot pigment in the lungs of all city dwellers is by definition a pneumoconiosis, but it causes minimal tissue damage and does not impair lung function. The dusts that most frequently produce tissue damage and may affect lung function are silica and asbestos. These inert materials are indigestible by pulmonary alveolar macrophages, producing damage to the macrophages with resultant release of factors that cause scar formation and neutrophil attraction. The granulocytes release enzymes that result in tissue damage.

Inhaled silica particles are engulfed by phagocytes and carried to the pulmonary lymph nodes (Fig. 2-8). These particles evoke a marked proliferation of scar-tissue cells, forming silicotic nodules with extensive fibrosis. As scar tissue contracts it causes overdistention of the surrounding lung tissue, resulting in emphysema. Silicosis is sometimes complicated by pulmonary tuberculosis.

Inhaled asbestos fibers become lodged in the bronchioles, where they set up foci of chronic irritation. The fibers produce peribronchiolar, and then diffuse, scarring and thickening of alveolar walls. Complications include lung cancer and cancer of the pleura, known as *mesothelioma*.

CWP is the accumulation of coal dust in the lungs. The respiratory bronchioles become surrounded by aggregates of coal dust, macrophages, fibroblasts, and connective tissue. The uncomplicated disease does not usually alter

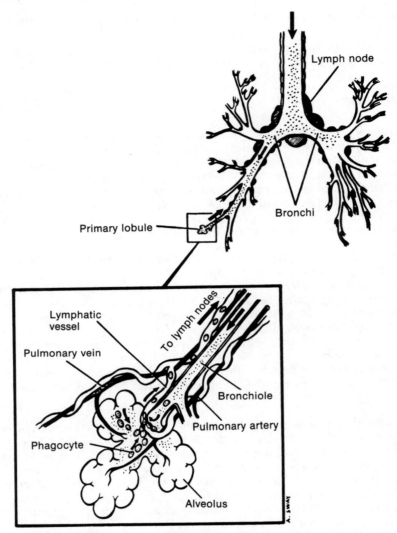

**Fig. 2-8.** Pneumoconiosis: Route of dust particles. Finer dust particles reach the alveoli and are carried by phagocytes to lymph nodes along the bronchi. (American Lung Association: Introduction to Lung Diseases, 5th ed, p 89. New York, American Lung Association, 1973)

pulmonary function. Approximately 2% of coal workers develop complicated CWP with larger areas of black fibrous tissue, which may form cavities. Pulmonary function is affected in this severe form of CWP. *Black lung disease* is a legal term that refers to CWP or chronic obstructive pulmonary disease in people who had been exposed to coal dust.

## LABORATORY FINDINGS

Usually found only in complicated or advanced disease

Leukocytosis and increased sedimentation rate when an associated infection is present

Secondary erythrocytosis if hypoxemia is severe and of long duration

Normocytic anemia—chronic-disease type

Sputum may contain mycobacteria, tumor cells, or asbestos fibers

Increased serum $\gamma$-globulin due to chronic disease

Decreased arterial $PO_2$ and oxygen saturation in long-standing cases with impaired gas exchange

Biopsy of lung or neck lymph node shows inhaled dust particles

## *SARCOIDOSIS*

Sarcoidosis is a multisystem, granulomatous disorder of unknown etiology; it most commonly affects young adults. The patient usually presents with enlarged lymph nodes adjacent to the lung, pulmonary infiltration, or lesions of the skin or eyes. The diagnosis is most firmly established when clinical and x-ray findings are supported by tissue biopsies that show histologic evidence of widespread, noncaseating granulomas (Fig. 2-9). Granulomas are circumscribed inflammatory foci comprising mononuclear cells; they are reported to be activated T-lymphocytes.[3] Immunologic manifestations include raised or abnormal immunoglobulins and depression of delayed hypersensitivity, which suggests impaired cell-mediated immunity. Progressive pulmonary sarcoidosis with significant impairment of pulmonary function develops in fewer than one third of patients, but represents the major cause of disability and death.

## LABORATORY FINDINGS

Increased serum angiotensin-converting enzyme—this enzyme converts angiotensin I to angiotensin II and normally occurs within the pulmonary capillary endothelial cells. Increased activity of this enzyme in sarcoidosis is believed to be the result of an increased rate of enzyme synthesis by epithelioid cells of the sarcoid granulomas and of release of the enzyme into the bloodstream. In a recent report, 83% of patients with active disease had elevated enzyme levels.[10] The enzyme level tends to fall during spontaneous or steroid-induced remission of the disease.

Increased sedimentation rate and serum fibrinogen indicate active disease.

Decreased serum albumin reflects chronic disease.

Increased serum globulins; stepwise increase of $\alpha_2$-, $\beta$-, and $\gamma$-globulins, especially IgG; this reflects humoral immunologic response of chronic inflammation

Leukopenia ($<5,000/\mu l$) in 40% of patients

Hyaline center

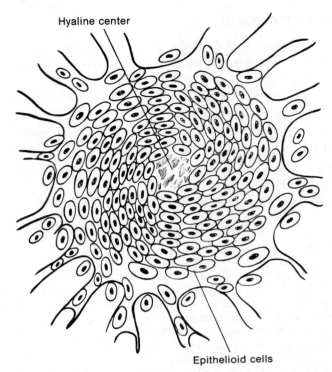

Epithelioid cells

**Fig. 2-9.** Sarcoidosis: Tubercle formation in sarcoid with no central caseation necrosis. (American Lung Association: Introduction to Lung Diseases, 5th ed, p 101. New York, American Lung Association, 1973)

Mild normocytic anemia—chronic-disease type

Decreased lymphocytes

Increased serum uric acid

Increased urine calcium as a result of increased intestinal absorption due to increased sensitivity to vitamin D.

Laboratory findings reflecting specific organ involvement of lungs, liver, spleen, central nervous system, pituitary, or kidneys

## PLEURAL EFFUSION

*Pleural effusion* refers to the accumulation of excessive amounts of fluid in the pleural space. It is a frequent manifestation of serious pulmonary or cardiac disease and occasionally is the first evidence of a systemic disease.

Normally, there are fewer than 10 ml to 20 ml of fluid in the pleural space, allowing the parietal (chest-wall) and visceral (lung) pleural surfaces to slide easily over one another. The normal balance of hydrostatic and osmotic pressures results in the flow of fluid from the chest wall, through the pleural space, into the lungs. Fluid flow into the lungs is also enhanced by the greater vascularity of lung pleura than of chest-wall pleura.

Pleural effusion may occur as a result of circulatory disorders, pulmonary infectious diseases, neoplasms, collagen disease, trauma, intra-abdominal disorders, and miscellaneous other processes.

## CIRCULATORY DISORDERS

### Congestive Heart Failure

Congestive heart failure is the most frequent cause of pleural effusion. Left ventricular failure or constrictive pericarditis increases systemic venous pressure, capillary pressure in the chest wall, and filtration pressure across the parietal pleura. Increased pulmonary capillary pressure decreases the reabsorptive capacity of the vessels on the surface of the lungs. Increased filtration pressure, combined with decreased reabsorptive capacity, results in accumulation of fluid in the pleural cavities. The pleural effusion is a transudate, which is low in protein content.

### Pulmonary Embolism or Infarction

An embolus that blocks a pulmonary vessel results in damage to the pleura overlying the affected area of lung. As a consequence, there is leakage of blood-tinged exudate fluid into the pleural space. This may occur without infarction of the lung. The amount of effusion from embolism is usually small, and it clears spontaneously if no further emboli occur. In contrast, pleural effusion following pulmonary ischemia or infarction is usually greater in volume and takes more time to clear.

### Hypoalbuminemia

A decrease in serum albumin may result from nephrotic syndrome, malabsorption, malnutrition, or cirrhosis. This hypoalbuminemia diminishes vascular osmotic pressure. Consequently, there is fluid accumulation in tissues and body cavities throughout the body, including the pleural space. The pleural fluid is a transudate.

## PULMONARY INFECTIOUS DISEASES

Various lung inflammations affect the overlying pleura, increasing its permeability. This results in an exudative effusion, which has a high protein content. An acute process has a predominance of polymorphonuclear leukocytes, whereas a chronic process shows mostly mononuclear leukocytes. A parapneumonic effusion is a purulent pleural effusion, without microorganisms, which occurs as a reaction to an inflammatory focus in the lung. Empyema (pus in the pleural space) is an infected purulent effusion that contains microorganisms in addition to leukocytes. Bacteria usually enter the pleural cavity from the lung. They may also enter through the bloodstream or, rarely, through injury to or perforation of the diaphragm, chest wall, or esophagus.

Viral pneumonias that often produce pleural effusions are those caused by coxsackievirus or echovirus. The pyogenic bacteria that usually cause empyema include *Staphylococcus aureus*, streptococci (aerobic and anaerobic), mixed anaerobic bacteria, *Klebsiella pneumoniae, Pseudomonas aeruginosa, Escherichia coli,* and *Streptococcus pneumoniae.* Infections with *Nocardia* and *Actinomyces* may produce empyemas. Effusions caused by mycobacteria usually contain mononuclear, rather than polymorphonuclear, leukocytes. The inflammatory reaction responsible for tuberculous effusion depends on the development of hypersensitivity to tuberculoprotein rather than to the presence of tubercle bacilli. The bacilli are scarce and difficult to identify in the effusion fluid, although numerous tubercle granulomas (localized foci of inflammation) are often present on the pleural surfaces. Of the three common systemic mycoses, only coccidioidomycosis has a propensity for production of pleural effusion. Of all the parasitic infestations that involve the lung and chest wall, only amebiasis frequently results in pleural effusions.

## NEOPLASMS

Bronchogenic carcinoma is the most common neoplasm to cause pleural effusion. The effusion may be secondary to tumor implants on the pleural surfaces, to pneumonia, or to decreased pleural lymphatic drainage. Diffuse mesotheliomas are tumors of the pleural surfaces associated with recurrent and intractable pleural effusions. Metastatic carcinomas of the pleura cause effusions. The most common primary site of pleural metastasis is the breast. Other primary sites are the ovary, kidney, stomach, and pancreas. Malignant lymphomas such as Hodgkin's disease, lymphosarcoma, and histiocytic malignant lymphoma may involve the pleura and cause effusion.

## COLLAGEN DISEASES

Pleural effusions have been reported in up to 55% of patients with lupus erythematosus but in only 5% of patients with rheumatoid arthritis.

## TRAUMA

Wounds of the chest wall, tearing of pleural adhesions when the lung collapses, and rupture of the esophagus all produce pleural effusion.

## INTRA-ABDOMINAL DISORDERS

### Abscess

When inflammation is located in the abdomen near the diaphragm, pleural effusions frequently occur. Examples include abscesses in the subdiaphragmatic space, in the dome of the liver, near the spleen, and around the kidneys.

### Pancreatitis

Acute or chronic pancreatitis with rupture and inflammation around the pancreas is frequently associated with pleural effusion.

### Cirrhosis of the Liver

Peritoneal effusion, known as *ascites,* commonly occurs in the late stage of cirrhosis. Pleural effusion may accompany ascites. This is the result of the passage of fluid from the abdomen to the pleura through lymphatic channels and spaces between diaphragmatic muscle fibers.

### Meigs' Syndrome

This syndrome includes the presence of pleural effusion and ascites associated with various ovarian tumors. When the ovarian tumor is removed, the fluids disappear. Apparently the tumor elicits a peritoneal effusion, which migrates across the diaphragm and involves the pleural space.

### MISCELLANEOUS

### Uremia

Pleural effusions, pericardial effusions, and ascites occur in patients with uremia. Although the pathogenesis of the fluid accumulation is not known, its exudative character suggests that an increase in vascular permeability is responsible.

### Myxedema

Patients with severe hypothyroidism and myxedema exhibit generalized fluid retention in body tissues and body cavities.

## LABORATORY FINDINGS

Effusions are often subdivided into transudates, which are ultrafiltrates of plasma and have a low concentration of protein, and exudates, which result from capillary damage or lymphatic blockage and have a high concentration of protein. The traditional differentiating factor between the two types of effusions has been that an exudate has greater than 3.0 g/dl of protein and a transudate has less than 3.0 g/dl of protein. This has resulted in too great an overlap between the two categories. The following criteria are now widely used to define an exudate:

1. A pleural fluid–serum ratio of total protein of 0.5 or greater
2. A pleural fluid lactate dehydrogenase (LDH) of 20 IU or greater
3. A pleural fluid–serum ratio of LDH of 0.6 or greater

Values below these indicate that the fluid is a transudate.

Conditions causing pleural transudates are congestive heart failure, cirrhosis, and hypoalbuminemia. The most common causes of pleural exudates are pulmonary embolism and infarction, malignant tumor involving the pleura, empyema, pneumonia, and tuberculosis.

## LUNG ABSCESS

An abscess of the lung is a necrotic lesion filled with pus. When bacteria reach a high enough density in a localized tissue site, the surrounding host cells die and suppuration results, forming an abscess. Abscesses are usually due to aspiration of infected material from the upper air passages by a patient who is unconscious from alcohol intoxication or excessive sedation. The presence of aspirated food particles or of a chemical injury to the airway epithelium impairs clearance of microorganisms and increases the likelihood of abscess formation. Bronchial obstruction by a tumor can result in abscess formation.

Pneumonia due to large numbers of one or more species of necrotizing bacteria is often complicated by abscess formation. Most community-acquired infections are due to anaerobic bacteria. Most hospital-acquired infections are due to mixtures of aerobic and anaerobic bacteria. The aerobic bacteria are predominantly *Staphylococcus aureus* and gram-negative bacilli. Abscesses may also occur with tuberculosis or with infection from *Coccidioides immitis* or *Histoplasma capsulatum*. The abscess may be putrid and foul smelling when it is due to anaerobic bacteria. In most instances the abscess ruptures into a bronchus and its contents are expectorated.

## LABORATORY FINDINGS

Sputum—abundant, foul, purulent; Gram's stain and acid-fast stain rarely show pathogenic organisms; cultures may show one or more aerobic and anaerobic bacteria, *Mycobacterium tuberculosis,* or fungi

Blood culture may be positive in the acute stage.

Leukocytosis (15,000/$\mu$l–30,000/$\mu$l)—this is often absent in elderly or debilitated patients.

Increased sedimentation rate reflects acute inflammation.

Normocytic anemia—chronic-disease type

Frequent albuminuria

Decreased serum albumin; polyclonal gammopathy in abscesses of long duration

Positive serologic tests for antibodies to *C. immitis* and *H. capsulatum* when these infections are responsible for abscess formation

## *ALLERGIC PULMONARY PARENCHYMAL DISEASES*

In contrast to asthma, which may also have an allergic etiology, allergic pulmonary parenchymal diseases predominantly involve the lung tissues, rather than the bronchi. There are two categories of these diseases.

### *HYPERSENSITIVITY PNEUMONITIS*

Hypersensitivity pneumonitis (extrinsic allergic alveolitis) is a diffuse interstitial lung disease caused by an immune-complex type of allergic response to a variety of inhaled organic dusts. Farmer's lung, associated with the contamination of moldy hay by thermophilic *Actinomyces,* is the prototype of numerous identical lung diseases that are associated with specific antigens. These antigens include a variety of saprophytic bacteria and fungi found in bark, barley, cork, cheese mold, and many other sources. The acute stage may include a hemorrhagic pneumonia, edema, inerstitial pneumonia, or vasculitis. Granulomas are frequently found. This disease often results in pulmonary fibrosis.

## EOSINOPHILIC PNEUMONIAS

Eosinophilic pneumonias (pulmonary infiltrates with eosinophilia; Löffler's syndrome) may be caused by parasites, drugs, or fungi. Most eosinophilic pneumonias, however, are of unknown etiology, although a hypersensitivity mechanism is suspected. Many patients have coexisting bronchial asthma. The lungs show extensive infiltration with eosinophils, mononuclear cells, mucous plugging of bronchioles, and edema.

### LABORATORY FINDINGS

Marked increase of eosinophils in blood (to 10%–70%)

Increased sedimentation rate

Increased serum $\gamma$-globulin

Leukocytosis during acute febrile episodes; lymphopenia

Decreased $PO_2$ and $O_2$ saturation as a result of impaired gas exchange

Decreased $PCO_2$ and increased $pH$ (respiratory alkalosis) as a result of compensatory hyperventilation

## PULMONARY EDEMA

Pulmonary edema indicates that there is an increased amount of extravascular water in the lungs. In contrast to that in pleural effusion, this fluid is not in the pleural space.

The factors controlling fluid filtration across all vascular membranes including those in the lungs are the permeability of the membrane; the hydrostatic (outward) pressures within and around capillaries; the osmotic (inward) pressure within and around capillaries; and the removal of fluid by the pulmonary lymphatic vessels. The direction of fluid flow across the alveolocapillary membranes is the net result of all of these factors and forces. Normally, there is a net outward filtration pressure of 4 mm Hg.

Pulmonary edema develops when one or more of the above factors are significantly altered. When fluid filtration exceeds the rate of fluid removal, liquid accumulates progressively in the following sites: pericapillary spaces, peribronchovascular spaces, and alveolar air spaces. The major causes of pulmonary edema are increased hydrostatic pressure secondary to various cardiac disorders and increased permeability of the pulmonary capillaries. *Adult respiratory distress syndrome* (ARDS) is a term used to describe the clinical, laboratory, and pathologic consequences of widespread damage to the alveolocapillary membranes resulting in pulmonary edema (see Respiratory Distress Syndrome).

### LABORATORY FINDINGS

Early decrease in arterial $PO_2$, which becomes more marked as pulmonary edema progresses

Arterial $PCO_2$ may be decreased, normal, or increased. A decrease reflects compensatory hyperventilation and an increase reflects impaired gas exchange in severe edema.

Arterial $pH$ is usually normal or increased, but occasionally decreased. Increased $pH$ usually reflects decreased $PCO_2$; decreased $pH$ reflects increased $PCO_2$ or lactic acidosis.

## PULMONARY EMBOLISM AND INFARCTION

Pulmonary embolism (*i.e.*, the plugging of pulmonary arteries) is a consequence of clots that form most frequently in the deep peripheral venous circulation, break loose, and obstruct pulmonary arteries (see Peripheral Venous Disease, Chap. 1). Because the lung has a double blood supply, most emboli do not cause infarction. Pulmonary infarcts rarely develop when the bronchial circulation is intact and normal (*i.e.*, in the absence of congestive heart failure or underlying chronic pulmonary disease). The combination of shock and congestive heart failure appears to be the most significant risk factor in the development of pulmonary infarction.[15]

Pulmonary infarcts are firm, hemorrhagic, wedge-shaped areas of necrosis, which extend from the point of complete artery obstruction to the surface of the lung (Fig. 2-10). The pleural surface over the infarct becomes covered with fibrin. The air spaces of the infarcted lung are filled with RBC and clotted blood. Phagocytes clear up the exudate within a few weeks. The vascular blood clots begin to disintegrate shortly after they reach the lungs. Complete clot lysis occurs within a few days to weeks. Infarcts heal following restoration of blood flow through the occluded vessel. As the pulmonary circulation becomes less obstructed, the physiologic effects diminish.

The most important physiologic alteration following embolization is the development of pulmonary hypertension, which results from increased pulmonary vascular resistance. The increased resistance is due to arterial obstruction by the thrombi and accompanying pulmonary vasoconstriction. Significant pulmonary hypertension usually occurs only when more than 30% to 50% of the pulmonary arterial tree is occluded, which is uncommon. Pulmonary hypertension forces the heart to work harder. The right ventricle may begin to fail, producing congestive heart failure. This is termed *pulmonary heart disease*, or *cor pulmonale*. Arterial oxygenation is characteristically diminished because of right-to-left shunting, secondary to small areas of lung collapse and ventilation–perfusion imbalances.

### LABORATORY FINDINGS

Decreased arterial $PO_2$ (usually to 60 mm Hg–80 mm Hg) is the most constant laboratory finding.

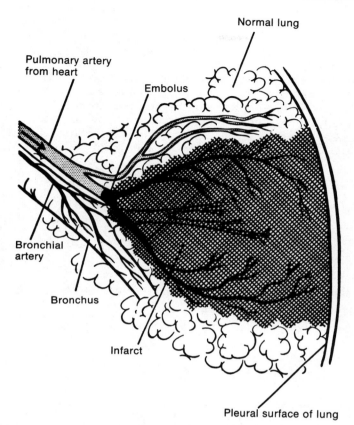

Normal lung

Pulmonary artery
from heart

Embolus

Bronchial
artery

Bronchus

Infarct

Pleural surface of lung

**Fig. 2-10.** Embolism and infarction: An infarct resulting from occlusion of a pulmonary artery near the surface of the lung. (American Lung Association: Introduction to Lung Diseases, 5th ed, p 105. New York, American Lung Association, 1973)

Decreased $PCO_2$ and increased $pH$ (respiratory alkalosis) due to increased ventilation as compensation for hypoxemia; this depends on the size and duration of the infarction

Leukocytosis of up to 15,000/$\mu$l

Increased sedimentation rate

Increased serum LDH (especially $LDH_2$ and $LDH_3$)—rises on the first day, peaks on the second day, normal by the tenth day

## FAT EMBOLISM

Fat embolism is the phenomenon of fat particles entering the venous circulation, usually from fractured bones of the legs or pelvis. The fat particles lodge in the lungs and other organs. The pathogenesis of the widespread damage to various organs clearly relates to the presence of fat in the bloodstream. It is not known, however, whether the fat droplets enter the venous system at the site of the injury or whether they are formed by aggregations of chylomicrons and platelets. The presence of microscopic evidence of fat emboli in patients with nontraumatic disorders such as burns, diabetes mellitus, and pancreatitis suggests the latter mechanism. It is likely that both mechanisms are operative. Once fat droplets impact in the lungs or other organs, the action of lipases presumably releases free fatty acids, which are toxic to the endothelium and capillary membranes. Because the lungs filter a large proportion of the droplets, they suffer the most damage. ARDS may be a result of fat embolism.

## LABORATORY FINDINGS

Marked decrease in arterial $PO_2$ and oxygen saturation

Normal or decreased $PCO_2$—the latter reflects the effect of hyperventilation in response to hypoxemia

Fat droplets in urine and in blood

Increased serum lipase and triglycerides

Decreased hemoglobin—sudden drop in the absence of bleeding

Marked decrease in platelet count

Possible findings of disseminated intravascular coagulopathy

## *RESPIRATORY DISTRESS SYNDROME*

Respiratory distress syndrome (RDS) of the newborn occurs when an infant is delivered prematurely, before there is maturation of the enzymes that produce pulmonary surfactant in the lung. Surfactant consists of several phospholipids, primarily lecithin. Lacking surfactant to stabilize the alveoli, the air sacs collapse on the infant's expiration. This results in *atelectasis,* which is collapse of lung tissue. Edema fluid then leaks into the alveoli and accumulates along the alveolar septa, forming what are called *hyaline membranes.* This disorder is also known as *hyaline membrane disease.* As a consequence of atelectasis, edema fluid in the alveoli, and hyaline membranes, there is interference with normal alveolocapillary oxygen exchange. The blood perfusing the lungs is not fully oxygenated and the infant becomes hypoxemic and cyanotic.

When similar pathologic changes occur in adults, they are known as ARDS.[4] This syndrome occurs as a consequence of acute diffuse alveolar injury from a wide variety of causes. Some precursors of ARDS include shock, trauma, burns, infections, sepsis, disseminated intravascular coagulation, fat or amniotic-fluid embolism, aspiration, near drowning, toxic gas inhalation, and drug abuse. These conditions all produce increased pulmonary capillary permeability, resulting in pulmonary edema. The protein-rich fluid that fills the alveoli is not a consequence of heart failure, which is the most common cause of pulmonary edema. There are increased pulmonary vascular resistance and pulmonary hypertension due to hypoxia, vasoconstriction, increased interstitial fluid pressure, or intravascular blood clots.

Because there is no single diagnostic test representing a marker of the syndrome, one must define the syndrome by its description. The criteria for the diagnosis of ARDS include the following:

1. A clinical history of a catastrophic event
2. Clinical respiratory distress
3. Diffuse pulmonary infiltrates on chest x-ray film
4. Arterial hypoxemia less than 50 mm Hg while the patient is breathing more than 60% oxygen

### LABORATORY FINDINGS

#### RDS

Determination of lecithin and sphingomyelin in amniotic fluid is the single most accurate test of fetal lung maturity. The lecithin–sphingomyelin ratio (L/S ratio) is lower in prematurity than at maturity. RDS is unlikely when the ratio is high, indicating lung maturity. When a mixture of amniotic fluid and ethanol is shaken, the mixture will produce foam if an adequate amount of surfactant is present. If amniotic fluid is not available, the L/S ratio may be determined through analysis of the gastric aspirate of the infant.

#### RDS and ARDS

The following are cumulative findings occurring in order of increasing severity of pulmonary insufficiency:

Decreased $PO_2$ and oxygen saturation, probably due to decreased ventilation–perfusion ratio and to shunts

Increased $PCO_2$ and decreased $pH$ (respiratory acidosis), due to decreased ventilation and impaired compensatory response to hypoxemia

Decreased bicarbonate and greater decrease in $pH$ (metabolic acidosis) secondary to tissue hypoxia and lactic acidosis

## *RESPIRATORY FAILURE*

*Respiration* refers to the exchange of oxygen and $CO_2$ between the alveoli and the pulmonary capillaries. *Respiratory failure* is defined as the presence of decreased arterial $PO_2$ and normal or increased arterial $PCO_2$. Respiratory insufficiency or failure is a disorder of function; it is not necessarily accompanied by tissue damage or disease. It is analogous to heart failure, kidney failure, and liver failure, each of which may result from varied disease processes. The disorders associated with respiratory failure may be classified in the following categories: diseases causing airway obstruction, lung inflammation, or pulmonary edema; pulmonary vascular diseases; diseases of the chest wall and pleura; and diseases affecting neuromuscular control of breathing. Each of the disorders requires complete clinical evaluation for diagnosis. The laboratory findings provide limited, but important, information in understanding the severity of pulmonary impairment.

## LABORATORY FINDINGS

Arterial $PO_2$ and $PCO_2$ are the only clinical laboratory indicators of pulmonary function. ($pH$ is altered with changes in $PCO_2$, but this also reflects changes in bicarbonate.) Decreased arterial $PO_2$ is an early and sensitive indicator of respiratory insufficiency. Hypoxemia occurs in the following circumstances:

1. Hypoventilation: impaired movement of air in and out of the lungs. This may be seen following sedative or narcotic drug depression of respiration; impaired cerebral control of respiration due to stroke, brain tumor, or injury; weakness of respiratory muscles; or obesity.
2. Diffusion abnormality: impaired exchange of $O_2$ and $CO_2$ between alveoli and pulmonary capillaries. This may occur owing to injury to the alveolar membranes, such as following prolonged use of certain cytotoxic drugs.
3. Ventilation–perfusion abnormality: diminished ventilation to areas of the lung that continue to receive normal blood flow. Associated with this abnormality are many forms of lung disease, including pulmonary edema, viral pneumonia, pulmonary embolism, and RDS.
4. Right-to-left shunt: flow of venous blood through portions of the lungs that are completely unventilated. This could occur with lung collapse (atelectasis); extensive filling of the lungs with edema fluid, pus, blood, or inflammatory cells as in pneumonia; or with accumulation of air or fluid in the pleural cavity.

The four abnormalities that cause hypoxemia may be differentiated by determining the patient's arterial $PCO_2$ and $PO_2$ while he is breathing room air and again while he is breathing 100% oxygen. The basis for this differentiation is shown in Table 2-1.

Arterial $PCO_2$ is the single most important measurement of alveolar ventilation. $CO_2$ retention (hypercapnia) occurs less frequently than does hypoxemia and indicates a serious ventilatory problem. Hypercapnia is accompanied by acidosis

**Table 2-1.** Pulmonary Causes of Hypoxemia and Their Differentiation

| ABNORMALITY | ARTERIAL $PCO_2$ | ARTERIAL $PO_2$ (ROOM AIR) | ARTERIAL $PO_2$ (100% $O_2$) |
|---|---|---|---|
| Hypoventilation | Increased | Decreased | Normal |
| Diffusion abnormality | Normal or decreased* | Normal at rest; decreased during exercise | Normal |
| Ventilation–perfusion abnormality | Normal, increased, or decreased* | Decreased | Normal |
| Right-to-left shunt | Normal or decreased* | Decreased | Low |
| Fall in cardiac output in patient with right-to-left shunt | Normal, increased, or decreased* | Decreased | Low |

* Attributable to hyperventilation from secondary causes
(Adapted from Hyde RW: Clinical interpretation of arterial oxygen measurements. Med Clin North Am 54:617–629, 1970)

and hypoxemia unless the patient is receiving oxygen. This occurs acutely following sudden airway obstruction, pulmonary edema, sedative overdose, or cardiac arrest. This also may occur following long-standing severe pulmonary or alveolar hypoventilation, as seen in emphysema and chronic bronchitis.

Decreased $PCO_2$ (hypocapnia) is due to hyperventilation and occurs more frequently than does hypercapnia. Hypocapnia is accompanied by alkalosis. Hyperventilation is seen as a response to hypoxemia in many pulmonary diseases including pneumonia, atelectasis, pulmonary embolism, and acute RDS.

## BRONCHOGENIC CARCINOMA

Most primary cancers of the lung originate from the cells that line the major bronchi. Some may grow into and along the bronchial lumina, causing varying degrees of narrowing and obstruction. Other carcinomas may perforate the bronchial wall, destroying cartilage and invading adjacent lung tissue. Many invade lymphatic vessels and involve regional lymph nodes (Fig. 2-11). Some invade blood vessels and metastasize or disseminate throughout the body, especially to the brain and adrenal glands. The major histologic types are squamous carcinoma, undifferentiated small-cell carcinoma, undifferentiated large-cell carcinoma, and adenocarcinoma. Undifferentiated small-cell carcinoma is also known as *oat cell carcinoma*, reflecting the microscopic appearance of the tumor cells. Lung cancer is usually diagnosed by symptoms of the tumor in the chest, of distant metastases, or of systemic complications, by chest x-ray examination, and finally by biopsy.

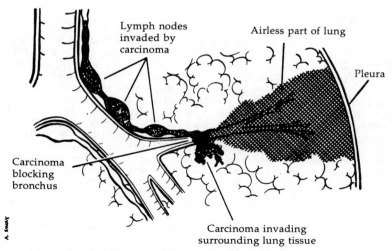

**Fig. 2-11.** Bronchogenic carcinoma. (American Lung Association: Introduction to Lung Diseases, 5th ed, p 81. New York, American Lung Association, 1973)

## LABORATORY FINDINGS

Evidence of tumor in a biopsy of the bronchus, lung, pleura, or mediastinal lymph nodes

Presence of tumor cells in cytologic exam of sputum or bronchial brushings

Laboratory findings of complications—pneumonia, lung abscess, pleural effusion

Laboratory findings due to metastases—adrenal insufficiency, impaired liver function

Hypercalcemia due to some squamous cell carcinomas

### Laboratory Findings of Ectopic Hormone Formation by Oat Cell Carcinomas
*Cushing's Syndrome*
Increased plasma cortisol

Hypochloremic and hypokalemic alkalosis.

*Inappropriate Antidiuretic Hormone Secretion*
Decreased serum sodium

Decreased serum osmolality

Increased urine osmolality

Increased urine sodium

*Carcinoid Syndrome*
Increased urinary 5-hydroxyindoleacetic acid or serotonin

Increased serum calcitonin

## REFERENCES

1. Benjamin SP, McCormack LJ: Structural abnormalities in COPD. Postgrad Med 62:101–106, 1977
2. Catanzaro A: Pulmonary coccidiodomycosis. Med Clin North Am 64:461–473, 1980
3. Crystal RG (mod): NIH Conference. Pulmonary sarcoidosis: A disease characterized and perpetuated by activated lung T-lymphocytes. Ann Intern Med 94:73–94, 1981
4. Divertie MB: The adult respiratory distress syndrome. Mayo Clin Proc 57:371–378, 1982
5. Editorial: Emphysema: Beginning of an understanding. Br Med J 1:961–962, 1980
6. Macher A: Histoplasmosis and blastomycosis. Med Clin North Am 14:447–459, 1980
7. Murray HW, Tuazon C: Atypical pneumonias. Med Clin North Am 64:507–527, 1980
8. Pennington JE: Aspergillus lung disease. Med Clin North Am 64:475–490, 1980
9. Reichman RC, Dolin R: Viral pneumonias. Med Clin North Am 64:491–506, 1980
10. Rohrbach MS, DeRemee RA: Measurement of angiotensin converting enzyme activity in serum in the diagnosis and management of sarcoidosis. In Homburger HA, Batsakis JB (eds): Clinical Laboratory Annual, Vol 1, pp 435–453. New York, Appleton-Century-Crofts, 1982
11. Sbarbaro JA: Tuberculosis. Med Clin North Am 64:417–431, 1980
12. Snider GL: Pathogenesis of emphysema and chronic bronchitis. Med Clin North Am 65:647–651, 1981
13. Tellis CJ, Putnam JS: Pulmonary disease caused by nontuberculosis Mycobacteria. Med Clin North Am 64:433–446, 1980
14. Tuazon CU: Gram-positive pneumonias. Med Clin North Am 64:343–362, 1980
15. Wilson JE: Pulmonary embolism, diagnosis and treatment. Clin Notes Respir Dis 19:1–15, 1981
16. Wolinsky E: Nontuberculous Mycobacteria and associated diseases. Am Rev Respir Dis 119:107–158, 1979

# BIBLIOGRAPHY

**American Lung Association:** Chronic Obstructive Pulmonary Disease, 5th ed. New York, American Lung Association, 1977

**American Lung Association:** Diagnostic Standards and Classification of Tuberculosis and other Mycobacterial Diseases, 14th ed. New York, American Lung Association, 1981

**American Lung Association:** Introduction to Lung Diseases, 5th ed. New York, American Lung Association, 1973

**Guenter CA, Welch MH:** Pulmonary Medicine. Philadelphia, JB Lippincott, 1977

**Hinshaw HC, Murray JF:** Diseases of the Chest, 4th ed. Philadelphia, WB Saunders, 1980

**Rose NR, Friedman H (eds):** Manual of Clinical Immunology, 2nd ed. Washington, American Society Microbiology, 1980

# 3
# GASTROINTESTINAL DISEASES

Reflux Esophagitis
Peptic Ulcer
Gastritis
Carcinoma of the Stomach
Regional Enteritis
Carcinoid Tumor
Acute Appendicitis
Ulcerative Colitis
Mesenteric Infarction
Intestinal Obstruction
   Fluid and Electrolyte Losses
   Distention
   Infarction
Diverticular Disease
Carcinoma of the Colon
Diarrhea
   Increased Delivery of Small-Intestinal
      Contents to Colon
   Small-Intestinal Hypersecretion
   Decreased Fluid Absorption by the
      Small Intestine

Small-Intestinal Transit
   Abnormalities
Intestinal Ischemia
Increased Accumulation of Colonic
   Contents
   Increased Colonic Secretions
   Exudation from Colonic Mucosa
   Decreased Colonic Absorption
   Other Causes
Intestinal Infections
   *Campylobacter* Enteritis
   Antibiotic-Associated
      Pseudomembranous Colitis
   Shigellosis
   Nontyphoidal Salmonellosis
   Typhoid Fever
Peritonitis
Gastrointestinal Bleeding
Impaired Intestinal Absorption
   Maldigestion
   Malabsorption
      Pathophysiology

## REFLUX ESOPHAGITIS

*Reflux esophagitis* refers to the regurgitation of gastric contents into the lower esophagus with resultant esophageal inflammation. This regurgitation occurs as a consequence of incompetence or weakness of the lower esophageal sphincter muscle. The specific etiology of sphincter incompetence is unknown. Several factors interact to produce reflux esophagitis. These include frequency of gastroesophageal reflux, gastric volume available for reflux, acidity of the gastric contents, efficacy of esophageal clearance mechanisms, and resistance of the esophageal tissue to injury.[5]

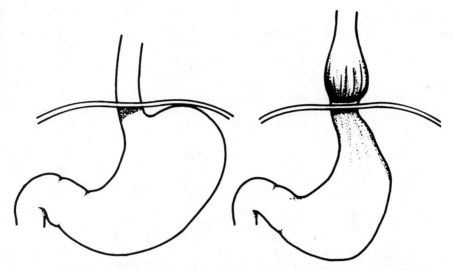

**Fig. 3-1.** Hiatus hernia showing displacement of the cardia of the stomach through the diaphragm into the thoracic cavity. (Given BA, Simmons SJ: Gastroenterology in Clinical Nursing, 3rd ed, p 121. St Louis, CV Mosby, 1979)

When there is regurgitation of gastric contents into the lower esophagus, esophageal inflammation may result. This causes edema, vascular engorgement, mucosal erosions, hemorrhage, and eventually fibrosis and narrowing. Another possible complication is pulmonary aspiration of the regurgitated gastric contents. This usually causes pneumonia.

It was once thought that upward displacement of the esophageal sphincter, such as that occurring in a hiatus hernia, diminished the sphincter's competence, with consequent regurgitation of gastric contents (Fig. 3-1). It has now been demonstrated that hiatus hernia and reflux esophagitis occur independently. Each condition may be found with or without the other.

## LABORATORY FINDINGS

Microcytic anemia due to chronic blood loss

Occult blood in stool due to esophageal erosions

## *PEPTIC ULCER*

*Peptic ulcer* is a general term for a circumscribed ulceration of the gastrointestinal (GI) mucosal surface in any area bathed by acid and pepsin. Approximately 75% of peptic ulcers occur in the proximal few centimeters of the duodenum, known as the *duodenal bulb*; they also occur along the lesser curvature of the stomach. These are known as *duodenal ulcers* and *gastric ulcers,* respectively. Other sites for ulcers are less frequent.

Patients with duodenal ulcers secrete more acid than do patients with gastric ulcers. Duodenal-ulcer patients empty food from their stomachs more rapidly than do persons without ulcers. This rapid emptying results in a large amount of acid in the duodenum. Gastric–peptic ulcerations appear to result from reduced mucosal resistance rather than from excessive acid secretion. Other pathophysiologic features in patients with gastric ulcers that do not appear with duodenal ulcers are inflammation of the stomach, fasting hypergastrinemia as a result of decreased gastric acid secretion, bile regurgitation into the stomach with bile-acid injury to the gastric mucosa, and abnormal gastric motility

Peptic ulcers of the lower esophagus occur as a result of reflux esophagitis due to gastroesophageal-sphincter incompetence. Peptic ulcers may also occur in the jejunum after inadequate partial gastric resection or inadequate vagotomy. Continued acid–pepsin hypersecretion damages the jejunal mucosa.

Acute ulcers are superficial, multiple, and transient, and they heal without scarring. A chronic peptic ulcer is usually deep, single, firm, and persistent and is associated with scarring of the gastric or duodenal wall (Fig. 3-2). The ulcerative process may erode into blood vessels in the base of the ulcer, resulting in bleeding. Other complications are perforation and gastric retention. The latter is usually due to scarring and obstruction in the region of the pylorus or duodenum.

The major digestive secretions of the gastric mucosa are hydrochloric acid, pepsinogens, and mucus. Acid converts pepsinogens into pepsin, which initiates the digestion of proteins. Gastric-acid secretion is stimulated by the vagus nerves and gastrin, a hormone produced in the distal stomach and pancreas. Gastric-acid secretion is inhibited by hormonal secretions of the stomach and small intestine. There are elements that normally protect the stomach mucosa from ulceration or autodigestion by acid and pepsin. These include the rapid rate of mucosal cell regeneration, the rate and quality of mucus formation by the gastric glands, barriers to mucosal permeability, and an adequate mucosal blood flow.

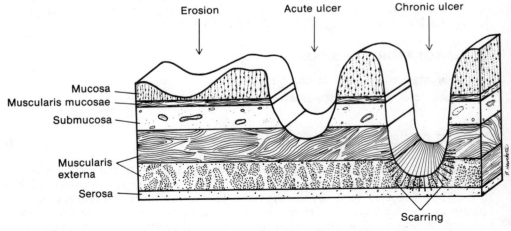

**Fig. 3-2.** Mucosal erosion, acute peptic ulcer, and chronic peptic ulcer.

The mechanism of ulcer formation is as follows: hydrochloric acid (HCl) penetrates the mucosa and disrupts mast cells, which liberate histamine. Histamine causes vasodilatation and stimulation of increased acid and pepsin secretion. Penetration of acid and pepsin through the damaged mucosal surface leads to erosions and ulcerations of the mucosa.

Gastric erosion due to aspirin may result from the direct effect of acetylsalicylic acid on the mucosa.

Erosions and stress ulcers occur after severe injuries or illnesses associated with hypotension or shock. Shock results in decreased mucosal blood supply and increased mucosal permeability to gastric acid. Patients with acute stress-type ulcers following intracranial injury develop gastric-acid hypersecretion and hypergastrinemia. Patients with stress ulcers associated with burns have acid hyposecretion and normal serum gastrin levels.

Gastrin is produced by G cells in the islets of Langerhans of the pancreas and in the distal stomach and duodenum. Tumors of these cells produce excessive amounts of gastrin, which stimulates hypersecretion of HCl. The excessive HCl causes intractable duodenal ulcers, recurrent gastric ulcers, or ulcers at the gastrojejunal anastomosis following partial gastrectomy. This disorder is known as the Zollinger–Ellison syndrome (see Chap. 6).

### LABORATORY FINDINGS

Peptic ulcer—normal or increased gastric acid; there is no correlation of the amount of gastric acid with the presence of peptic ulceration; lack of gastric acid excludes the diagnosis of peptic ulcer

Zollinger–Ellison syndrome—increased volume of gastric secretions, increased basal acid secretion (greater than 60% of the maximal acid secretion following betazole [Histalog] or pentagastrin stimulation), and increased fasting serum gastrin level

Pyloric obstruction with gastric retention and vomiting—dehydration and azotemia; decreased serum Na, Cl, K; increased $CO_2$ content and increased $p$H (metabolic alkalosis)

Perforation—leukocytosis with left shift, dehydration, increased amylase, increased lipase

Hemorrhage—acute, normocytic anemia; chronic, microcytic hypochromic anemia; occult blood in stool

## GASTRITIS

Gastritis is an inflammation of the gastric mucosa; it may be acute or chronic, diffuse or localized. Acute gastritis may follow the ingestion of an irritant such as alcohol, a corrosive poison, or aspirin. Chronic gastritis usually appears as a mild superficial inflammation in which there is vascular congestion and edema of the entire gastric mucosa. The severe form, or end stage, of chronic gastritis is termed *atrophic gastritis.* In this stage the gastric mucosa is thin and flattened.

Chronic gastritis appears to be the result of repeated acute injuries to the gastric mucosa that cannot be adequately dealt with by normal defense and repair mechanisms. Three types of chronic gastritis have been described: hypersecretory, autoimmune, and environmental.[4] In the case of hypersecretory chronic gastritis, the injurious agent appears to be an exaggerated acid–pepsin secretion by parietal cells. This overrides the defense mechanisms of the gastric antrum and damages the gastric mucosa. In autoimmune chronic gastritis, autoantibodies are directed against intrinsic factor and parietal cells. The parietal-cell loss results in hypochlorhydria, which stimulates antral G cells to hyperfunction and secrete gastrin in increased quantity. Intrinsic-factor antibodies interfere with the binding of vitamin $B_{12}$ to gastric intrinsic factor or with $B_{12}$ absorption in the ileum. A significant proportion of patients with this type of gastritis eventually develops pernicious anemia. The gastric mucosal injury in environmental chronic gastritis is probably based on dietary toxins and irritants, such as alcohol.

Parietal-cell antibodies are also found in association with many cases of thyroid and adrenal hypofunction, suggesting a more general relationship between disorders of the endocrine glands and atrophic gastritis, possibly through a common autoimmune mechanism.

Chronic gastritis eventually destroys the gastric acid-secreting cells so that the stomach is unable to secrete HCl, even after maximal stimulation with Histalog or pentagastrin. Another consequence of atrophic gastritis may be gastric carcinoma, which occurs with increased frequency after atrophic gastritis of approximately 10 to 20 years' duration.

### LABORATORY FINDINGS

Occult blood in stool due to gastric mucosal erosions

Hypochromic, microcytic anemia due to chronic blood loss

Macrocytic anemia due to pernicious anemia following atrophic gastritis of long duration

Early decrease in gastric acid due to decreased acid formation by injured and atrophic gastric parietal cells

Late absence of gastric acid which is unresponsive to Histalog or pentagastrin stimulation

Increased serum gastrin due to lack of gastric acid and loss of acid inhibition of gastrin secretion

Parietal-cell antibodies frequently occur in atrophic gastritis.

Intrinsic-factor antibodies occur in many cases of autoimmune chronic gastritis that result in pernicious anemia.

Decreased serum vitamin $B_{12}$ due to decreased formation of intrinsic factor by atrophic gastric parietal cells (see Pernicious Anemia, Chap. 8).

## CARCINOMA OF THE STOMACH

Factors that contribute to the development of gastric cancer include pernicious anemia, chronic gastritis with gastric atrophy and achlorhydria, gastric polyps, and perhaps diet. Peptic ulcers of the stomach do not predispose the patient to the development of gastric cancer. It is often difficult, and sometimes impossible, to grossly distinguish a benign gastric ulcer from an ulcerated carcinoma. A biopsy is required to make this important distinction.

Sites of metastases are the following, in order of frequency: regional lymph nodes, liver, lung.

## LABORATORY FINDINGS

Gastroscopic biopsy and cytology—essential for diagnosis

Hypochromic, microcytic anemia due to chronic blood loss

Occult blood in stool

Blood in gastric contents

Gastric analysis—50% of patients have no gastric acid, even following stimulation; 50% have normal or decreased gastric acid

Increased serum gastrin due to hypochlorhydria

## *REGIONAL ENTERITIS*

Regional enteritis is also known as *Crohn's disease*. This is an inflammatory disease of unknown etiology. It usually affects the ileum but often involves the colon, upper small intestine, and occasionally other parts of the GI tract.[7] Frequently, multiple segments of intestine are involved at the same time and are separated by areas of uninvolved intestine. All layers of the bowel wall are involved by edema, lymphocytic infiltration, fibrosis, and occasionally granulomas. These changes result in mucosal ulcers, thickening and rigidity of the bowel wall, and narrowing of the bowel lumen. Partial bowel obstruction frequently occurs.

Inflammation of the outer walls of the intestine results in adherence of loops of diseased intestine to normal intestine, urinary bladder, vagina, or peritoneum. Cracks or fissures penetrate deeply into the diseased loops of bowel wall, allowing the inflammation to spread through the entire wall. This often results in the formation of communicating fistulous tracts between the diseased intestine and the adherent organs.

The inflammatory process frequently results in intestinal loss of protein, mild to moderate steatorrhea, and impaired absorption of vitamin $B_{12}$, bile acids, and other nutrients.

Various extraintestinal disorders are often associated with regional enteritis:

1. Disorders that parallel the activity of the intestinal disease and that are possibly immunologically related (*e.g.,* arthritis, mouth inflammation, erythema nodosum [an inflammatory skin disease characterized by tender red nodules])
2. Disorders that run an independent course (*e.g.,* ankylosing spondylitis [rigidity of the spine], sacroiliitis, uveitis [eye inflammation], and various forms of liver inflammation)

3. Disorders that reflect complications of disrupted bowel physiology (*e.g.*, renal stones resulting from increased oxalate absorption, gallstones resulting from impaired ileal absorption of bile salts)
4. Amyloidosis, which is secondary to the long-standing inflammatory and suppurative disease

In children with regional enteritis, the predominant manifestations are growth retardation, arthritis, fever, and anemia.

### LABORATORY FINDINGS

Leukocytosis and increased sedimentation rate occur during the acute inflammatory phase.

Hypochromic, microcytic anemia due to chronic blood loss

Occult blood in stool due to intestinal mucosal bleeding

Decreased serum albumin and total protein due to loss of protein from the intestinal mucosa and to impaired dietary intake

Increased alkaline phosphatase, serum glutamic-oxaloacetic transminase (SGOT) (AST [aspartate aminotransferase]) or bilirubin due to associated liver disease

Increased urine oxalate and calcium oxalate renal calculi due to increased colonic absorption of dietary oxalate

#### Laboratory Findings of Complications

Peritonitis

Gastrointestinal bleeding

Impaired intestinal absorption

Amyloidosis*

Arthritis—synovial fluid similar to that of rheumatoid arthritis, but with negative rheumatoid factor

Ankylosing spondylitis†

## *CARCINOID TUMOR*

Carcinoid tumors arise from cells that are located chiefly in the appendix and small intestine, but may rarely also be found in the colon, stomach, pancreas, ovary, or bronchus. The cells are called *argentaffin cells* because they are stainable with silver (*argentum* is silver).

The cells produce serotonin (5-hydroxytryptamine), histamine, bradykinin, and prostaglandins. These substances act on blood vessels, causing a characteristic clinical syndrome that consists of episodes of bright red flushes over the

* See Chapter 10.
† See Chapter 9.

face and upper chest, diarrhea, and occasionally asthma. Right-sided valvular heart disease also occurs. Carcinoid tumors that arise in the intestinal tract do not produce the clinical syndrome unless hepatic metastases have occurred. This is because the endocrine products released by the tumor into the portal circulation are rapidly destroyed by liver enzymes. Hepatic metastases of the tumor, however, release these vasoactive substances through the hepatic veins directly into the systemic circulation, producing symptoms. Primary pulmonary and ovarian carcinoid tumors also secrete their products directly into the systemic circulation and often produce symptoms before metastasizing.

Serotonin and prostaglandins act on intestinal smooth muscle to produce colicky pain, increased intestinal secretion, and diarrhea. Serotonin also affects the pulmonary and tricuspid valves in the right side of the heart. Left-sided heart lesions are rare because serotonin is destroyed during passage through the lungs. Histamine and bradykinin are responsible for cutaneous flushing by causing vasodilatation. Histamine may also play a role in producing asthmatic attacks.

## LABORATORY FINDINGS

Increased urine 5-hydroxyindoleacetic acid (5-HIAA), a metabolite of serotonin—occurs only when hepatic metastases are present

Increased blood and urine serotonin, found only after hepatic metastases of intestinal carcinoid tumor and in gastric carcinoid tumors

Laboratory findings of diarrhea

## *ACUTE APPENDICITIS*

Inflammation of the appendix is usually preceded by obstruction of the appendiceal lumen by kinking, swelling of the lymphoid tissue in the appendiceal wall, or calcified fecal material. Inflammation causes increased secretion and intraluminal pressure. This results in swelling and impaired circulation in all layers of the appendix. Mucosal ulceration is followed by infection of the entire appendiceal wall; this leads to necrosis, perforation, and peritonitis.

## LABORATORY FINDINGS

Early increase in WBC (to 12,000/$\mu$l–14,000/$\mu$l; later up to 20,000/$\mu$l); more than 75% neutrophils with a "shift to the left"

Normal sedimentation rate

### Laboratory Findings of Complications

Dehydration—decreased urine volume; increased blood urea nitrogen (BUN), hematocrit, and urine specific gravity

Abscess formation—increased sedimentation rate

Peritonitis

## ULCERATIVE COLITIS

Ulcerative colitis is a chronic inflammatory and ulcerative disease of the colon and rectum. It is of unknown etiology and is characterized most often by bloody diarrhea. The disorder begins in the rectum and progresses proximally, frequently involving the entire colon. The mucosal surface has many bleeding points and increased friability. There are also areas of sloughing of the inflamed mucosa; these leave ulcerations, which are covered by a purulent exudate. Later, the lengths of the colon and rectum are reduced owing to muscle hypertrophy.

When the acute inflammatory and ulcerative process penetrates deeply into the colonic wall, the organ may become nonperistaltic and massively dilated. This complication is called *toxic megacolon.* In this disorder, there is increased danger of perforation of the colon. The loss of proteins, fluid, electrolytes, and RBC from the oozing mucosal surface is greatly increased.

A complication of ulcerative colitis of many years' duration is carcinoma of the colon. There are also several associated extracolonic complications: arthritis, ankylosing spondylitis, erythema nodosum, pyoderma gangrenosum (an ulcerating skin inflammation), uveitis, and various types of liver and bile-duct inflammation.

### LABORATORY FINDINGS

Definitive diagnosis requires a colonic mucosal biopsy.

Normocytic anemia (acute blood loss) or microcytic anemia (iron deficiency due to chronic blood loss)

Gross or occult blood in stool; WBC in stool

Leukocytosis during acute exacerbation

Increased sedimentation rate—indicates active inflammation

Decreased serum K, Na, Cl—due to diarrheal loss

Decreased serum albumin due to loss of protein from the diseased bowel wall; the degree of hypoalbuminemia parallels the severity of the disease

Increased alkaline phosphatase, SGOT(AST) and bilirubin due to associated liver disease

#### Laboratory Findings of Complications

Carcinoma of the colon

Gastrointestinal bleeding

Arthritis (see Chap. 9)

## MESENTERIC INFARCTION

Mesenteric infarction occurs when there is a sudden decrease in the flow of intestinal arterial or venous blood. Gradual narrowing of vessels by atherosclerosis may not result in bowel infarction, because collateral vessels develop. Infarcted intestine deposits a bloody, infected exudate into the peritoneal cavity. The bowel may eventually perforate in one or several sites, leading to the formation of localized abscesses or to widespread peritonitis.

Arterial thrombosis usually results from atherosclerosis of the mesenteric artery at its point of origin from the aorta. Arterial occlusion might also result from emboli originating in the left side of the heart. Venous thrombosis usually is secondary to portal hypertension, thrombocytosis, intra-abdominal abscesses, or estrogens.

Infarction without thrombosis may occur as a complication of decreased circulation as in septicemia, congestive heart failure, constrictive pericarditis, or shock. The mechanism is decreased mesenteric blood flow, which leads to venous stasis, reduced intestinal blood flow, and impaired capillary circulation. Increased venous pressure may also lead to protein-losing enteropathy, which is characterized by diffusion of protein-rich fluid into the bowel lumen and its loss in the stool.

Because of its extensive collateral vascular supply, the colon is less likely than the small intestine to become infarcted. Colonic infarction occurs only when the collateral blood supply is reduced by a generalized decrease in blood flow or by extensive atherosclerotic vascular disease.

## LABORATORY FINDINGS

### Acute Infarction

Leukocytosis with a "shift to the left"

Decreased $pH$ and $CO_2$ content (metabolic acidosis) reflect lactic acidosis from the necrotic bowel.

Increased serum LDH, with all isoenzymes increased, reflects tissue necrosis.

Increased hematocrit and BUN reflect hemoconcentration following intestinal fluid loss.

Laboratory findings of intestinal bleeding, intestinal obstruction, and shock

### Chronic Ischemia

Laboratory findings of impaired intestinal absorption

## *INTESTINAL OBSTRUCTION*

*Intestinal obstruction* indicates interference with the normal progression of intestinal contents from the mouth toward the anus. *Mechanical obstruction* denotes a physical barrier, which may be extrinsic or intrinsic. The latter may be due to a tumor or to scarring and narrowing following inflammation. This scarring and narrowing often occurs with ulcerative colitis, regional enteritis, and diverticulitis. Most intestinal obstructions in adults involve the small intestine and are secondary to adhesions, which are fibrous bands on the outer surface of the intestine. Adhesions develop as a late consequence of prior abdominal surgery.

*Paralytic ileus* refers to a disorder of intestinal motility that results in failure to propel intestinal contents. Peristalsis ceases and the intestine dilates. There is no mechanical blockage. This may be secondary to decreased bowel blood supply or it may be a reaction to nonintestinal abdominal disorders such as ureteral stones, peritonitis, or retroperitoneal hemorrhage.

The pathophysiologic abnormalities in obstruction depend on fluid and electrolyte losses, abdominal distention, and bowel infarction.

### FLUID AND ELECTROLYTE LOSSES

The obstructed bowel lumen becomes progressively distended with fluid as a result of the effects of rising intraluminal pressure. Distention increases intestinal secretion of water and electrolytes in the obstructed segment. The secretion results from a decreased flow of water and sodium from the intestinal lumen into the bloodstream and a normal or increased fluid flow from the bloodstream into the lumen. Increased intraluminal pressure also impairs venous drainage, resulting in fluid accumulation in the bowel wall. Some of this fluid exudes from the serosal surface into the peritoneal cavity. The final, and often major, source of fluid and electrolyte loss is vomiting. Large quantities of fluid and electrolytes are also lost following gastric or intestinal intubation and suction, which may be instituted in an attempt to relieve the obstruction. The cumulative effect of these multiple sites of fluid loss is a decrease in plasma volume, leading to hemoconcentration, reduced cardiac output, compensatory vasoconstriction, prerenal azotemia, decreased tissue perfusion, and metabolic acidosis. Prolonged vomiting results in loss of chloride, potassium, and sodium and in development of metabolic alkalosis. Vomiting is more common in obstruction of the gastroduodenal junction than in small-bowel obstruction.

### DISTENTION

Distention is due to accumulation of intestinal gas and secretions and is more severe in distal than in proximal obstructions. Distention results in a cycle of decreased fluid absorption and increased fluid secretion from the bowel wall. This leads to bowel-wall edema, impaired circulation and viability, and occasionally perforation. Abdominal distention may cause elevation of the diaphragm, which contributes to pneumonia, lung collapse, and respiratory failure.

### INFARCTION

Infarction usually results from twisting of the bowel or from entrapment of a loop of bowel in a hernia. The trapped loop of bowel has compromised vascularity and becomes first infarcted and then gangrenous. The leakage of bloody infected fluid from the bowel wall into the peritoneal cavity produces peritonitis. This fluid is absorbed into the bloodstream, resulting in bacteremia, septic shock, and respiratory failure.

## LABORATORY FINDINGS

Leukocytosis—counts <15,000/$\mu$l suggest simple obstruction; counts >15,000/$\mu$l suggest impaired circulation; counts >25,000/$\mu$l suggest infarction. Leukocytosis may not occur in older, debilitated patients or in those using corticosteroids or other immunosuppressive drugs.

Leukopenia with left shift suggests infarction with sepsis.

Increased serum amylase indicates bowel infarction, secondary pancreatitis, and leakage of pancreatic amylase into the peritoneum and bloodstream.

Decreased $pH$ and $CO_2$ content (metabolic acidosis) reflect lactic acidosis occurring with bowel infarction

Increased $pH$ and $CO_2$ content (metabolic alkalosis) secondary to vomiting with loss of fluid, $H^+$, Cl, and K

Increased BUN suggests dehydration, blood in the intestine, or renal damage.

Increased LDH (all isoenzymes) suggests infarction of the intestine.

Decreased serum K and Cl secondary to vomiting

Ascitic fluid—infarction is suggested by bloody fluid, fetid odor, bacteria, elevated amylase

Gastric contents—presence of blood suggests infarction of the small intestine

Rectal contents—presence of blood is common due to bleeding from infarcted bowel

**Laboratory Findings of Dehydration**

Decreased urine volume occurs early

Increased hemoglobin and hematocrit

Increased urine specific gravity

Increased BUN

## DIVERTICULAR DISEASE

Diverticula are small, saccular mucosal herniations through the muscular wall of the colon (Fig. 3-3). High intraluminal pressure forces the mucosa through the muscular coat at weak points, usually where the colonic blood vessels pierce the muscle wall. Diverticula most frequently occur in the sigmoid colon, which is located between the descending colon and the rectum. Muscular spasm precedes and contributes to the formation of diverticula. Other contributing factors are low-fiber diet and constipation.

Diverticula may erode into adjacent blood vessels, resulting in hemorrhage. In diverticulosis, both the circular smooth muscle and the longitudinal smooth muscle of the colon become thickened. This results in shortening and narrowing of the colon, which may produce segmental partial obstruction and extremely high localized intraluminal pressures (Fig. 3-4).

Perforation of an inflamed diverticulum results in inflammation of the diverticulum; this condition is known as *diverticulitis*. Inflammation is probably due to inability of the narrow-mouthed, nonmuscular diverticula to empty accumulated mucus, intestinal contents, and cellular debris. High intraluminal pressure precipitates perforation, which leads to bacterial or fecal contamination of the adjacent pericolic tissues, and an abscess develops. The inflamed bowel segment often adheres to the bladder or to other nearby pelvic organs, and a communicating fistulous tract may develop. With repeated inflammation, the colonic wall becomes thickened and the lumen narrows, often resulting in ob-

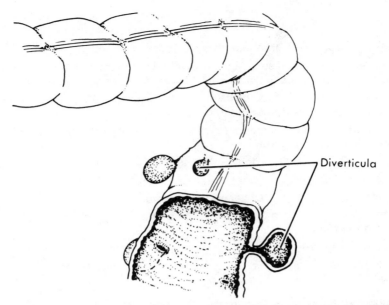

**Fig. 3-3.** Diverticula of colon. (Given BA, Simmons SJ: Gastroenterology in Clinical Nursing, 3rd ed, p 272. St Louis, CV Mosby, 1979)

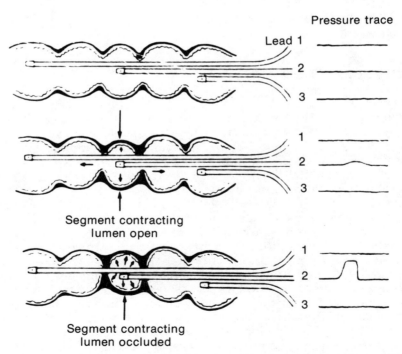

**Fig. 3-4.** Mechanism of production of localized increased intracolonic pressure. Open-ended recording tubes indicate intraluminal pressure at various sites. (Painter NS, Truelove SC, Ardran GM, Tuckey M: Segmentation and the localization of intraluminal pressures in the human colon, with special reference to the pathogenesis of colonic diverticula. Gastroenterology 49:169–177, 1965)

struction. One of the most dangerous complications is perforation into the peritoneal cavity with leakage of purulent or fecal material and the development of peritonitis.

### LABORATORY FINDINGS

Leukocytosis and increased sedimentation rate reflect acute inflammation.

Occult blood in stool due to mucosal bleeding

**Laboratory Findings of Complications**

Intestinal hemorrhage

Peritonitis due to perforation

Obstruction of colon

Pyelonephritis or cystitis due to inflammation from adherent diverticulitis

## CARCINOMA OF THE COLON

Carcinoma of the colon arises from the colonic mucosal epithelium, usually in the rectum and sigmoid colon. It may arise in a benign adenomatous polyp or villous adenoma. The tumor grows as a mass protruding into the bowel lumen or as an ulcerating lesion that invades the bowel wall. The latter is often associated with rectal bleeding. As the cancer penetrates into the bowel wall, it may gain access to lymphatic vascular channels and involve adjacent viscera. Lymphatic-vessel involvement results in spread or metastasis of the tumor to regional lymph nodes and then to the liver. It may subsequently spread to the lungs.

Cancers of the ascending colon frequently bleed slowly and are a common cause of iron-deficiency anemia in older people. There is an increased incidence of colonic cancer among patients with ulcerative colitis of long duration and among patients with familial polyposis.

Complications include intestinal hemorrhage, obstruction, perforation with peritonitis, abscesses, and formation of fistulae to adjacent organs.

### LABORATORY FINDINGS

Biopsy of colonic tumor is necessary for definitive diagnosis.

Occult or gross blood in stool

Leukocytosis and increased sedimentation rate indicate inflammation or necrosis of the tumor.

Microcytic anemia, iron-deficiency type, due to chronic blood loss

Decreased serum potassium as a result of potassium loss from mucus-secreting villous tumor of the rectum

Increased serum carcinoembryonic antigen—this test is used to monitor the adequacy of treatment and evidence of recurrence

Decreased serum protein reflects protein loss in stool or poor dietary intake.

**Laboratory Findings of Complications**

Intestinal hemorrhage

Peritonitis due to perforation

Obstruction of the colon

# DIARRHEA

Many different disorders of the small and large intestine may produce diarrhea.[6] Bloody diarrhea may occur in ulcerative colitis, shigellosis, or amebiasis. Conditions producing diarrhea may be divided into those that result from delivery of an increased volume of small-intestinal contents to the colon and those that result from colonic hypersecretion or inflammation. In both situations there are increases in colonic contents.

## INCREASED DELIVERY OF SMALL-INTESTINAL CONTENTS TO COLON

### Small-Intestinal Hypersecretion

Whenever intestinal secretion exceeds absorption, fluid accumulates within the intestinal lumen.

Infectious causes include *Vibrio cholera* bacilli, which attach to jejunal epithelial cells and elaborate a toxin that stimulates secretion of a bicarbonate-rich fluid into the small intestine. A similar toxin is produced by certain toxigenic strains of *Escherichia coli,* which is responsible for many cases of traveler's diarrhea, and by *Shigella dysenteriae.* Nontoxigenic bacterial diarrheas are caused by *Salmonella, Campylobacter,* and some strains of *E. coli.* Ingestion of staphylococcal or clostridial enterotoxin in contaminated food has a similar effect. Secretory diarrhea may also be caused by viruses or parasites.

Hormonal causes include a nonbeta-cell pancreatic adenoma, which produces hormones that cause a syndrome of watery diarrhea, hypokalemia, and achlorhydria. Elevated levels of the following hormones have been identified in patients with this syndrome: vasoactive intestinal peptide (VIP), gastric inhibitory peptide (GIP), gastrin, secretin, and glucagon. In the Zollinger–Ellison syndrome, increased gastrin and gastric acidity inactivate pancreatic enzymes, producing diarrhea. Increased gastric secretion stimulates pancreatic secretion, which enhances diarrhea. Carcinoid tumor produces serotonin, and medullary carcinoma of the thyroid produces calcitonin; both of these cause secretory diarrhea.

Other agents that have been shown to cause fluid accumulation in the intestinal lumen include alcohol, prostaglandins, caffeine, and laxatives.

### Decreased Fluid Absorption by the Small Intestine

Decreased small-intestinal fluid absorption may be due to decreased surface area, as in intestinal resection. It may also be due to disease of the intestinal mucosa, such as gluten enteropathy, tropical sprue, regional enteritis, Whipple's disease, or amyloidosis. It may be due to osmotic diarrhea, in which lactase deficiency results in the accumulation of lactose in the small intestine. Lactose is an osmotically active nonabsorbable disaccharide that causes fluid retention in the intestinal lumen. Lactose metabolites, which are acidic, further exacerbate the diarrhea.

### Small-Intestinal Transit Abnormalities

Shortened transit time may be partially responsible for the diarrhea seen in medullary carcinoma of the thyroid, carcinoid syndrome, and irritable bowel syndrome. Transit time is affected in disorders of neural innervation such as that occurring in diabetes mellitus and scleroderma. Choleraic and salmonellal toxins increase intestinal motility, contributing to diarrhea.

### Intestinal Ischemia

When two of the three major mesenteric arteries are blocked, malabsorption and diarrhea result.

#### INCREASED ACCUMULATION OF COLONIC CONTENTS

### Increased Colonic Secretions

Villous adenoma is a tumor of the rectosigmoid colon. The tumor often secretes large amounts of mucoid, potassium-rich fluid. Small-bowel resection and regional ileitis impair ileal absorption of fatty acids and bile acids. The acids increase colonic secretions and motility.

### Exudation From Colonic Mucosa

Inflammatory diarrhea occurs in ulcerative colitis, amebiasis, shigellosis, and pseudomembranous colitis. The latter disorder occurs following treatment with broad-spectrum antibiotics, which allows intestinal overgrowth of *Clostridium difficile.* The clostridial toxin causes the colitis and diarrhea.

### Decreased Colonic Absorption

There is decreased colonic surface area following colon resection. Colonic mucosal disease and decreased absorption occur following radiation and with ulcerative colitis. Osmotic diarrhea follows the use of certain laxatives.

### Other Causes

Rapid transit through the colon may be caused by laxatives or irritable bowel syndrome.

## LABORATORY FINDINGS

Culture of stool yielding *Salmonella, Shigella, Yersinia,* or *Campylobacter*

Neutrophils in stool—ulcerative colitis, amebiasis, pseudomembranous colitis, invasive bacterial enteritis due to *Salmonella, Shigella,* or *Yersinia*

Blood in stool—ulcerative colitis, amebiasis, pseudomembranous colitis, enteritis due to *Shigella, Campylobacter, Salmonella*

Presence in stool of *Entamoeba histolytica* or *Giardia lamblia*

Increased hemoglobin, hematocrit, and BUN reflect hemoconcentration due to loss of fluid and electrolytes in stool.

Decreased urine sodium and volume due to marked fluid and electrolyte loss in stool

Decreased $pH$ and $CO_2$ content (metabolic acidosis) due to intestinal loss of bicarbonate; less commonly, metabolic alkalosis occurs as a result of loss of fluid, acid, potassium, and chloride in the stool. This occurs with congenital acid diarrhea and with villous adenoma.

Increased stool fat due to malabsorption or maldigestion

Biopsy of small- or large-intestinal mucosa may show diagnostic pathologic changes.

# INTESTINAL INFECTIONS

Infections of the intestinal tract are usually due to bacteria but may also be caused by viruses. The relative frequency of each infectious agent is related to the age group affected. Patients less than two years of age are primarily infected by *Salmonella* and rotavirus.[2] In patients from two to ten years of age, *Shigella* infection predominates. In persons older than ten years, the commonly occurring organisms include *Salmonella, Shigella, Campylobacter* and parvoviruslike agents, the most common of which is Norwalk virus.[2] (*Salmonella* and *Shigella* infections are further discussed in this chapter.)

Intestinal infection is manifested by diarrhea. Organisms cause disease either by elaborating toxin, by invading the intestinal epithelium, or by attaching to the surface of the intestinal epithelium. *V. cholera*, certain strains of *E. coli*, and *Clostridium difficile* cause toxigenic diarrhea. The enterotoxins bind to specific receptor sites on the mucosal cells of the small intestine and stimulate hypersecretion of fluid and electrolytes. The diarrheal fluid contains abundant fluid and mucus but no inflammatory cells and very little protein. The toxin of *C. difficile* also causes intestinal bleeding.

Invasive diarrheas are characterized by loss of intestinal mucosa and often by presence of leukocytes and blood in the stool. This condition is known as *dysentery. Salmonella, Shigella, Entamoeba histolytica,* and probably *Campylobacter* belong in this group of organisms (see Amebiasis in Chap. 11).

Agents that cause disease by attaching to the intestinal epithelium include rotavirus, parvoviruslike agents, and *G. lamblia.* There are varying degrees of damage to the intestinal villi with resultant disaccharidase deficiency and electrolyte and fat malabsorption. Viruses usually cause upper-GI symptoms, vomiting, and upper respiratory infection.

## CAMPYLOBACTER ENTERITIS

*Campylobacter fetus* subspecies *jejuni* causes an acute gastroenteritis characterized by rapid onset of chills, fever, and cramping abdominal pain.[3] Within 24 hours of onset, diarrhea commences. The stools initially are loose and may progress to become mucoid, watery, or frankly bloody. This organism is the most common cause of bacterial diarrhea. The disease usually is self-limiting and is similar to viral gastroenteritis, lasting three to six days. Occasionally there are severe symptoms that mimic salmonellosis, shigellosis, or ulcerative colitis. The disease may be recurrent and may last for a month or longer. Relapses are reported in 25% of patients.

## LABORATORY FINDINGS

Presence of fecal leukocytes and gross or occult blood

Stool culture yields *Campylobacter.*

Phase-contrast microscopy of stool may reveal *Campylobacter.*

### ANTIBIOTIC-ASSOCIATED PSEUDOMEMBRANOUS COLITIS

Antibiotic-associated pseudomembranous colitis is characterized by severe diarrhea, dehydration, fever, leukocytosis, abdominal pain, and gastrointestinal bleeding.[1] A characteristic membrane or patchy white material may be adherent to the colonic mucosa. The membranes are composed of fibrin, sloughed epithelial cells, mucin, and inflammatory cells. This condition may occur during, or within four weeks following, use of various antimicrobial agents. In recent years it has been demonstrated that when the indigenous intestinal flora is disturbed by antibiotic therapy, there is overgrowth of *Clostridium difficile.* The disease produced is due to the action of a cytotoxin produced by *C. difficile.* The enterotoxin results in damage to the large-bowel mucosa identical to the injury produced by an invasive organism such as *Shigella.*

## LABORATORY FINDINGS

Presence of fecal leukocytes and gross or occult blood

Presence of toxin of *C. difficile*

### SHIGELLOSIS

Shigellosis is also known as *bacillary dysentery.* All species of the genus *Shigella* produce an acute inflammation of the intestinal tract in which there is diarrheal passage of blood and mucus. *S. dysenteriae* causes a particularly severe form of dysentery. There is a high incidence in infants and children below the age of 5 years. Acquired antibodies are protective in older persons.

Following ingestion, *Shigella* organisms reach the intestinal lumen, where they proliferate. Bacteria penetrate the epithelial cells lining the terminal ileum and entire colon and then multiply in the mucosa and submucosa. Penetration beyond the submucosa is rare. Following invasion of the epithelium, *Shigella* produces a toxin that severely depresses protein synthesis and results in mucosal cell death. Clumps of necrotic mucosal cells are sloughed, resulting in mucosal ulcerations, superficial abscesses, and bleeding. In contrast to salmonella infection, in shigellosis bacterial invasion of the bloodstream is extremely rare.

## LABORATORY FINDINGS

Culture of *Shigella* from stool, rectal swab, or sigmoidoscopic swab

Smear of stool shows mucus, leukocytes, macrophages, and gross or occult blood

### NONTYPHOIDAL SALMONELLOSIS

*Salmonella* species are a common cause of infections. The nontyphoidal diseases are usually brief, self-limited, and mild. Relatively large numbers of organisms must be ingested to induce illness. The most commonly incriminated species is *S. typhimurium.* Although foods of animal origin are probably the source of most human salmonellal infections, the exact vehicle of transmission is unknown in most cases. Organisms invade the mucosa of the distal small intestine and proximal colon, resulting in intestinal inflammation. Diarrheal fluid and electrolyte loss occurs. If salmonella are not impeded by the mucosa, lymphoid follicles, and mesenteric lymph nodes, they gain access to the bloodstream. The resulting bacteremia may be transient and inconsequential or it may lead to widespread extraintestinal focal infections. The organisms may also give rise to typhoidlike fever, in which there are both enteric and systemic disease. Paratyphoid fever tends to be a milder illness than is typhoid fever. The bacterial serotypes vary greatly in their virulence. *S. choleraesius* is highly virulent, frequently producing bacteremia and serious salmonellal infections. *S. typhimurium* is of intermediate virulence and accounts for most cases of enterocolitis.

Subtotal gastrectomy, gastroenterostomy, and vagotomy predispose a patient to salmonellal gastroenteritis. This could be a consequence of diminished gastric acid, rapid passage of organisms into the small intestine, or altered intestinal flora. Intestinal bacteria normally protect against salmonellal infections by producing fatty acids that are bacteriostatic to *Salmonella.* There is an increased incidence of infections with salmonella in infants and in patients with depressed resistance to infection. This is seen in cirrhosis, lupus erythematosus, leukemia, lymphoma, and other neoplastic diseases. Patients with sickle-cell disease have diminished immune defenses and consequently are unusually susceptible to salmonellal septicemia. Devitalized, damaged tissue and sites of prosthetic devices have predilections for salmonellal infections.

### LABORATORY FINDINGS

**Enterocolitis**

Stool culture, usually positive for *S. typhimurium*, for 1–4 weeks

Stool may contain leukocytes.

No systemic leukocytosis

**Paratyphoid Fever**

Stool and bloodstream cultures usually positive for *S. paratyphi B* or *S. typhimurium*

**Bacteremia**

Intermittently positive blood cultures, usually of *S. choleraesuis*

Negative stool cultures

Leukocytosis

**Local Infections**

Meningitis, especially in infants

Positive culture of organisms from local abscesses at various sites

## *TYPHOID FEVER*

Typhoid fever is caused by *Salmonella typhi*. The disease is characterized by fever, headache, apathy, prostration, cough, splenomegaly, rash, and leukopenia. The course of the illness is usually severe and prolonged.

Typhoid bacilli in the small intestine quickly pass through the intestinal mucosa into the regional lymphatics, where they are phagocytized. Neutrophils are unable to kill ingested typhoid bacilli. Some bacilli escape engulfment in the regional nodes, entering the bloodstream and producing a transient bacteremia. These organisms are quickly removed by reticuloendothelial cells in the liver, spleen, bone marrow, and lymph nodes. Bacteria invade cells at various sites, multiply, and reenter the bloodstream. At this time clinical features of the disease become evident. During this phase of sustained bacteremia, there is characteristically infection of the biliary tract. Multiplication of typhoid bacilli in bile results in continued bacterial seeding of the intestinal tract. Entry of infected bile into the intestine is responsible for the increase in *S. typhi* in the feces during the second and third weeks of disease. The ability of *Salmonella* to persist in the biliary tract results in a chronic carrier state with continued bacterial excretion in the feces. Organisms in the bloodstream are excreted in the urine.

Involvement of lymphoid tissue in the distal ileum leads to mucosal necrosis, ulceration, and erosion of blood vessels, resulting in intestinal bleeding. Involvement of the liver, spleen, and mesenteric lymph nodes commonly occurs.

Mechanisms other than circulating bacterial endotoxin appear to account for the sustained fever and toxemia in typhoid fever. Immunity in typhoid fever is not related to the presence of antibodies against the common antigens of *S. typhi*. The intracellular persistence of bacteria requires cellular immune mechanisms for complete eradication of the organism.

## LABORATORY FINDINGS

Positive blood culture for *S. typhi* during the first 10 days (90%); fewer than 30% are positive at the end of the third week

Positive bone marrow culture for *S. typhi* occurs even when blood cultures are negative.

Positive stool culture for *S. typhi* after 10 days, especially during third to fifth week (85%); stool culture may remain positive for more than 1 year in 3% of patients, who are termed chronic enteric carriers. The bacilli are harbored in the gallbladder.

Positive urine culture for *S. typhi* during third to fourth week (25%)

Leukopenia—4000/$\mu$l–6000/$\mu$l in first two weeks; 3000/$\mu$l–5000/$\mu$l in second two weeks

Normochromic, normocytic anemia—chronic-disease type

Proteinuria during febrile period

No increase in sedimentation rate

Serologic tests are nonspecific

**Laboratory Findings of Complications**

Liver involvement—increased serum LDH (especially LDH$_5$), alkaline phosphatase, SGOT (AST)

Intestinal ulceration—blood in stool during second to third week

Relapse—positive blood culture

## PERITONITIS

Peritonitis is inflammation of the peritoneum. The peritoneum is the membrane that lines the abdominal cavity. It consists of the outer, parietal peritoneum, which covers the inside of the abdominal wall, and the inner, visceral peritoneum, which covers the intestines and mesentery and abdominal organs. The most common underlying conditions of peritoneal inflammation include perforated peptic ulcer, ruptured appendix, gangrene of the bowel, gangrenous cholecystitis, and perforated diverticula. Other causes include inflammation of the fallopian tubes, abdominal trauma, peritoneal dialysis, bile peritonitis, and penetrating wounds. The most likely cause following surgery is bowel-content leakage due to breakdown of an anastomosis. This refers to the site of suturing of the GI tract.

The major factors that contribute to the establishment of peritonitis are a continued source of infection and the presence of a foreign material, such as bile, feces, or necrotic tissue, that interferes with host defense mechanisms.

Normal bacterial flora, which are harmless in the intestinal tract, become a source of infection when they reach the peritoneal cavity. When peritonitis occurs, multiple organisms are characteristically encountered in the peritoneal cavity. The most common bacteria involved are *Escherichia coli, Klebsiella, Streptococcus, Pseudomonas, Bacteroides,* and *Clostridium perfringens.* Inflammation due to soilage from the stomach, pancreas, and upper small intestine is caused more often by acid, bile, and enzyme action than by bacteria. The process may be acute or gradual and localized or widespread. Fluid diffuses from the vascular system into the peritoneal cavity. This may result in shock. Paralytic ileus (dilatation and loss of motility of the intestine), septicemia, and oliguria occur not long after the onset of widespread peritonitis. Death results from circulatory, respiratory, or renal failure, fluid and electrolyte imbalance, or septicemia.

## LABORATORY FINDINGS

Ascitic fluid—turbid, bloody, may contain fat globules; increased WBC; Gram's stain and aerobic and anaerobic cultures show multiple organisms; increased amylase; increased mononuclear cells and decreased glucose occur in tuberculous peritonitis

Leukocytosis—up to 50,000/$\mu$l with 80%–90% neutrophils; may not occur in older patients

Increased hemoglobin, hematocrit, and BUN—reflect hemoconcentration secondary to extracellular fluid loss into the peritoneal cavity

Laboratory findings of any of the underlying conditions listed above

# GASTROINTESTINAL BLEEDING

Bleeding into the GI tract is manifested by gross or occult blood in the feces or vomitus. Hematemesis, or vomiting of blood, indicates that the bleeding is above the duodenal–jejunal junction. Vomited blood that has been exposed to gastric acid becomes brown or black; this indicates a slower rate of bleeding than does red or maroon blood.

Melena is the passage of black, tarry stools; it usually indicates a bleeding site in the stomach or small intestine. Burgundy stools are usually associated with bleeding from the ascending colon. Bright red rectal bleeding usually indicates that the bleeding is from the descending colon or lower. Occult blood in the stool indicates that there is at least 30 ml of blood from some level of the alimentary tract.

The most common underlying conditions of GI bleeding are peptic ulcer, gastritis, dilated esophageal veins (varices), colonic carcinoma, bleeding colonic diverticula, gastric carcinoma, colonic polyps, ulcerative colitis, and hemorrhoids.

## LABORATORY FINDINGS

Gross or occult blood in stool, vomitus, or gastric contents

Hypochromic, microcytic anemia, iron-deficiency type, due to chronic blood loss

Altered liver function tests suggest cirrhosis of the liver with esophageal varices as the source of bleeding.

Increased BUN due to breakdown of blood in the colon by bacteria resulting in increased nitrogen formation

Laboratory findings or any of the underlying conditions listed above

# IMPAIRED INTESTINAL ABSORPTION

Failures of intestinal absorption may be divided into two broad categories: maldigestion of nutrients in the intestinal lumen and malabsorption of properly digested nutrients as a result of damage to the intestinal mucosa.

## MALDIGESTION

The digestion of nutrients depends on the proper coordination of the following: the presence of conjugated bile salts to increase the solubility of fat molecules; adequate concentrations of fat-, protein-, and carbohydrate-splitting enzymes; an optimal alkaline environment for digestive enzyme activity; and adequate intestinal motility. Impairment of any of these elements leads to maldigestion and steatorrhea (increased fat in the stool).

Disorders leading to maldigestion include the following:

1. Gastric surgery
2. Pancreatic insufficiency
3. Hepatobiliary disorders, which result in diminished concentration of bile acids
4. Intestinal disorders, which produce impaired enterohepatic circulation or bacterial overgrowth, resulting in decreased intestinal bile acids

## MALABSORPTION

Properly digested nutrients may be incompletely absorbed as a result of various types of damage to the intestinal mucosa. As with maldigestive syndromes, impaired absorption of fat and steatorrhea are the principal clinical features of malabsorption disorders because digestion and absorption of fat require an intricate series of steps.

Disorders leading to malabsorption include the following:

1. Intestinal diseases
   *Gluten-sensitive enteropathy*, which is also known as *celiac disease* and as *celiac sprue*, is an immunologic disorder. It is thought to result from sensitivity to gliadin, a protein constituent of the grain protein gluten. The immunologic response leads to epithelial-cell damage and rapid turnover of epithelial cells, resulting in atrophy of small intestinal villi (Fig. 3-5). Atrophic intestinal villi impair absorption.
   *Tropical sprue* also causes villous atrophy and malabsorption. This syndrome is possibly due to viral or nonspecific enteritis, which is followed by colonization of the upper small bowel by *Klebsiella, Enterobacter,* or *E. coli.* These bacteria produce enterotoxins that damage intestinal epithelium.
   *Regional enteritis* produces malabsorption as a consequence of transmural inflammation of the small intestine (see Regional Enteritis).
   *Radiation* produces intestinal fibrosis and small-vessel inflammation, resulting in malabsorption.
2. Intestinal resection of greater than 100 cm
3. Impaired intestinal circulation due to congestive heart failure or arteriosclerosis of mesenteric arteries
4. Giardiasis and strongyloidosis, in which parasites attach to intestinal epithelial cells, may lead to malabsorption when infestation is severe.

### Pathophysiology

The most prominent and significant finding in patients with malabsorption is steatorrhea. This occurs because fat digestion and absorption require a complex

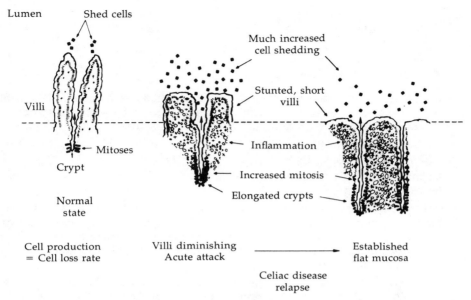

Lumen    Shed cells

Much increased
cell shedding

Villi

Stunted, short
villi

Mitoses

Inflammation

Crypt

Increased mitosis

Elongated crypts

Normal
state

Cell production
= Cell loss rate

Villi diminishing
Acute attack

Established
flat mucosa

Celiac disease
relapse

**Fig. 3-5.** Normal balance between cell loss from villous tips and cell replacement by mitosis in crypts. During an acute attack of celiac disease, cells are shed faster than they are replaced; atrophic flattened villi result. (Brooks, FP: Gastrointestinal Pathophysiology, 2nd ed, p 280. New York, Oxford University Press, 1978)

functioning interrelationship among the pancreas, liver, jeunal mucosa, and intestinal lymphatics. Disorders of any of these elements may result in impaired lipid absorption.

Impaired protein absorption, or increased protein loss, is known as *protein-losing enteropathy*. This leads to hypoproteinemia, a fall in plasma osmotic pressure, subcutaneous edema, ascites, and pleural effusions.

Anemia may result from defective absorption and subsequent depletion of body stores of iron, folic acid, and vitamin $B_{12}$. Because iron is principally absorbed in the duodenum, iron malabsorption occurs in duodenal mucosal diseases and following gastric surgery. Folic-acid deficiency results from various intestinal mucosal diseases, such as tropical sprue. Vitamin-$B_{12}$ deficiency may result from pernicious anemia, intestinal bacterial overgrowth with binding of vitamin $B_{12}$ by bacteria, ileal diseases with impaired $B_{12}$-intrinsic-factor absorption, or pancreatic insufficiency (see Megaloblastic Anemias, Chap. 8).

Malabsorption of fat may be accompanied by malabsorption of vitamin K; this, in turn, leads to low levels of prothrombin and plasma clotting factors V, VII, IX, and X. Bleeding may result.

Impaired absorption of fat-soluble vitamin D interferes with calcium absorption. Excessive calcium is lost in the stool. This results in poorly calcified bones, a condition known as *osteomalacia* (see Chap. 10). Hypocalcemia is a stimulus for secondary hyperparathyroidism (see Chap. 6). Impaired protein absorption may result in softened bones, a condition known as *osteoporosis*.

The presence in the colon of unabsorbed bile salts and of long-chain fatty acids inhibits normal colonic water and electrolyte absorption. This results in diarrhea.

## LABORATORY FINDINGS

Increased number and size of fat globules in stool; increased neutral fat (unsplit fats) indicates impaired fat digestion; increased free fatty acids (split fats) indicates normal fat digestion but impaired fat absorption

Increased quantity of fat in 72-hr stool sample after the patient has been on a 100-g-fat diet daily for three days

Decreased serum carotene indicates fat malabsorption or decreased dietary intake of carotene.

Impaired D-xylose tolerance test (decreased urinary excretion of a measured amount of ingested xylose) indicates impaired jejunal mucosal absorption of xylose. Because this carbohydrate does not require digestion by pancreatic enzymes, the tolerance test is normal in pancreatic insufficiency and does not indicate maldigestion.

Decreased serum levels of total protein, albumin, $\gamma$-globulin, iron, folate, vitamin $B_{12}$, calcium, phosphorus, magnesium, and cholesterol result from impaired intestinal absorption.

Anemia—macrocytic, due to impaired absorption of folate or vitamin $B_{12}$; microcytic, due to iron deficiency

Increased urine oxalate accompanying steatorrhea indicates an increase in colonic absorption of oxalates and their excretion in urine.

Prolonged prothrombin time results from impaired vitamin-K absorption.

Intestinal biopsy may show mucosal villous atrophy, tumor, or inflammation.

## REFERENCES

1. Bartlett JG: Antibiotic-associated pseudomembranous colitis. Hosp Pract 16:85–95, 1981
2. Blacklow NR, Cukor G: Viral gastroenteritis. N Engl J Med 304:397–406, 1981
3. Blaser MJ, Reller LB: Campylobacter enteritis. N Engl J Med 305:1444–1452, 1981
4. Correa P: The epidemiology and pathogenesis of chronic gastritis: Three etiologic entities. Front Gastrointest Res 6:98–108, 1980
5. Dodds WJ, Hogan WJ, Helm JF, Dent J: Pathogenesis of reflux esophagitis. Gastroenterology 81:376–394, 1981
6. Gianella RA: Pathogenesis of acute bacterial diarrheal disorders. Annu Rev Med 32:341–357, 1981
7. Kirsner JB, Shorter RG: Recent developments in "nonspecific" inflammatory bowel disease. N Engl J Med 306:775–782, 1982

## BIBLIOGRAPHY

**Brooks FP:** Gastrointestinal Pathophysiology, 2nd ed. New York, Oxford University Press, 1978
**Given BA, Simmons SJ:** Gastroenterology in Clinical Nursing 3rd ed. St Louis, CV Mosby, 1979

# 4
# *HEPATOBILIARY AND PANCREATIC DISEASES*

Hepatic Failure
Alcoholic Liver Disease
Viral Hepatitis
Chronic Hepatitis
Cirrhosis
   Classification and Pathogenesis
   Pathophysiology
Primary Biliary Cirrhosis

Pyogenic Liver Abscess
Hepatoma (Hepatocellular Carcinoma)
Metastatic Carcinoma of the Liver
Acute Cholecystitis
Cholangitis
Major Bile-Duct Obstruction
Acute Pancreatitis
Chronic Pancreatitis

## *HEPATIC FAILURE*

A variety of toxic agents such as alcohol, viruses, drugs, and toxins may damage liver cells to varying degrees. Viral hepatitis accounts for about 50% of cases of liver damage, drugs account for about 25%, and all other conditions account for about 25%. The most severe degree of injury results in hepatic failure. Liver failure may occur acutely or as an end stage of cirrhosis. Lipid accumulation in the liver cells (fatty liver) is a common consequence of liver-cell injury. Cell death or necrosis is the ultimate consequence of severe hepatocellular injury. Necrosis may involve only individual hepatic cells, scattered throughout the liver, or it may be extensive, with varying degrees of destruction of the hepatic lobules. Localized necrosis is readily repaired by hepatocellular regeneration. Widespread necrosis, however, results in the collapse of the hepatic supporting framework and the consequent obliteration of the reparative process. Extensive damage also affects hepatic circulation and biliary excretion. If the regenerative activity is insufficient to replace the destroyed liver tissue, hepatic failure will ensue.

    Severe neurologic disturbance, known as *hepatic encephalopathy*, frequently accompanies liver failure. The exact mechanism is uncertain but some possibilities include impaired metabolism of ammonia, short-chain fatty acids, and amino acids. Other factors include impaired metabolism of drugs and increased cerebral sensitivity to toxins.

**97**

Another complication of severe liver disease is oliguric hepatic failure, also known as *hepatorenal syndrome* or *hepatic nephropathy*. The precise cause of this disorder has not been established. The most consistent finding is decreased renal blood flow, associated with renal vascular constriction. The cause of the vasoconstriction is unknown. Renal failure is the result of functional derangement. No specific glomerular or tubular changes have been described.

## LABORATORY FINDINGS

Markedly increased bilirubin (up to 40 mg/dl) reflects impaired bilirubin excretion.

Markedly decreased albumin reflects decreased protein synthesis.

Decreased cholesterol reflects decreased hepatic synthesis of cholesterol

Serum glutamic-oxaloacetic transaminase (SGOT) (AST [aspartate aminotransferase]) and serum glutamic-pyruvic transaminase (SGPT) (ALT [alanine aminotransferase])—rapid fall from previously elevated levels indicates massive loss of liver cells

Decreased blood urea nitrogen (BUN) reflects decreased protein metabolism

Increased BUN and creatinine and oliguria reflect oliguric hepatic failure (hepatorenal syndrome)

Decreased glucose reflects decreased glycogen storage in liver

Prolonged prothrombin time reflects decreased hepatic synthesis of prothrombin and factors VII, IX and X

Decreased fibrinogen reflects decreased hepatic synthesis of fibrinogen

Increased ammonia reflects decreased hepatic urea synthesis.

Increased $pH$, decreased $PCO_2$ (respiratory alkalosis) reflects hyperventilation associated with cerebral edema

Leukocytosis indicates massive liver-cell necrosis.

## *ALCOHOLIC LIVER DISEASE*

Chronic alcohol ingestion leads to multiple interferences with normal liver-cell metabolism. Important effects are increased synthesis of fatty acids, decreased utilization of fatty acids, and increased incorporation of dietary fat into hepatic lipids. These disturbances result in a hepatic accumulation of lipids known as *fatty liver*. A more severe stage of alcoholic liver disease is liver-cell necrosis, which is often accompanied by bile stasis and jaundice. This condition is termed *alcoholic hepatitis*.[5] *Hepatitis* indicates inflammation associated with liver-cell necrosis but does not imply an infectious etiology or component. It is not evident which factors determine the development of fatty liver in some alcoholics and of alcoholic hepatitis in others, all of whom have been drinking comparable amounts of alcohol. In the chronic stage of alcoholic liver disease there are varying degrees of hepatic fibrosis, which often leads to portal cirrhosis (Fig. 4-1). The factors that determine whether the lesion of alcoholic hepatitis progresses to portal cirrhosis are not well understood. Severe alcoholic hepatitis and Laennec's portal cirrhosis can lead to hepatic failure and death.

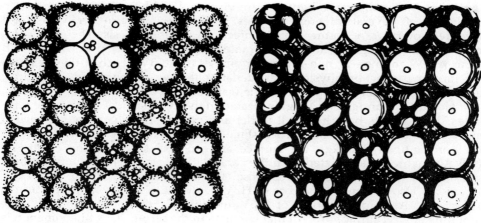

Alcoholic necrosis　　　　　　Portal cirrhosis

**Fig. 4-1.** Diagrammatic relationship between alcoholic necrosis and portal cirrhosis, which is an example of micronodular cirrhosis. (Schiff L [ed]: Diseases of the Liver, 4th ed, p 842. Philadelphia, JB Lippincott, 1975)

## LABORATORY FINDINGS

Increased SGOT (AST), SGPT (ALT)—reflect liver-cell necrosis

Ratio of SGOT–SGPT (AST–ALT) >2 occurs in 70% of patients with alcoholic liver disaese.[2]

Increased $\gamma$-glutamyl transpeptidase (GGT)—this enzyme is a sensitive indicator of chronic alcohol consumption

Increased alkaline phosphatase reflects cholestasis but does not correlate with the severity of alcoholic hepatitis.

Increased serum bilirubin reflects cholestasis.

Increased serum immunoglobulins reflect chronic hepatic injury.

Increased prothrombin time reflects decreased hepatic synthesis of prothrombin and factors VII, IX, X; this indicates severe hepatic injury.

Macrocytic anemia due to folic acid deficiency, which is the most frequent cause of anemia in alcoholic liver disease (see Chap. 8)

Macrocytosis occurs in liver disease, even in the absence of folate deficiency; this is due to excessive lipids in red blood cell (RBC) membranes.

Microcytic anemia due to iron or pyridoxine deficiency

Leukocytosis reflects severe hepatic inflammation.

## *VIRAL HEPATITIS*

Hepatitis may be caused by noninfectious as well as infectious agents. The noninfectious causes include toxins, alcohol, and drugs. The infectious agents that most frequently cause hepatitis are viruses. Viral hepatitis may be due to any one of several different viruses, including Epstein-Barr virus and cytomegalovirus. The former causes infectious mononucleosis. The most common viruses causing hepatitis are designated hepatitis A virus (HAV), hepatitis B virus (HBV) and non-A, non-B virus or viruses (NANBV). Each of these viruses has its own distinct biophysical characteristics, its own antigens and antibodies, and its own clinical and epidemiologic features.[1,7]

Hepatitis A antigen (HA Ag) is located in the cytoplasm of infected hepatocytes. HBV infects both liver cell nuclei and cytoplasm. It is a double-shelled structure known as the Dane particle (Fig. 4-2). This has three distinct antigens: the core antigen ($HB_cAg$); the surface antigen ($HB_sAg$); and the e antigen ($HB_eAg$), which is associated with the core of the virus. Each of the three antigens elicits its own antibody response. DNA polymerase, which is not antigenic, is also present in the core of HBV. Only the complete Dane particle is infectious. A unique feature of HBV infection is the production of large amounts of viral surface protein that circulate in the serum. This phenomenon is not observed in any other known viral disease. Circulating $HB_sAg$, derived from the plasma of noninfectious carriers, is the source for preparation of hepatitis B vaccine. At this time NANBV has not been identified.

HAV is shed in the stool early in the infection, prior to onset of symptoms (Fig. 4-3). The disease is transmitted by oral contact with contaminated material. Because viremia is of short duration, blood is not a source of disease transmission. HBV and NANBV are primarily transmitted through blood and blood products. NANBV is the major cause of posttransfusion hepatitis, accounting for 85%–90% of cases.

HAV differs from HBV and NANBV in that it is completely eliminated from the liver and does not cause chronic hepatitis, chronic carrier states, or cirrhosis. It rarely causes massive hepatic necrosis.

The most frequent response to HBV exposure is an asymptomatic infection. The large majority of patients (80%–85%) with clinically evident acute viral hepatitis recover completely. These patients have no evidence of residual liver dysfunction or liver damage (Fig. 4-4). Approximately 1% to 3% of patients

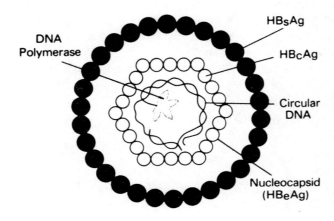

DNA Polymerase

HBsAg

HBcAg

Circular DNA

Nucleocapsid (HBeAg)

**Fig. 4-2.** Schematic representation of hepatitis B virus. (Overby LR (ed): Hepatitis Forum. Chicago, Abbott Laboratories, Diagnostics Division, 1980. Reproduced with permission of Abbott Diagnostics Division)

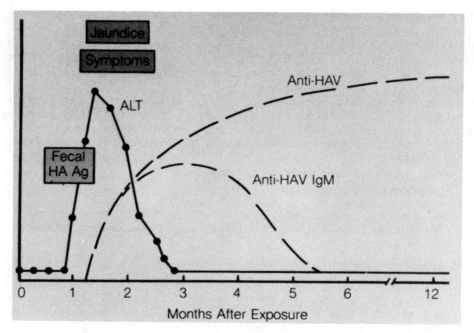

**Fig. 4-3.** The clinical, serologic, and biochemical course of typical type A hepatitis. (HA Ag: hepatitis A antigen; ALT: alanine aminotransferase; Anti-HAV: antibody to hepatitis A virus IgG class; Anti-HAV IgM: antibody to HAV IgM class) (Hoofnagle JH: Types A and B Viral Hepatitis—Perspectives on Viral Hepatitis, No. 2, p 4. Chicago, Abbott Diagnostics Division, 1981)

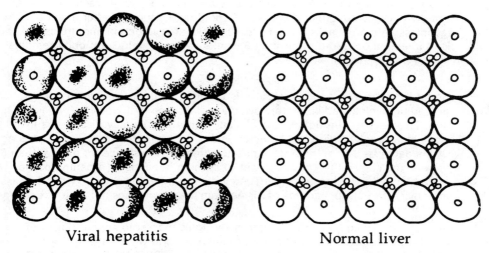

**Fig. 4-4.** Necrosis in acute viral hepatitis of average severity involves individual cells diffusely throughout the lobule (*left*). The basic lobular architecture of the liver is unimpaired. Healing takes place by regeneration and no scar tissue is formed. After recovery the liver is normal (*right*). (Schiff L [ed]: Diseases of the Liver, 4th ed, p 841. Philadelphia, JB Lippincott, 1975)

develop overwhelming hepatitis, sustain hepatic failure, and usually die. Five percent to ten percent of patients with HBV develop chronic hepatitis, whereas 20% to 40% of patients with NANBV develop chronic hepatitis (see Chronic Hepatitis).

Immune complexes composed of $HB_sAg$, immunoglobulin, and complement appear to play a role in the pathogenesis of various extrahepatic manifestations of viral hepatitis. HBV immune complexes have been demonstrated at various sites, accounting for hives, arthritis, glomerulonephritis, and polyarteritis.

## LABORATORY FINDINGS

In interpreting serologic tests for hepatitis, remember that all patients with jaundice do not have hepatitis and that all cases of heapatitis are not due to viruses.

### Serologic Tests[3,4]

*Hepatitis A[8]*
*Hepatitis A antigen* (HA Ag) is found in the stool 5 days to 6 days before the onset of symptoms or hepatic biochemical abnormalities. The antigen disappears from the stool immediately after the appearance of the antibody (Fig. 4-3).

*Hepatitis A antibody* (anti-HAV) appears in the serum soon after onset of the acute illness; its appearance coincides with an increase in serum transaminases (Fig. 4-3). Detection of anti-HAV indicates that the patient has had the infection in the past, will be resistant to subsequent hepatitis A infections, and is no longer infective. The IgM class of anti-HAV appears 1 week to 6 weeks after infection and indicates that HAV infection occurred within the prior 4 weeks to 8 weeks. Anti-HAV IgM is no longer detectable 3 months to 6 months after infection. The IgG class antibody peaks 5 weeks to 10 weeks after infection and indicates that HAV infection occurred more than 8 weeks earlier. The IgG antibody remains elevated indefinitely.

*Hepatitis B*
*Hepatitis B Surface Antigen* ($HB_sAg$) is the first serologic marker to appear, preceding clinical and laboratory evidence of disease by 1 week to 6 weeks (Fig. 4-5). This persists throughout the clinical illness and usually disappears in 1 week to 13 weeks. This is not detected in 5%–10% of patients. In general, $HB_sAg$ disappears just before the transminases increase. Persistence for greater than 6 months indicates either development of chronic hepatitis or a benign carrier state (Fig. 4-6). The presence of $HB_sAg$ indicates infection with HBV and implies infectivity. The disappearance of $HB_sAg$ from the serum does not assure recovery from infection.

*Antibody to $Hb_sAg$* (anti-$HB_s$) is the last serologic marker to appear (Fig. 4-5). It is not detected until the end of convalescence, several weeks after $HB_sAg$ disappears. During this "serologic gap" period, neither $HB_sAg$ nor anti-$HB_s$ is present in the serum. Antibody to $HB_cAg$ (anti-$HB_c$) must be identified at this stage in order to establish hepatitis B infection. The rate of anti-$HB_s$ appearance may depend on the rapidity of $HB_sAg$ clearance. Detectable antibody is present for at least 18 months after its appearance and may persist indefinitely.

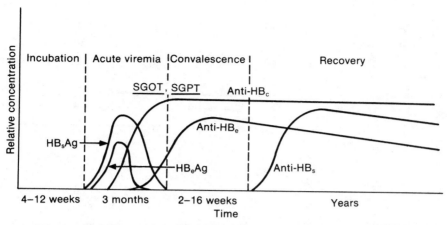

**Fig. 4-5.** Typical sequence of serologic markers in patients with *acute* type B hepatitis following exposure to HBV. This serologic sequence occurs in about 75% of patients with acute type B hepatitis. Most of the remaining patients show a later appearance of anti-HB$_e$. (Reproduced with permission of Abbott Diagnostics Division. Data from which this graph was generated came from clinical studies using Abbott assays of known sensitivity and specificity.)

Development of anti-HB$_s$ connotes recovery from hepatitis B infection, absence of infectivity, and immunity from future HBV infection.

*Hepatitis B Core Antigen* (HB$_c$Ag) is not found in the serum. This antigen is present in liver cell nuclei at the same time that HB$_s$Ag is present in the serum and in liver cell cytoplasm.

*Antibody to HB$_c$Ag* (anti-HB$_c$) appears in the serum shortly after the appearance of HB$_s$Ag (Fig. 4-5). This is the first antibody to appear, filling the "serologic gap" described above. Its presence implies a recent HBV infection. High serum titers correlate well with the continuing presence of viral antigens in the liver. The highest levels of anti-HB$_c$ are found in the chronic HB$_s$Ag carrier state (Fig. 4-6). This can be lifelong but it does not confer immunity as does anti-HB$_s$.

*Hepatitis B e Antigen* (HB$_e$Ag) is found only in serum that is reactive for HB$_s$Ag. The biophysical characteristics and origin of HB$_e$Ag remain unknown. It appears in the serum of all patients with acute hepatitis B at about the same time HB$_s$Ag appears and before the appearance of any detectable biochemical abnormality (Fig. 4-5). At this time the patient is most infectious. The antigen usually lasts for 2 weeks to 6 weeks and disappears before clearance of HB$_s$Ag. Disappearance of HB$_e$Ag may be interpreted as probable recovery and clearance of HB$_s$Ag. The detection of HB$_e$Ag in serum for 10 weeks or more after the onset of illness implies progression of the hepatitis B infection to chronic liver disease (Fig. 4-6). In some patients with chronic hepatitis, HB$_e$Ag eventually disappears from the blood; in others, it persists. The presence of HB$_e$Ag indicates that the patient's blood is infectious.

*Antibody to HB$_e$Ag* (anti-HB$_e$) develops after the detection of anti-HB$_c$ but before the appearance of anti-HB$_s$. It usually appears when HB$_e$Ag disappears (Fig. 4-5). The seroconversion from HB$_e$Ag to anti-HB$_e$ indicates that the

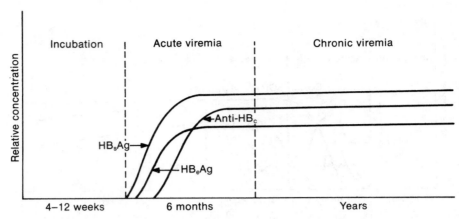

**Fig. 4-6.** Typical sequence of serologic markers in patients with *chronic* type B hepatitis following exposure to HBV. Some patients with chronic hepatitis show disappearance of HB$_e$Ag and appearance of anti-HB$_e$; these patients are less infectious than patients with persistence of HB$_e$Ag. (Reproduced with permission of Abbott Diagnostics Division. Data from which this graph was generated came from clinical studies using Abbott assays of known sensitivity and specificity.)

infection and the disease are on the wane. In the chronic carrier state, presence of anti-HB$_e$ is a favorable sign and indicates decreased infectiousness.

A tabulation of the five serologic tests for hepatitis B and their clinical correlation is shown in Table 4-1. It must be emphasized that exact identification of the stage of the disease cannot be made from one determination of serologic tests alone, because identical serologic patterns may be found in different clinical stages. Therefore, the clinical stage may be established only by using the patient's history, physical findings, sequential liver function tests, and sequential serologic tests.

*Non-A, Non-B Hepatitis*
At the present time, there is no specific serologic test for the non-A, non-B form of hepatitis. This is a diagnosis of exclusion. It should be considered in a patient who develops hepatitis 5 weeks to 10 weeks following blood transfusion and who is negative for anti-HAV, HB$_s$Ag, anti-HB$_s$, and anti-HB$_c$.

**Other Laboratory Findings**

Markedly increased SGOT (AST) and SGPT (ALT) (from 10 times to 100 times normal) indicates severity of liver cell damage; both enzymes are usually increased to the same degree; a fluctuating course of the transminases is frequently seen in non-A, non-B hepatitis.

Increased γ-glutamyl transpeptidase

Slightly increased alkaline phosphatase (1–3 times normal) indicates mild cholestasis.

Slightly increased lactate dehydrogenase (LDH) (1–3 times normal), especially LDH$_5$

**Table 4-1.** Serologic Interpretation in Type B Hepatitis*

| HB$_s$Ag | HB$_e$Ag | ANTI-HB$_c$ | ANTI-HB$_e$ | ANTI-HB$_s$ | INTERPRETATION |
|---|---|---|---|---|---|
| + | − | − | − | − | Late incubation period of hepatitis indicative of onsent of viremic state |
| + | + | − | − | − | Very early acute phase of hepatitis, very infectious, within 3–5 days after onset of viremic state |
| + | + | + | − | − | Acute phase of hepatitis, very infectious, usually 7–14 days after onset of viremic state. The same profile is found in serum of patient who is a chronic carrier (Fig. 4-9) |
| + | − | + | − | − | Acute or chronic hepatitis B infection |
| + | + | + | + | − | Patient is undergoing HB$_e$Ag/anti-HB$_e$ sero-conversion; is prognostic for resolution of viral disease. This profile may also be found in chronic hepatitis. |
| + | − | + | + | − | Acute phase of hepatitis; low infectivity; resolution of viremic state. This profile may indicate continued viral replication. |
| − | − | + | − | − | This may occur: (1) in "silent carriers of HBV in whom HB$_s$Ag is below the threshold of detectability; (2) in the "convalescence window," a period between the decay of HB$_s$Ag to below detectability and prior to seroconversion to anti-HB$_s$ (likelihood of infectivity exists); (3) representing remote past infection with HBV (*i.e.,* a long persistence of anti-HB$_c$; or (4) because of a cross-reacting antibody (false-positive) |
| − | − | + | + | − | May represent either a current or recent past infection with HBV |
| − | − | + | + | + | Patient is in recovery state of disease, indicates past infection and persisting immunity |
| − | − | + | − | + | Patient is in recovery state of disease; anti-HB$_e$ levels are no longer detectable; persisting immunity |

* The most frequently encountered serologic profiles are listed.
(Data from Mushahwar IK, Dienstag JL, Polesky HF et al: Interpretation of various serological profiles of Hepatitis B virus infection. Am J Clin Pathol 76:773–777, 1981)

Normal sedimentation rate and complete blood count (CBC)

Severe liver-cell necrosis may result in decreased serum albumin, decreased serum cholesterol, prolonged prothrombin time, and serum bilirubin > 25 mg/dl.

Liver biopsy is used to differentiate among the various stages of hepatitis: protracted acute hepatitis, chronic persistent hepatitis, and chronic active hepatitis.

**Findings by Stage of Disease**

*Anicteric Period*
Increased urine bilirubin

Increased urine urobilinogen

Increased SGOT (AST), SGPT (ALT)—level reflects the severity of liver damage; usually precedes jaundice

Decreased white blood cell (WBC) count with relative lymphocytosis; some atypical lymphocytes

Normal sedimentation rate

Retention of indocyanine green (Cardio-Green)

*Icteric Period (occurs about 5%–15% as frequently as anicteric hepatitis)*
Increased serum bilirubin (8 mg/dl–15 mg/dl)—rises in 10–14 days, then declines in 2–4 weeks

Slightly increased serum alkaline phosphatase reflects mild cholestasis.

Decreased urine urobilinogen; absent urobilinogen at the peak of disease.

Fall in SGOT (AST) and SGPT (ALT) indicates diminishing liver-cell necrosis.

Increased sedimentation rate

Increased serum iron reflects release from damaged liver cells.

Proteinuria might indicate immune-complex damage of the kidney

*Recovery Period*
Bilirubinuria disappears before bilirubinemia disappears.

Urine urobilinogen reappears.

Normal sedimentation rate

Slight decrease in serum albumin and mild elevation in $\gamma$-globulin


# CHRONIC HEPATITIS

Viral infections and drug-induced injury are the most common causes of chronic, as well as of acute, hepatitis. *Chronic hepatitis* is arbitrarily defined as clinical liver disease persisting for more than 6 months after the onset of acute hepatitis or as pathologic evidence of chronic inflammation seen on liver biopsy. Chronic hepatitis may last from 1 year to several decades.

Hepatitis A does not cause chronic hepatitis. Five percent to ten percent of patients with hepatitis B and twenty percent to forty percent of patients with non-A, non-B hepatitis develop chronic liver disease.

Autoimmune mechanisms may play a role in initiating or maintaining chronic hepatitis. Chronic inflammation of the liver is often associated with immune-complex disorders such as polyarteritis nodosa, glomerulonephritis, vasculitis, and arthritis. The similarity of human leukocyte antigen (HLA) typing in patients with chronic hepatitis and with a variety of autoimmune diseases may explain the presence of these diseases in approximately 20% of patients with chronic hepatitis.

Approximately 70% of patients with chronic hepatitis have a benign disorder called chronic persistent hepatitis, which heals completely. The remainder develop chronic active hepatitis with focal or extensive liver-cell necrosis. The greater the necrosis, the greater the likelihood of progression to cirrhosis and death in an average of 4 years to 5 years.

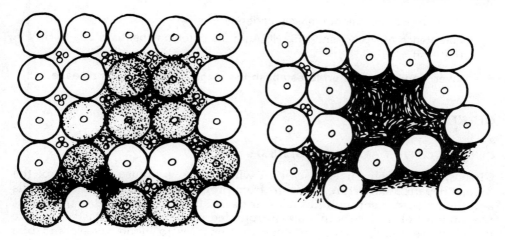

Subacute
hepatic necrosis

Postnecrotic cirrhosis

**Fig. 4-7.** Diagrammatic relationship between subacute hepatic necrosis and postnecrotic cirrhosis, which is a type of macronodular or multilobular cirrhosis. (Schiff L [ed]: Diseases of the Liver, 4th ed, p 841. Philadelphia, JB Lippincott, 1975)

The liver has a great capacity for regeneration, but when this is outstripped by the rate of necrosis, lobular collapse occurs and postnecrotic scars are formed. Cirrhosis that follows viral hepatitis is the multilobular or postnecrotic type (Fig. 4-7).

## LABORATORY FINDINGS

### Chronic Active Hepatitis

Increased SGOT (AST) and SGPT (ALT) (5–10 times normal)

Increased γ-globulin (2 times normal), especially IgG

Increased serum bilirubin (>4 mg/dl).

Increased alkaline phosphatase

Decreased serum albumin

Presence of smooth-muscle antibody (70%–90%)

Persistence of $HB_sAg$, anti-$HB_c$, $HB_eAg$ if the chronic hepatitis is due to HBV (Fig. 4-6)

### Chronic Persistent Hepatitis

Variable increase in SGOT (AST) and SGPT (ALT) (< 5 times normal)

Increased serum bilirubin (<4 mg/dl)

Variable increase in alkaline phosphatase

Increased γ-globulin, slight

Negative test for smooth-muscle antibody

Persistence of $HB_sAg$, anti-$HB_c$, $HB_eAg$ if the chronic hepatitis is due to HBV (Fig. 4-6)

**Liver biopsy is required to establish the stage of chronic liver disease**

# CIRRHOSIS

## CLASSIFICATION AND PATHOGENESIS

Cirrhosis is a chronic liver disease in which there is diffuse alteration of the normal hepatic architecture. It results from progressive destruction of liver cells and their replacement with fibrous scar tissue. It is characterized by regenerative nodules of liver cells that are surrounded by bands of fibrous connective tissue. These nodules have abnormal relationships to blood vessels and bile ducts, causing alterations in the circulation and in various hepatic functions.

Cirrhosis may be classified according to histologic findings or according to its cause. Unfortunately, there is not an absolute correlation between cause and pathology. Thus, one cannot ascertain the cause of cirrhosis with certainty from the pathologic findings.

The morphologic types of cirrhosis are micronodular (uniform small nodules, divided by thin fibrous septa [Fig. 4-1]), macronodular (variously sized nodules, divided by thin or thick fibrous septa), and multilobular (variously sized nodules, divided by very prominent fibrous septa; some areas of the liver show a normal pattern [Fig. 4-7]).

The various causes of cirrhosis include alcoholism, viral hepatitis, biliary obstruction, drugs and toxins, heavy metals, metabolic disorders, and congestive heart failure. In the United States, alcoholism is the most common cause of cirrhosis and viral hepatitis is the second most common cause. Although the pathogenesis of cirrhosis varies with each agent, the end results and effects are similar.

The reason why some, but not all, chronic alcoholics progress through the stages of fatty liver and alcoholic hepatitis to cirrhosis has not been determined. Studies suggest that most chronic drinkers will develop cirrhosis if given a regular dosage of alcohol over a long enough period of time. In alcoholic liver disease the following sequence of events occurs:

1. Central lobular damage
2. Portal fibrosis
3. A combination of the above two
4. Diffuse fibrosis

Fibrous bands connect portal and central areas of the hepatic lobules, disrupting the normal lobular architecture. Hepatic regeneration then causes uniform, small nodules to form. Micronodular cirrhosis results. This is also known as *portal cirrhosis* and as *Laennec's cirrhosis* (Fig. 4-8). Patients with long-standing Laennec's cirrhosis may also develop the histologic picture of postnecrotic cirrhosis (Fig. 4-7).

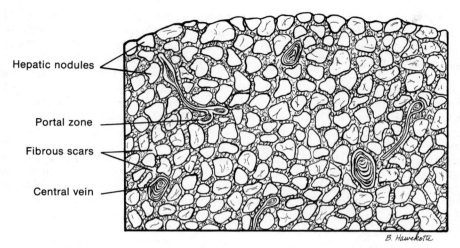

**Fig. 4-8.** Cut section of liver showing Laennec's cirrhosis.

Approximately 3% of the clinical cases of viral hepatitis progress to chronic active hepatitis. Approximately 50% of these patients develop cirrhosis. Incomplete septal or multilobular cirrhosis is the morphologic type of cirrhosis that usually follows hepatitis (Fig. 4-7).

Cirrhosis may also result from exposure to any one of many different drugs, chemicals, or toxins. Postnecrotic or macronodular cirrhosis then develops. Biliary cirrhosis results from long-standing bile stasis due either to major bile-duct obstruction or to primary biliary cirrhosis, a condition of intrahepatic bile-duct destruction of unknown cause. Other, rarer, causes of cirrhosis include hepatic deposition of heavy metals such as iron and copper (see Hemochromatosis and Wilson's Disease, Chap. 10).

## PATHOPHYSIOLOGY

Fibrosis, which is similar to scar formation, occurs in cirrhosis chiefly as the result of increased formation of connective tissue by the liver. This is a consequence of stimulation by a toxic agent, such as alcohol. Fibrosis also occurs as a response to the collapse of the hepatic architecture following liver necrosis.

Irregular hepatic nodules and widespread fibrous septa reduce the effective blood flow through the liver. Diminished hepatic blood flow and loss of liver cells may impair any of the following hepatic functions:

1. Synthesis of albumin, blood-clotting factors, cholesterol, triglycerides, fatty acids, and glycogen
2. Secretion of bile acids into the intestinal tract, which may lead to impaired intestinal absorption and steatorrhea; increased circulating bile acids, which may cause itching
3. Excretion of bilirubin, Cardio-Green, and gallbladder dyes
4. Inactivation of estrogens, ammonia, and drugs

Portal hypertension is a major and serious consequence of cirrhosis. The portal vein drains blood from the sinusoids of the spleen and from the vessels in the pancreas, stomach, and intestines. After penetrating the liver, the portal vein divides progressively into smaller and smaller branches, which finally end in the hepatic sinusoids. These sinusoids are a network of intercommunicating vascular spaces between the liver cells. The sinusoids contain a mixture of portal venous and arterial blood. In the normal liver, blood exits from the sinusoids into the central veins of the hepatic lobules, and then to the hepatic veins and the inferior vena cava (Fig. 4-9A). In cirrhosis, the normal vascular communication between the hepatic and portal venous systems are obstructed. Both the contracting scar tissue and the regenerating hepatic nodules compress and block the hepatic veins, resulting in an increase in portal venous pressure, termed *portal hypertension* (Fig. 4-9B). The increased resistance to blood flow through the liver leads to the development of an alternate or collateral circulation, ascites, and splenomegaly. The collateral circulation develops where the portal and systemic venous systems communicate (Fig. 4-9B). Increased portal venous pressure is reflected as increased pressure in the systemic circulation at these sites. As a consequence, these patients have hemorrhoids and dilated esophageal and gastric veins. These dilated veins are known as *varices*. Esophageal varices are serious complications of portal hypertension, especially when they bleed. Bleeding results from increased venous pressure in the varices and from irritation of the esophageal mucosa.

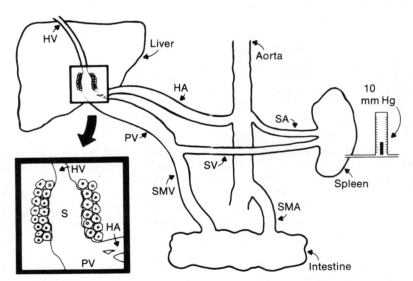

**Fig. 4-9A.** Schematic outline of normal hepatosplanchnic circulation with inset illustrating the dual hepatic blood supply converging in the hepatic sinusoid. (HV, hepatic vein; SV, splenic vein; PV, portal vein; SA, splenic artery; HA, hepatic artery; SMA, superior mesenteric artery; SMV, superior mesenteric vein; S, hepatic sinusoid.) (Reprinted from Becker FF [ed]: The Liver: Normal and Abnormal Functions, p 13. New York, Marcel Dekker Inc., 1974, by courtesy of Marcel Dekker Inc.)

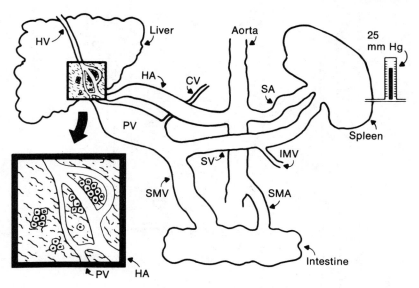

**Fig. 4-9B.** Schematic outline of the hypothesized hepatosplanchnic circulation in portal hypertension from hepatic cirrhosis. Portal blood flow is restricted by obliterated hepatic sinusoids and diverted into portasystemic venous collaterals (CV, IMV). Coronary veins drain into esophageal veins, which form varices. Increased venous pressure is seen as dilated vessels and increased splenic pressure. (HV, hepatic vein; SV, splenic vein; PV, portal vein; SA, splenic artery; HA, hepatic artery; SMA, superior mesenteric artery; IMV, inferior mesenteric vein; SMV, superior mesenteric vein; CV, coronary vein.) (Reprinted from Becker FF [ed]: The Liver: Normal and Abnormal Functions, p 39. New York, Marcel Dekker Inc., 1974, by courtesy of Marcel Dekker, Inc.)

*Ascites* is the accumulation of fluid in the peritoneal cavity. Although this may result from various mechanisms, cirrhosis is its most common cause. Ascites is the consequence of a combination of portal hypertension and hypoalbuminemia. The latter results in decreased plasma colloid oncotic pressure, contributing to the leakage of fluid out of capillaries and into the peritoneal cavity. Increased hepatic venous pressure leads to increased formation of hepatic lymph. When the capacities of the lymphatic system and the portal venous system cannot absorb the increased lymph, ascites develops. Another factor contributing to the formation of ascites is an impaired ability of cirrhotic patients to excrete sodium and water. These mechanisms are depicted in Figure 4-10.

As indicated in Figure 4-9B, portal hypertension increases the vascular pressure within the spleen, producing enlargement and congestion of the spleen. Its normal function as the site of blood-cell removal is accentuated. There is increased trapping and destruction of all blood cell components in the splenic pulp. This is called *hypersplenism* and it results in pancytopenia (*i.e.*, decreased RBC, WBC, and platelets).

Advanced cirrhosis may be complicated by progressive and irreversible renal failure. This is referred to as the *hepatorenal syndrome,* or *oliguric hepatic*

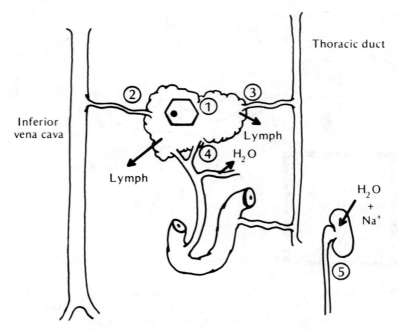

**Fig. 4-10.** Origin of ascitic fluid.
1. Liver-cell damage leads to hypoalbuminemia and decreased oncotic pressure.
2. Postsinusoidal block develops to produce *3*.
3. Lymph production increases.
4. Presinusoidal block to portal flow develops to produce increased hydrostatic pressure.
5. Water and sodium reabsorption by the kidneys increases.
(Reprinted from Ascites formation in cirrhosis and its management by Sherlock S from Scand J Gastroenterol 5 [Suppl] 7, 9–15, 1970, by permission of Universitetsforlaget, Oslo)

*failure*. Complete understanding of the mechanism of this syndrome is not presently available. Some clues may be found in the altered handling of sodium and water by the kidney in patients with liver disease. Bleeding, infection, and dehydration may also play a role in this syndrome. (Hepatic encephalopathy, which may be a complication of advanced cirrhosis, is described in the section on Hepatic Failure in this chapter.) Other complications of cirrhosis include an increased incidence of infections, hypogonadism, carbohydrate intolerance, hypoxemia, and gastrointestinal bleeding.

Cirrhosis that follows hepatitis B infection is associated with an increased incidence of hepatocellular carcinoma. The mechanism is unknown.

## LABORATORY FINDINGS

Biopsy of the liver shows nodules and fibrous septa.

Increased nonconjugated and conjugated bilirubin—impaired bilirubin excretion is a major defect in cirrhosis

Increased SGOT (AST) and SGPT (ALT) reflect the degree of liver cell necrosis. These are increased to a lesser degree than in hepatitis.

Increased alkaline phosphatase, 5-nucleotidase, and leucine aminopeptidase reflect cholestasis.

Slightly increased LDH, especially $LDH_4$ and $LDH_5$.

Increased γ-glutamyl transpeptidase

Retention of Cardio-Green is a sensitive index of impaired liver function in the absence of jaundice.

Decreased serum albumin reflects decreased synthesis, contributes to ascites, and indicates advanced liver disease

Increased β- and γ-globulins; gamma globulins are polyclonal and reflect chronic inflammation.

Decreased iron-binding capacity reflects decreased hepatic synthesis of transferrin.

Increased blood ammonia reflects impaired hepatic detoxification of proteins and occurs in hepatic failure or coma and after surgical anastomosis of the portal vein to the inferior vena cava.

Decreased serum sodium reflects dilution by increased plasma volume in association with ascites.

BUN is often decreased with severe liver disease owing to impaired protein metabolism; it may be increased with gastrointestinal (GI) hemorrhage

Decreased urine volume usually occurs when ascites and edema are present.

Increased urine bilirubin and urobilinogen reflect impaired bilirubin excretion and impaired hepatic metabolism of urobilinogen.

Microcytic hypochromic anemia reflects chronic GI blood loss; this is the most common type of anemia in cirrhosis.

Normocytic anemia reflects dilution by increased plasma volume, chronic inflammation, or hypersplenism.

Macrocytic anemia, nonmegaloblastic is due to excessive lipid in the RBC membrane; these red cells are more susceptible to hemolysis.

Macrocytic anemia, megaloblastic is due to folic acid deficiency.

WBC is increased with massive hepatic necrosis or GI hemorrhage; it is decreased with hypersplenism or folic-acid deficiency.

Decreased platelet count reflects hypersplenism; if severe, this suggests disseminated intravascular coagulopathy.

Prolonged prothrombin time is due to impaired hepatic formation of the vitamin-K dependent clotting factors (prothrombin and factors VII, IX, and X).

Decreased fibrinogen and factor V reflect impaired hepatic synthesis

## PRIMARY BILIARY CIRRHOSIS

Primary biliary cirrhosis is a disease of unknown etiology; it usually affects middle-aged women and is very slowly progressive.[10] In this disorder there is chronic bile stasis. The small intrahepatic bile ducts in the portal zones of the liver become progressively destroyed and gradually disappear. This is followed by portal-zone scar formation, cirrhosis, and portal hypertension. There is also intrahepatic biliary obstruction, with elevation of alkaline phosphatase and impaired bile excretion. Retained bile salts cause the chief clinical symptom of itching.

Although the etiology remains unknown, immunologic mechanisms are believed to play a key role. A current theory is that an antigen, possibly of bile-duct origin, is absorbed from the bile, combines with an antibody derived from the portal circulation, and fixes complement. Theoretically, this could then result in immune-complex formation within the bile-duct wall and eventual bile-duct destruction. Circulation of immune complexes might account for the frequent association of other immunologic diseases, such as Sjögren's syndrome and scleroderma. The common findings of antimitochondrial antibodies and increased serum IgM levels reflect the immunologic origin of this disorder. Hormonal, genetic, and environmental factors may play roles in the pathogenesis of primary biliary cirrhosis, possibly through their effects on immune responses.

### LABORATORY FINDINGS

Marked increase in serum alkaline phosphatase reflects increased synthesis of alkaline phosphatase proximal to the site of intrahepatic obstruction and also indicates impaired excretion of the enzyme.

Markedly increased conjugated (direct) bilirubin, $\gamma$-glutamyl transpeptidase, 5-nucleotidase, and serum cholesterol all reflect intrahepatic obstruction and impaired excretion.

Presence of antimitochondrial antibodies is a characteristic finding and reflects the immunologic nature of the disorder.

Increased $\alpha_2$-, $\beta$-, and $\gamma$-globulins, especially IgM, reflect the immunologic basis of this disorder.

Slightly decreased albumin occurs early; later it is markedly decreased.

Increased urine bilirubin and urobilinogen

Increased urine and hepatic copper reflect impaired hepatic metabolism of copper.

## PYOGENIC LIVER ABSCESS

Liver abscess is caused by bacteria which may enter the liver through the portal vein, the bile ducts, the bloodstream, or a penetrating wound or may be spread from an adjacent septic focus. The most common infecting organisms are gram-negative bacilli, especially *Escherichia coli,* and anaerobes such as *Bacteroides fragilis.*

### LABORATORY FINDINGS

Marked leukocytosis reflects inflammation.

Abnormal liver function tests:

Decreased albumin; increased globulin and alkaline phosphatase
Bilirubin might be elevated

Normocytic anemia, mild to moderate, reflects inflammation.

Positive aerobic or anaerobic culture of liver abscess


## HEPATOMA (HEPATOCELLULAR CARCINOMA)

There is a close association of liver-cell carcinoma with cirrhosis. About 50% of patients with hepatoma have had cirrhosis. Possibly the toxic factor that initially caused the cirrhosis, such as alcohol, virus, or iron, continues stimulating the hepatic cells until they become malignant. Cirrhosis that follows hepatitis B infection is associated with an increased incidence of hepatoma. A patient has a 22-times-greater chance of developing hepatoma if he is $HB_s Ag$-positive rather than $HB_s Ag$-negative. A current theory postulates that the tumor arises from a single transformed clone of infected liver cells.

This tumor frequently secretes a protein that is normally present only during fetal life—$\alpha_1$-fetoprotein. Although this protein may also be found in patients with gonadal and other tumors, very high blood levels suggest hepatoma as its most likely source. Serial measurement of $\alpha_1$-fetoprotein is helpful in evaluating the response of a hepatoma to treatment. A hepatoma may also secrete physiologically active peptides, having the effects of insulin, erythropoietin, parathormone, or gonadotropins.

### LABORATORY FINDINGS

Biopsy of the liver is necessary to establish the diagnosis.

Sudden worsening of laboratory findings in a patient with cirrhosis (see Cirrhosis)

Increased serum $\alpha_1$-fetoprotein is a frequent finding.

Increased serum carcinoembryonic antigen

Positive $HB_s Ag$ in a patient with cirrhosis suggests the possibility of hepatoma.

Blood in ascitic fluid

Laboratory findings reflecting possible hormonal activity of the tumor, having the effects of insulin, parathormone, erythropoietin, or gonadotropins


## METASTATIC CARCINOMA OF THE LIVER

Metastatic carcinoma of the liver indicates that the tumor originated at another site and has spread to the liver, usually through the bloodstream. This occurs 20 times more commonly than does primary hepatic malignancy. The liver is a very frequent site of tumor metastases because it receives a large amount of venous blood from the GI tract and the pelvis. Metastases through the hepatic artery also occur from primary sites in the breast, lung, kidney, ovary, and testes. Tumor cells may also spread directly from the gallbladder, colon, pancreas, or stomach. Metastatic tumor nodules in the liver are usually multiple.

## LABORATORY FINDINGS

Biopsy of liver showing tumor is necessary for definitive diagnosis.

Increased serum alkaline phosphatase occurs in 80% of patients. This reflects liver infiltration by tumor.

Marked increase in carcinoembryonic antigen

Increased LDH; isoenzymes do not show specific tissue localization

Normal serum bilirubin is a common finding.

## *ACUTE CHOLECYSTITIS*

Cholecystitis is inflammation of the wall of the gallbladder and cystic duct. This results from obstruction by stones lodged in the neck of the gallbladder or in the cystic duct. The stones interfere with bile drainage.

In the first stage of cholecystitis, the gallbladder mucosa or entire wall shows vascular congestion and edema. This is due to obstruction of the gallbladder outlet, which causes distention of the gallbladder and blockage of venous blood flow. In the second stage, inflammation occurs. It is presumed that the entrapped, concentrated bile acts as a chemical irritant to the gallbladder wall, bringing about the inflammatory cellular response. This toxic effect, along with the impaired circulation, edema, and distention, produces mucosal sloughing, gangrene, and an inflammatory exudate on the serosal surface. If the inflammation is unresolved, almost all patients will have secondary bacterial growth in the gallbladder and, possibly, generalized septicemia. The most commonly encountered bacteria are enteric organisms, especially *E. coli.* A necrotic gallbladder may perforate.

There is a close association between cholecystitis and gallstone formation. Obstruction of the cystic duct by a gallstone usually results in inflammation of the gallbladder. When gallstones become lodged in the common bile duct they may cause obstructive jaundice and inflammation of the common bile duct (Fig. 4-11). Disorders of bile-acid and cholesterol metabolism lead to cholesterol gallstones, which account for 75% of all gallstones. Pigment gallstones, in contrast, are composed of calcium salts of unconjugated bilirubin, carbonate and phosphate. Except for the fact that there is a frequent occurrence of pigment stones in patients with chronic hemolysis, particularly sickle-cell disease, there is no diagnostic laboratory characteristic of patients with gallstone disease.

## LABORATORY FINDINGS

Leukocytosis (12,000/$\mu$l–15,000/$\mu$l) and increased sedimentation rate reflect acute inflammation.

Increased SGOT (AST), alkaline phosphatase, 5-nucleotidase, and $\gamma$-glutamyl transpeptidase reflect slight hepatic inflammation and partial biliary obstruction.

Increased amylase might occur in the absence of clinically evident pancreatitis.

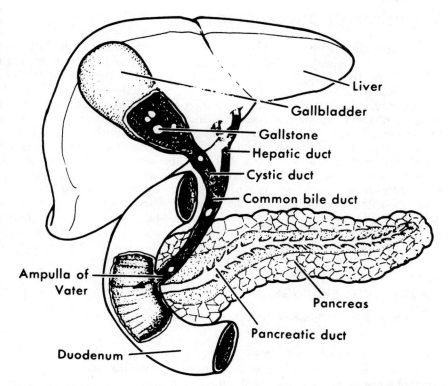

**Fig. 4-11.** Common sites of gallstones. (Given BA, Simmons SJ: Gastroenterology in Clinical Nursing, 3rd ed, p 196. St Louis, CV Mosby, 1979)

## CHOLANGITIS

*Cholangitis* refers to inflammation of the biliary tract resulting from obstruction, usually by gallstones or strictures. Obstruction predisposes the duct to bacterial infection proximal to the site of blockage. Septicemia may then occur. The infection rapidly ascends upward along the bile ducts into the liver, where single or multiple abscesses may form. Altered liver-function tests commonly occur.

### LABORATORY FINDINGS

Leukocytosis, up to 30,000/μl, indicates inflammation.

Frequently, positive blood cultures. *Escherichia coli* is the most frequently encountered organism. Other commonly encountered organisms include *Klebsiella, Enterobacter, Streptococcus fecalis,* and *Bacteroides fragilis.*

Increased serum bilirubin, 5-nucleotidase, alkaline phosphatase, γ-glutamyl transpeptidase, leucine aminopeptidase, SGOT (AST), and SGPT (ALT) reflect partial biliary obstruction.

## MAJOR BILE-DUCT OBSTRUCTION

Major bile-duct obstruction involves the hepatic ducts or common bile duct. When this occurs, conjugated bilirubin cannot enter the intestinal tract and regurgitates into the tissue fluid and bloodstream. The increased circulating conjugated bilirubin is excreted in the urine. Unconjugated bilirubin may also rise in the blood as a result of associated damage to hepatic cells and impairment of conjugation. Obstruction also results in increased hepatic synthesis and impaired hepatic excretion of alkaline phosphatase. Consequently, there is marked elevation of this enzyme in the blood. Another biochemical consequence of a completely obstructed biliary tract is a lack of urobilinogen in the urine, because no bilirubin reaches the intestine for bacterial conversion to urobilinogen.

Major bile-duct obstruction may be caused by carcinoma of the head of the pancreas, the bile ducts, or the ampulla of Vater. The ampulla is the duodenal opening of the common bile duct and pancreatic duct. Other causes of obstruction are gallstones within the bile duct, chronic pancreatitis, or strictures of the bile duct following prior gallbladder surgery (Fig. 4-12). Long-standing obstruction may result in a form of cirrhosis known as *biliary cirrhosis*.

### LABORATORY FINDINGS

Increased serum conjugated (direct) bilirubin

Increased urine bilirubin

Decreased or absent urine urobilinogen

Increased serum 5-nucleotidase, leucine aminopeptidase, and alkaline phosphatase reflect bile-duct obstruction.

Increased $\gamma$-glutamyl transpeptidase shows a faster and greater rise than does alkaline phosphatase or leucine aminopeptidase.

Prolonged prothrombin time is the result of impaired intestinal absorption of vitamin K and impaired hepatic synthesis of prothrombin and factors VII, IX, and X.

Increased amylase reflects possible accompanying pancreatitis.

Increased serum cholesterol and triglycerides

Increased $\alpha_2$- and $\beta$-globulins correspond to increased serum lipids.

Leukocytosis (10,000/$\mu$l–15,000/$\mu$l)

## ACUTE PANCREATITIS

Acute pancreatitis is a potentially lethal, inflammatory and necrotizing process. It is most commonly associated with alcoholism or gallstone disease. Less common causes of acute pancreatitis are the postoperative state, penetrating duodenal ulcers, metabolic disorders, infections, certain drugs, and trauma.

The association between hyperlipidemia and pancreatitis is well recognized. The mechanism by which increased lipids produce pancreatitis remains to be defined.

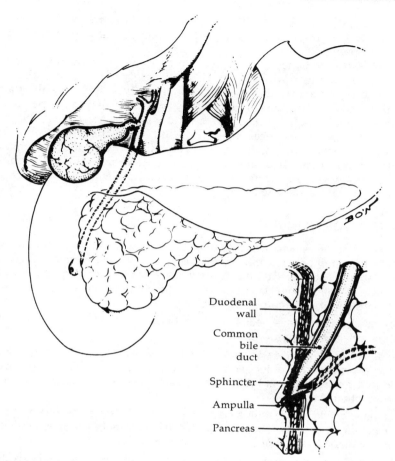

Duodenal
wall

Common
bile
duct

Sphincter

Ampulla

Pancreas

**Fig. 4-12.** Anatomic course of the common bile duct. This shows possible sites of extrahepatic bile-duct obstruction. (Sodeman WA Jr, Sodeman WA: Pathologic Physiology, 5th ed, p 803. Philadelphia, WB Saunders, 1974)

Pancreatic inflammation results from leakage of enzymes from the pancreatic ducts into the substance of the gland, with autodigestion of pancreatic tissues. Some proposed mechanisms include direct toxic effects of alcohol or drugs, dietary overstimulation of the gland, ductal obstruction, or reflux of bile and intestinal fluid into the pancreatic duct. Chronic alcohol consumption is followed by increased concentration of protein and decreased concentration of bicarbonate in pancreatic secretions. This results in precipitation of pancreatic-juice proteins and obstruction of the pancreatic ducts.[9] Under normal circumstances, the pancreas is protected against the action of its own enzymes by their secretion in an inactive form and also by the action of enzyme inhibitors. Activated pancreatic enzymes produce the following effects upon the pancreas: edema, liquefaction, necrosis, hemorrhage, fat necrosis, and vascular thrombosis. Proteolytic enzymes are primarily responsible for pancreatic autodigestion and for systemic toxicity. Lipase may contribute to the fat necrosis. Although elevated serum amylase is important diagnostically, it is not believed to contribute to pancreatic injury.

Acute attacks of pancreatitis may result in complete recovery, may recur without leaving permanent damage, or may progress to chronic pancreatitis. Shock, which may occur with severe acute pancreatitis, is the result of a shift of large volumes of fluid and protein from the vascular system to the peripancreatic tissues, peritoneal and pleural cavities, and dilated intestines. The systemic effects of pancreatitis are presumed to result from the absorption into the bloodstream of activated pancreatic enzymes and the products of pancreatic digestion. Severe pancreatitis may result in acute renal failure. Complications may involve the following systems: pulmonary, cardiovascular, neurologic, GI, hematologic, renal, and endocrine.

## LABORATORY FINDINGS

Increased serum amylase begins after 3–6 hr, peaks at 20–30 hr, persists for 48–72 hr; some patients with severe disease may have normal values; no correlation exists between the severity of pancreatitis and the degree of serum amylase elevation. Amylase passes from the inflamed pancreas directly into the bloodstream or into the peritoneal cavity.

Increased serum lipase peaks at 72–96 hr and persists up to 14 days after serum amylase has returned to normal.

Increased urine amylase occurs 6–10 hr after serum amylase elevation; urine levels are higher and of longer duration than serum levels. This is believed to be due to a reversible renal tubular defect, which results in decreased amylase reabsorption.

Increased amylase–creatinine clearance ratio; amylase clearance by the kidneys is accelerated in acute pancreatitis; this also occurs in nonpancreatic diseases, such as diabetic ketoacidosis and extensive burns

Decreased serum calcium occurs in severe acute pancreatitis; this is the result of calcium binding to fatty acids in fat, which undergoes necrosis from pancreatic enzyme action.

Leukocytosis (10,000/$\mu$l–20,000/$\mu$l)

Increased hematocrit reflects hemoconcentration.

Increased blood glucose, transient—probably due to decreased release of insulin, increased release of glucagon, and increased output of glucocorticoids and catecholamines

Hypertriglyceridemia, usually in association with alcoholism

Increased sedimentation rate reflects acute inflammation.

Ascitic or pleural fluid with increased amylase and albumin; presence of blood in ascitic fluid occurs in hemorrhagic pancreatitis

Poorer prognosis exists when three or more of the following are present:[6]
    Initial WBC > 16,000/$\mu$l
    Initial blood glucose > 200 mg/dl
    Decreased serum calcium < 8 mg/dl

Fall in hematocrit > 10%
Rise in BUN > 5 mg/dl
Arterial PO₂ < 60 mm Hg
Metabolic acidosis with base deficit > 4 mEq/l
Initial serum LDH > 350 IU/l
Initial serum SGOT > 250 IU/l

## CHRONIC PANCREATITIS

Chronic pancreatitis is usually the result of chronic relapsing pancreatitis, in which there are frequent exacerbations of acute inflammatory disease in the setting of a previously injured gland. In this disorder the pancreatic acini, which are the sites of digestive-enzyme production, are destroyed and replaced by fibrous scar tissue. Pancreatic ducts become dilated and filled with protein deposits and calcifications. Inflammation is minimal to moderate.

In children, the most common cause of chronic pancreatitis is cystic fibrosis. In adults, most cases are the result of chronic alcoholism. A minority of cases results from trauma and metabolic disorders such as hyperlipidemia, hyperparathyroidism, and hemochromatosis. Other causes include hereditary pancreatitis and biliary tract disease, usually caused by gallstones.

In alcohol-induced pancreatitis, there is damage to the pancreas even before the first clinical attack occurs. Pathologic changes include focally calcified protein plugs in the pancreatic ducts, decreased acinar cells, dilated ducts, and fibrosis. Scarring of the acini and obstruction of the pancreatic ducts cause a gradual decrease in the ability of the pancreas to secrete water, electrolytes, and digestive enzymes. The flow of pancreatic juice and the concentration of bicarbonate and enzymes fall. At least 90% of the pancreas must be destroyed in order to impair intestinal digestion of proteins and lipids. Diminished output of lipase results in impaired digestion of fat, with resultant steatorrhea. Decreased output of proteolytic enzymes leads to impaired protein digestion and, eventually, to hypoalbuminemia and edema. Carbohydrate digestion is not usually impaired. Patients with maldigestion resulting from chronic pancreatitis rarely manifest malabsorption of vitamins or minerals, perhaps because there are adequate bile acids in the intestinal lumen and an adequate intestinal absorptive surface. In far-advanced chronic pancreatitis, diabetes mellitus is the consequence of decreased insulin reserve.

### LABORATORY FINDINGS

Abnormal secretin test—following intravenous administration of secretin, decreased volumes of amylase and bicarbonate are secreted into the duodenum

Abnormal Lundh test—following a fat meal, decreased trypsin is secreted into the duodenum

Increased stool neutral fat (unsplit fats); increased total fat in 72-hour stool sample when the patient has been on a 100-g fat diet daily for three days

Increased stool nitrogen reflects impaired protein digestion.

Undigested muscle fibers in the stool reflects impaired protein digestion.

Increased serum bilirubin and alkaline phosphatase reflect obstruction of the intrapancreatic portion of the common bile duct.

Impaired oral glucose tolerance—diabetic curve may be seen in far-advanced disease

Increased ascitic fluid amylase reflects leakage from the injured pancreas.

Laboratory findings of maldigestion (see Chap. 3)

# REFERENCES

1. Bernstein LM, Siegel, ER, Goldstein CM: The hepatitis knowledge base. Ann Intern Med 93:191–222, 1980
2. Cohen JA, Kaplan MM: The SGOT/SGPT ratio—an indicator of alcoholic liver disease. Dig Dis Sci 24:835–838, 1979
3. Czaja AJ: Serologic markers of hepatitis A and B in acute and chronic liver disease. Mayo Clin Proc 54:721–732, 1979
4. Deinhardt F: Predictive values of markers of hepatitis virus infection. J Infect Dis 141:299–303, 1980
5. Mendenhall CL: Alcoholic hepatitis. Clin Gastroenterol 10:417–441, 1981
6. Ranson JHC, Rifkind KM, Turner JW: Prognostic signs and non-operative peritoneal lavage in acute pancreatitis. Surg Gynecol Obstet 143:209–219, 1976
7. Reed JS, Boyer JL: Viral hepatitis, epidemiologic, serologic and clinical manifestation. DM 25:1–61, 1979
8. Reinstone SM, Purcell RH: New methods for the serodiagnosis of hepatitis A. Gastroenterology 78:1092–1094, 1980
9. Sarles H, Laugier R: Alcoholic pancreatitis. Clin Gastroenterol 10:401–415, 1981
10. Sherlock S: Primary biliary cirrhosis. Am J Med 65:217–219, 1978

# BIBLIOGRAPHY

**Brooks FP (ed):** Gastrointestinal Physiology, 2nd ed. New York, Oxford University Press, 1978
**Given BA, Simmons SJ:** Gastroenterology in Clinical Nursing, 3rd ed. St Louis, CV Mosby, 1979
**Greenberger NJ:** Gastrointestinal Disorders: A Pathophysiologic Approach, 2nd ed. Chicago, Year Book Medical Publishers, 1981
**Stenger RJ:** Liver disease. Hum Pathol 8:603–619, 1977

# 5

# GENITOURINARY DISEASES

Acute Poststreptococcal
    Glomerulonephritis
Nephritis Due to Bacterial Endocarditis
Rapidly Progressive Glomerulonephritis
Nephrotic Syndrome
   Proteinuria
   Hypoalbuminemia
   Edema
   Hyperlipidemia and Lipiduria
Diabetic Nephropathy
Sickle Cell Nephropathy
Myeloma Nephropathy
Lupus Nephritis
Polyarteritis Renal Disease
Scleroderma Renal Disease
Toxemia of Pregnancy
Acute Renal Failure
  Prerenal Acute Renal Failure
  Intrarenal Acute Renal Failure
  Postrenal Acute Renal Failure
Chronic Renal Failure
  Azotemia
  Acidosis
  Sodium Wasting and Water Excretion

Calcium and Phosphorus Metabolism
Anemia
Bleeding Tendency
Hypertension
Ionic Disturbances
Neurologic Dysfunction
Renal Tubular Acidosis
  Proximal Renal Tubular Acidosis
  Distal Renal Tubular Acidosis
Pyelonephritis
Renal and Perinephric Abscesses
Renal Calculi
Renal Infarction
Renal-Vein Thrombosis
Polycystic Kidney Disease
Adenocarcinoma of the Kidney
Cystitis
Benign Prostatic Hyperplasia
Prostatitis
Carcinoma of the Prostate
Vaginitis
Ectopic Pregnancy
Hydatidiform Mole

## ACUTE POSTSTREPTOCOCCAL GLOMERULONEPHRITIS

Acute poststreptococcal glomerulonephritis is a fairly common glomerular disease that occurs most often in children between the ages of three and seven. The glomerular manifestations usually appear 1 week to 2 weeks after a streptococcal infection. Acute glomerulonephritis more commonly follows streptococcal skin infection than streptococcal pharyngitis. Elevated antistreptolysin titers during the nephritic stage indicate prior streptococcal infection. The onset is usually abrupt and is manifested by the appearance of smoky-colored urine, reflecting hematuria; edema, usually limited to swelling around the eyes; mild proteinuria; and mild to moderate hypertension.

Most cases may be ascribed to specific nephritogenic strains of Group A streptococcus. The bacteria do not enter the blood, urine, or kidneys. However, streptococcal antigen circulates and elicits the formation of antibody, which combines with antigen to form immune complexes. The complexes deposit in the glomeruli and activate complement, attracting granulocytes, which damage glomerular basement membranes. Streptococcal infection does not lead to the formation of antibodies against glomerular basement membrane. Through immunofluorescent and electron microscopy, immunoglobulins and complement have been demonstrated to be deposited in a granular fashion along the glomerular capillaries and basement membranes.

The glomerular filtration rate (GFR) is moderately or markedly depressed owing to obstruction of the glomerular capillaries by endothelial proliferation and swelling. Tubular function is less severely impaired than is glomerular function. More than 95% of the children stricken with this disease heal spontaneously or with conservative therapy. A small minority of pediatric patients develops a rapidly progressive form of glomerulonephritis, and another small group undergoes slow progression to chronic glomerulonephritis with chronic renal failure. In adults there are both a higher mortality during the acute phase of the disease and a higher incidence of progression to rapidly progressive glomerulonephritis (RPGN). RPGN rapidly terminates in chronic renal failure.

## LABORATORY FINDINGS

### Evidence of Streptococcal Infection

Throat culture—Group A streptococcus

Increased antistreptolysin O (ASO) titer appears 1–3 weeks after infection and peaks at 3–5 weeks; 50% of patients show no rise in ASO titer; height of the titer does not reflect severity of the renal disease

Increased DNase B—this streptococcal antibody is more frequently elevated than is ASO following streptococcal skin infections.

### Urine

Hematuria, gross or microscopic, occurs during the initial upper respiratory infection and then reappears with nephritis in 1–2 weeks. It lasts 2–12 months.

Leukocyturia

Casts—red blood cell (RBC), white blood cell (WBC), granular, fatty, hyaline

Proteinuria (usually <3 g/day) disappears before hematuria occurs

Oliguria

Increased specific gravity occurs early in the disease.

### Blood

Increased blood urea nitrogen (BUN), creatinine

Decreased creatinine clearance

Increased sedimentation rate

Leukocytosis with increased neutrophils

Mild normocytic anemia due to hemodilution, marrow depression, or increased RBC destruction

Decreased albumin, increased $\alpha_2$-globulin; the former reflects urinary loss; the latter indicates acute inflammation.

Decreased serum complement occurs 24 hours before the onset of hematuria, rises to normal when hematuria subsides, and lasts for 2–12 weeks. This reflects transient depletion of complement when immune complexes deposit in the kidney.

## NEPHRITIS DUE TO BACTERIAL ENDOCARDITIS

In bacterial endocarditis, the kidney may be affected in one of three ways: diffuse glomerulonephritis, focal glomerulonephritis, or renal infarction. Because bacteria are rarely found in the glomeruli, the microscopic thrombi seen in focal glomerulonephritis are considered to be the result of formation of bacterial antigen–antibody complexes. The accompanying depression of serum complement levels supports this concept.

Clinically, findings indicative of glomerular involvement may range from asymptomatic proteinuria or hematuria to the nephrotic syndrome or acute renal failure.

### LABORATORY FINDINGS

Proteinuria is usually present.

Microscopic hematuria

Renal insufficiency—increased BUN and creatinine; decreased urine specific gravity

Decreased serum complement during the acute phase

## RAPIDLY PROGRESSIVE GLOMERULONEPHRITIS

In rapidly progressive glomerulonephritis (RPGN), the glomerular injury is accompanied by a rapid and progressive decline in renal function, frequently with oliguria or anuria, usually resulting in irreversible renal failure within weeks or months. Hematuria is a common finding, but proteinuria is variable, and hypertension and edema may or may not be present.

The disease is histologically characterized by widespread proliferation of cells in Bowman's space of the glomerulus with conspicuous "crescent" formation (Fig. 5-1). Whatever the pathogenesis of glomerular crescents, their formation correlates well with the severity of renal insufficiency. When present in large numbers, they are a poor prognostic sign.

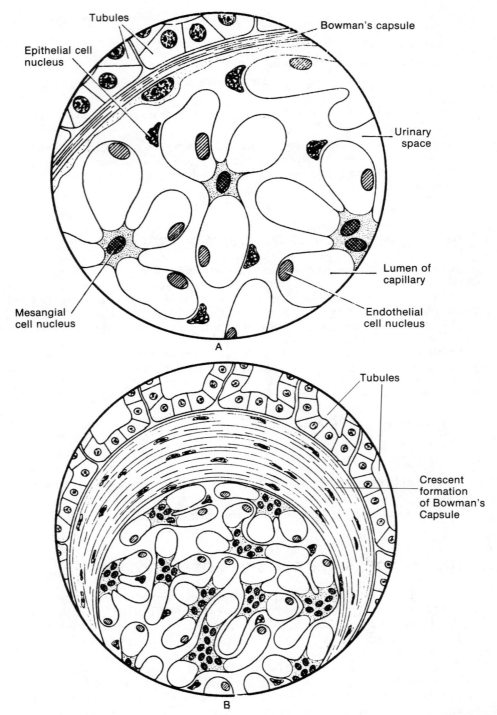

Tubules

Epithelial cell
nucleus

Bowman's capsule

Urinary
space

Lumen of
capillary

Mesangial
cell nucleus

Endothelial
cell nucleus

A

Tubules

Crescent
formation
of Bowman's
Capsule

B

**Fig. 5-1.** (*A*) Normal glomerulus showing thin Bowman's capsule. (*B*) Diffuse proliferative glomerular nephritis with crescent formation at the site of Bowman's capsule. (de-
Wardener HE: The Kidney, 4th ed, p 267. Edinburgh, Churchill Livingstone, 1973)

This syndrome may occur in any of the following glomerular diseases:

Poststreptococcal glomerulonephritis
Goodpasture's syndrome
Wegener's granulomatosis
Lupus erythematosus
Periarteritis nodosa
Henoch-Schönlein purpura
Idiopathic RPGN

More than 50% of the patients with RPGN have none of these antecedent or underlying disorders. These cases probably represent a heterogeneous group with different causes. They have in common rapid progression, poor prognosis, and extensive glomerular crescent formation.

Goodpasture's syndrome is characterized by rapidly developing renal insufficiency and recurrent lung hemorrhages. Although rare, the condition is of great interest because the pathogenetic mechanism of glomerular damage has been documented to be the result of antiglomerular basement membrane antibodies. These antibodies may be demonstrated in the glomeruli, in the circulation, and along the pulmonary alveolar basement membranes by immunofluorescence and elution studies. It is thus assumed that the pulmonary and renal lesions are due to the deposit of circulating antibodies that are directed against antigens common to both the pulmonary and glomerular basement membranes. It is not known which factors stimulate the formation of the autoantibodies to the basement membranes.

## LABORATORY FINDINGS

Marked increase in serum BUN and creatinine

Urine—gross and microscopic hematuria, WBC, casts of all types

Proteinuria, usually >3 g/day

Decreased urine specific gravity

Decreased urine volume—often <400 ml/day

Normocytic anemia, may be severe

Renal biopsy shows characteristic glomerular crescents.

## *NEPHROTIC SYNDROME*

The nephrotic syndrome is not a single disease entity but rather a group of findings characterized by marked proteinuria, decreased plasma protein, generalized edema, and a rise in serum lipids.

Many renal and systemic diseases might be associated with the nephrotic syndrome:

Glomerulonephritis (*e.g.,* membranous, membranoproliferative)
Lipoid nephrosis
Systemic diseases (*e.g.,* diabetes, amyloidosis, lupus erythematosus)
Circulatory disturbances (*e.g.,* renal vein thrombosis)

Toxins
Infections
Malignancy

The most common primary renal disease causing adult nephrotic syndrome is membranous nephritis.[9]

The characteristic features of the syndrome follow.

### Proteinuria

Although glomerular protein leakage is the principal source of urinary protein, failure of tubular protein reabsorption may contribute to the proteinuria. Glomerular injury results in proteinuria through some combination of effects on both the size of the basement membrane pores and the charge on the glomerular capillary wall. The largest proportion of protein lost in the urine consists of albumin, but about one third of the urinary protein is IgG.

### Hypoalbuminemia

Decreased serum albumin and IgG primarily reflect the result of renal protein loss. Another mechanism for hypoalbuminemia is the renal breakdown of albumin, probably through tubular reabsorption and degradation of large quantities of filtered protein.

### Edema

Hypoproteinemia results in the loss of colloid oncotic pressure of the blood, which causes fluids to leak from blood vessels into the interstitial space. This reduces plasma volume and cardiac output. The kidney responds to the stimulus of arterial hypovolemia by releasing renin, which stimulates aldosterone production by the adrenal cortex. Aldosterone enhances retention of sodium and water. In the presence of low oncotic pressure, the retained salt and water leak into the interstitial space, producing edema (Fig. 5-2). In this situation, the normal blood volume protecting mechanisms are frustrated because most of the retained sodium and water do not remain in the plasma, but escape into the interstitial tissues.

### Hyperlipidemia and Lipiduria

Increased plasma lipids appear to be due to increased lipid synthesis and also to decreased lipid degradation. In the nephrotic syndrome, lipiduria presumably results from increased glomerular permeability. Proximal tubular cells reabsorb a fraction of the filtered lipoprotein and slough into the urine as oval fat bodies.

### LABORATORY FINDINGS

Increased urine proteins, especially albumin (>3.5 g/24 hr; may be >20 g/24 hr)

Decreased serum albumin (usually <2.5 g/dl)

Increased serum cholesterol (>350 mg/dl), triglycerides, lipoproteins; decreased or normal serum cholesterol occurs with poor nutrition and suggests a poor prognosis

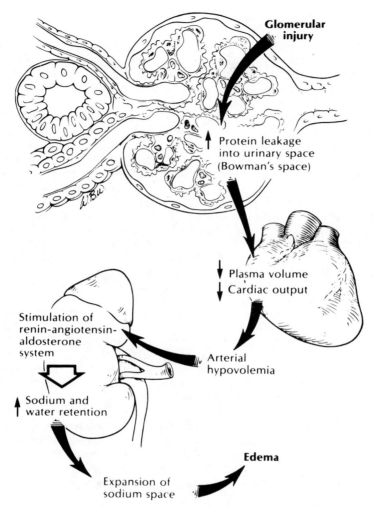

**Fig. 5-2.** Nephrotic syndrome and edema formation. (Knox FG: Textbook of Renal Pathophysiology, p 210. Hagerstown, Harper & Row, 1978)

Increased serum $\alpha_2$- and $\beta$-globulins, marked; decreased $\gamma$-globulin, especially IgG

Urine—free fat droplets, fatty casts, and oval fat bodies; when examined by polarized light, the lipids in casts are seen as being doubly refractile or birefringent and they display a symmetric "Maltese-cross" pattern. Oval fat bodies are lipid-containing renal tubular epithelial cells.

Increased sedimentation rate due to increased fibrinogen

Decreased serum calcium reflects fall in serum albumin; ionized calcium is usually normal.

## *DIABETIC NEPHROPATHY*

About one third of all diabetic patients have some form of renal involvement. In juvenile-onset diabetes, glomerulosclerosis is more prevalent; in adult-onset diabetes, atherosclerotic vascular disease and hypertensive renal changes are predominant. Approximately 50% of juvenile diabetics and 6% of adult-onset diabetic patients become uremic.

In glomerulosclerosis, the glomeruli are primarily affected and they show diffuse or nodular zones of dense sclerosis. Renal vessels of all sizes show varying degrees of sclerosis and narrowing of their lumina. The interstitial renal tissues frequently show scarring and chronic inflammatory cells, which become more prominent as the arterial and arteriolar narrowing worsens. These cellular changes do not imply infection.

The pathogenesis of diabetic glomerulosclerosis is poorly understood. The mechanism is related to the pathogenesis of systemic diabetic microangiopathy, which affects small vessels throughout the body, including the retina, skin, and muscles. Glomerulosclerosis develops in relation to the *duration* of diabetes rather than to its severity. The renal lesion usually occurs after 15 years to 20 years of insulin dependence. Involvement of larger vessels is often due to accelerated arteriosclerosis. The small vessel and glomerular lesions might be secondary to metabolic changes induced by insulin deficiency and hyperglycemia.

Proteinuria is an early manifestation of diabetic glomerulosclerosis, preceding other renal symptoms by many years. It correlates with the degree of glomerular involvement. Proteinuria is seen more frequently in juvenile-onset than in adult-onset diabetics. As the glomerular lesions worsen, proteinuria increases to nephrotic levels. This increase is followed by hypertension and, occasionally, by hematuria. Once proteinuria reaches nephrotic levels and hypertension occurs, there is usually progression to renal failure and death within 5 years to 7 years.

Patients with uncontrolled diabetes and glycosuria are predisposed to urinary infections and have an increased incidence of pyelonephritis. A fulminant form of pyelonephritis causes necrosis of the renal papillae. This is called *necrotizing papillitis* or *papillary necrosis*. Bits of necrotic renal tissue are sloughed and passed in the urine. These patients die of renal failure.

### LABORATORY FINDINGS

Laboratory findings of diabetes mellitus (see Chap. 6)

**Diabetic Glomerulosclerosis**

Proteinuria—often >5 g/24 hr

Hyaline and granular casts and oval fat bodies in urine

Decreased serum protein

Azotemia, late

**Papillary Necrosis**

Sudden decrease in renal function

Hematuria

Renal tissue fragments in the urine

**Urinary-Tract Infection**

Increased urine WBC

Positive urine cultures

## SICKLE CELL NEPHROPATHY

The principal manifestation of renal disease in patients with sickle cell trait or sickle cell anemia is recurrent hematuria. This is thought to be due to impaired renal medullary blood flow, with bleeding as a consequence of intravascular sickling.

Impaired renal concentrating ability is a consistent finding in sickle cell nephropathy. This occurs as a consequence of extensive tubular damage in the region of the medullary papillae, where capillaries have been blocked by sickled red blood cells. Impaired concentrating ability occurs despite normal, or even increased, glomerular filtration rate and renal plasma flow.

Increased tendencies toward pyelonephritis and papillary necrosis also occur in patients with sickle-cell disease.

### LABORATORY FINDINGS

Laboratory findings of sickle-cell disease (see Chap. 8)

Hematuria, gross and microscopic

Decreased renal concentrating ability

Proteinuria (in approximately 30% of patients)

## MYELOMA NEPHROPATHY

Multiple myeloma is a malignant disease of plasma cells of the bone marrow; it produces increased amounts of a single immunoglobulin, which is termed a *monoclonal protein.* When light chains of these immunoglobulins appear in the urine they are known as *Bence Jones proteins.* Bence Jones proteinuria indicates that the tumor cells are synthesizing light chains faster than they are synthesizing heavy chains and that they cannot form the complete immunoglobulin molecule. The excess of free light chains is readily filtered through the glomerulus because they are of low molecular weight. Bence Jones proteinuria occurs in 35% to 50% of patients with myeloma.

Renal involvement occurs in approximately 50% of patients with multiple myeloma and may take a variety of forms. Myeloma predominantly affects the tubules, because the light chains frequently precipitate in, and obstruct, renal tubules. The protein casts stimulate a foreign-body type of reaction, cause tubular atrophy, and sometimes cause tubular calcification. These findings are often called · *myeloma kidney.* The glomerular changes in myeloma consist of basement-membrane thickening. Chronic renal inflammation also occurs. All of these changes account for impairment of renal function. Death from uremia is a common occurrence in patients with multiple myeloma.

Fanconi's syndrome, manifested as proximal renal tubular acidosis, is probably due to the direct nephrotoxic effect of Bence Jones protein on the renal tubular epithelium. Nephrotic syndrome is commonly encountered in myeloma and probably results from both urinary protein losses and decreased albumin synthesis by the liver. Amyloidosis, which occurs in 5% to 15% of myeloma patients, is manifested by extensive amyloid deposits in the glomeruli (see Chap. 10). These glomerular deposits produce progressive renal impairment or the nephrotic syndrome.

### LABORATORY FINDINGS

Laboratory findings of multiple myeloma (see Chap. 8)

Proteinuria—albumin, globulins, and Bence Jones proteins

Azotemia and loss of urine concentrating ability

Increased serum calcium, seen in one third of patients, often accompanied by polyuria, and associated with rapidly progressive renal failure

Anemia, which is greater than expected for the degree of azotemia

Occasional proximal renal tubular acidosis—glycosuria, decreased serum uric acid, increased urine potassium, phosphaturia, decreased serum phosphorus, oliguria, aminoaciduria

## *LUPUS NEPHRITIS*

In systemic lupus erythematosus (SLE), the kidneys are involved in varying degrees in up to 90% of patients. Renal disease usually manifests itself within two years after the diagnosis of SLE is established. Occasionally, evidence of renal disease does not appear for many years. Virtually all clinical syndromes of glomerulonephritis may occur in SLE: acute nephritis, rapidly progressive nephritis, nephrotic syndrome, and chronic renal failure. In general, the severity of the clinical features correlates with the severity of the renal pathologic features.

The pathogenesis of glomerular damage has been well documented as a type of immune-complex nephritis, the lesion being induced by deposit of DNA–anti-DNA immune complexes in the glomeruli. Immunoglobulin, complement, and DNA may all be demonstrated in the glomeruli by immunofluorescent techniques. Furthermore, antinuclear antibody may be extracted from renal tissues. The immune-complex deposits involve different areas of the glomeruli and produce different clinical pictures.

### LABORATORY FINDINGS

Laboratory findings of lupus erythematosus (see Chap. 9)

Antinuclear antibody in nearly 100% of cases with active SLE

Anti-DNA antibody, usually present in active SLE and active renal disease

Serum complement, usually depressed in active lupus nephritis

LE test—positive in most cases

There are four pathologic subgroups of lupus nephritis, each of which has particular clinical and laboratory features. The pathologic characteristics are seen in a renal biopsy by light, immunofluorescence, and electron microscopy.

*Mesangial lupus nephritis*
Mildest glomerular involvement
Urine sediment—normal or slightly abnormal, slight hematuria
Proteinuria <1 g/day
No azotemia

*Focal proliferative glomerulonephritis*
Fewer than 50% of glomeruli involved
Proteinuria 1 g/day to 3 g/day
Recurrent hematuria

*Membranous glomerulonephritis*
Proteinuria in all patients—nephrotic syndrome in half of patients
Hematuria
Pyuria

*Diffuse proliferative glomerulonephritis*
Proteinuria >3.5 g/day in all patients
Urine—renal epithelial cells, hematuria, WBC, casts of all types

## POLYARTERITIS RENAL DISEASE

Polyarteritis nodosa is a systemic autoimmune disorder characterized by inflammation and necrosis of medium-sized arteries. Immune complexes of the hepatitis B antigen have been demonstrated in the circulation and in involved vessels of some of these patients. Whether or not other viruses play a role in the production of polyarteritis remains to be established. In 75% of patients with this disease, renal arterioles and glomerular capillaries are affected. When the kidney is involved, renal failure is often rapidly progressive. Other manifestations of renal involvement in polyarteritis are the nephrotic syndrome and hypertension.

### LABORATORY FINDINGS

Laboratory findings of polyarteritis nodosa (see Chap. 1)

Proteinuria—always present

Hematuria, gross or microscopic, very common

Urine sediment—WBC casts and oval fat bodies

Leukocytosis and increased sedimentation rate reflect systemic inflammation.

## SCLERODERMA RENAL DISEASE

Scleroderma is a steadily progressive disorder that involves the skin, heart, lungs, and kidneys. Clinical renal involvement occurs in up to 45% of patients; autopsy findings report that 50% to 90% have renal involvement. The renal lesions primarily involve the interlobular arteries, which show necrosis and intimal edema. The necrotizing vascular lesions extend into the glomeruli and produce microthrombi in the glomerular capillaries. Numerous microinfarcts occur in the renal cortex. Marked narrowing of arterial lumina leads to decreased renal blood flow. Many of the vascular changes precede the development of hypertension, which occurs in 25% to 35% of patients with scleroderma renal disease.

## LABORATORY FINDINGS

Laboratory findings of scleroderma (see Chap. 9)

Proteinuria (about one third of patients)—may be minimal and is usually <2 g/day

Azotemia (about one fifth of patients) indicates advanced renal disease

Oliguria and renal failure are a terminal occurrence.

## TOXEMIA OF PREGNANCY

Toxemia usually appears after 32 weeks' gestation, particularly in the presence of preexisting renal disease or hypertension. This disorder is characterized by edema and hypertension, followed by proteinuria. Postpartum acute renal failure may be accompanied by uremia, hypertension, and often microangiopathic hemolytic anemia.

One hypothesis for the development of toxemia is as follows: Diminished uteroplacental blood flow leads to altered prostaglandin E (PGE) and renin synthesis, causing release of renin from the uterus and, possibly, diminished PGE secretion. There is also increased sensitivity to angiotensin and norepinephrine. These factors all increase peripheral vascular resistance, resulting in hypertension.

The pathologic renal lesion consists of swelling of the glomerular endothelial cells and the deposit of fibrinlike material within and under the endothelial cells. Fibrin deposits in the glomeruli cause a reduction in the GFR. The absence of immunologic damage to the glomerulus suggests that the fibrin deposits are due either to direct endothelial cell injury or to intravascular coagulation. Disseminated intravascular coagulation (DIC) in toxemia is probably a result of the release of trophoblastic material from the placenta. The severity of the glomerular pathologic changes correlates with the degree of proteinuria. The renal lesion may resolve as early as 4 weeks after delivery, but occasionally it persists for as long as 2 years.

## LABORATORY FINDINGS

**Urine**

Proteinuria, variable degree—this is a characteristic finding

Increased urine specific gravity

Most patients have normal urine sediment, although a few will have microscopic hematuria and RBC casts

Oliguria in severe disease

### Serum

Increased serum uric acid (70% of patients) is the result of decreased tubular secretion and renal clearance of urates; the degree of increase correlates with the severity of the renal lesion.

Marked decrease in serum total protein and albumin is a common finding.

Decreased sodium excretion due to increased tubular reabsorption of sodium secondary to decreased effective circulating blood volume

Increased serum glutamic-oxaloacetic transaminase (SGOT) (AST [aspartate aminotransferase]), serum glutamic-pyruvic transaminase (SGPT) (ALT [alanine aminotransferase]) due to ischemic damage to liver cells; the degree of abnormality parallels the severity of the disease

Normal serum creatinine and BUN—there is reduced GFR in toxemia, which normalizes the increased GFR occurring in normal pregnancy

Increased hematocrit due to hemoconcentration, which is an index of the severity of disease

**Laboratory findings of disseminated intravascular coagulation (see Chap. 8)**

## ACUTE RENAL FAILURE

*Acute renal failure* refers to a diverse group of clinical conditions that are associated with sudden impairment of renal function, occurring within minutes, hours, or a few days. This impairment is characterized by increased urea and creatinine in the blood and, usually, by oliguria. The latter is defined as urine output of less than 400 ml/24 hr. Acute renal failure is classified as prerenal, intrarenal, or postrenal.

### PRERENAL ACUTE RENAL FAILURE

Prerenal acute renal failure results from diminished blood flow to the kidneys. It is the consequence of heart failure or a decrease in extracellular or vascular volume. These could occur following sodium depletion, dehydration, shock, or blood loss. If the pressure in the afferent glomerular artery falls below 60 mm Hg to 70 mm Hg then glomerular filtration drops significantly and only minimal urine is formed. The earliest physiologic response is water and sodium-chloride retention. This retention is reflected as decreased urine volume with low urine sodium concentration and high urine osmolality. These characteristic findings help to differentiate prerenal from intrarenal failure (Table 5-1). Prerenal failure is also characterized by a disproportionate elevation of BUN as compared with the level of serum creatinine. As filtration and flow through the tubules are diminished, the smaller urea molecules diffuse back into the bloodstream more readily than do the larger creatinine molecules. The BUN–creatinine ratio increases to greater than 20 : 1 (normal = 10–20 : 1). Urea and creatinine continue to be excreted; these contribute to the high urine osmolality in the presence of water reabsorption (Table 5-1). If impaired renal circulation is severe or prolonged, damage to the kidney will result, producing intrarenal renal failure superimposed upon prerenal renal failure.

**TABLE 5-1.** Urinary Indices in Oliguric Renal Failure

| LABORATORY MEASUREMENTS | PRERENAL | INTRARENAL |
|---|---|---|
| Urine osmolality, mOsm/Kg $H_2O$ | >500 | <350 |
| Urine sodium, mEq/liter | <20 | >40 |
| Urine/plasma (U/P) urea N | >8 | <3 |
| U/P creatinine | >40 | <20 |
| Renal failure index (urinary Na divided by U/P creatinine ratio) | <1 | >1 |
| Fractional excretion of filtered sodium $FE_{Na}$ (U/P sodium ratio divided by U/P creatinine ratio × 100) | <1 | >1 |

(Miller TR, Anderson RJ, Linas SL et al: Urinary diagnostic indices in acute renal failure. Ann Intern Med 89:47–50, 1978)

## INTRARENAL ACUTE RENAL FAILURE

Intrarenal acute renal failure may be caused by acute tubular necrosis, acute interstitial nephritis, acute glomerulonephritis, severe vasculitis, or hemolytic-uremic syndrome. The pathogenesis of acute renal failure is varied and depends on its cause.[6] The following mechanisms have been implicated: tubular obstruction, tubular fluid reflux, diminished glomerular blood flow, and decreased glomerular function. Glomerular damage and possible renal failure occur with acute glomerulonephritis and vasculitis on the basis of inflammatory and immunologic glomerular injury. Acute renal failure often follows acute tubular necrosis (ATN), which may result from severe underperfusion due to shock or sepsis or from renal poisons (Fig. 5-3). Ischemic injury occurs if the renal blood supply is blocked for more than 40 minutes. Renal poisons include metals, antibiotics, organic compounds, and various medications. Their effects are accentuated when they are administered under conditions of dehydration and reduced renal blood flow. The two mechanisms of renal tubular damage produce different tubular lesions: Nephrotoxins produce extensive necrosis of the renal tubular epithelium without damage to the tubular basement membranes; in contrast, ischemic injury to the kidney causes patchy necrosis of the renal tubular epithelium and, in addition, causes disruption of the tubular basement membranes (Fig. 5-3). Tubular contents leak into the capillaries that surround the tubules.

On the basis of clinical and experimental evidence, hypoperfusion appears to produce renal failure by four mechanisms.[1] It reduces renal blood flow directly, and, by increasing renal vascular resistance, causes a further decrease in renal blood flow. It also decreases glomerular permeability and produces tubular injury. All four factors together reduce the GFR and urine volume. Nephrotoxins produce renal failure by tubular injury and perhaps by reducing glomerular permeability.[1]

When acute tubular necrosis occurs, the kidneys can no longer retain sodium, but they do retain increased amounts of urea and creatinine. Plasma urea nitrogen and creatinine are increased. Urinary sodium is increased, whereas urine urea, creatinine, and osmolality are decreased. These findings are of value in differentiating prerenal from intrarenal acute renal failure (Table 5-1).

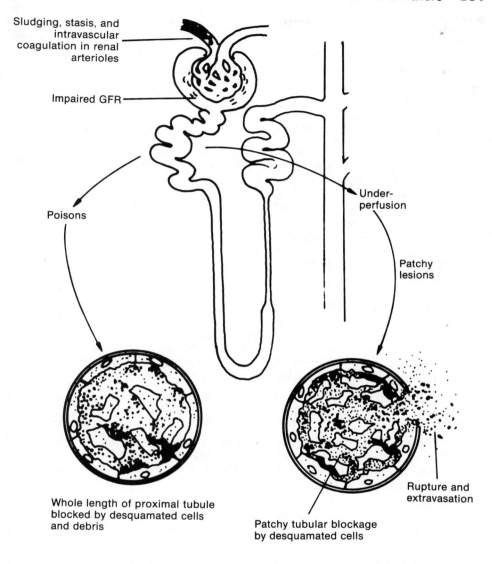

Sludging, stasis, and intravascular coagulation in renal arterioles

Impaired GFR

Poisons

Under-perfusion

Patchy lesions

Whole length of proximal tubule blocked by desquamated cells and debris

Patchy tubular blockage by desquamated cells

Rupture and extravasation

Poisons                                    Underperfusion

**Fig. 5-3.** Acute renal failure. The tubules are encircled by basement membranes, which rupture in underperfusion (ischemic) tubular necrosis. (Blandy J: Lecture Notes on Urology, p 121. Oxford, Blackwell Scientific Publications, 1976)

Recovery from acute tubular necrosis depends on the type of injury sustained. With nephrotoxic injury due to poison, regeneration of tubular epithelial cells takes place over the intact basement membrane, and normal renal function is restored. With disruption of the tubular basement membrane, which occurs following ischemia, some fibrosis and distortion of the renal tubule occur during recovery, resulting in a permanent reduction in renal function. Most patients who survive ATN, regardless of the mechanism, usually recover all or most of their renal function. Failure to recover completely is usually a consequence of superimposed urinary-tract infection. Maximal recovery may take as long as a year. Urinary concentrating ability rarely, if ever, is completely recovered.

### POSTRENAL ACUTE RENAL FAILURE

Postrenal acute renal failure may be caused by obstruction of the urinary collecting system anywhere from the renal pelvis to the urethral orifice. Blockage of urinary flow may be due to an enlarged prostate, calculi, or ureteral compression by a pelvic or retroperitoneal tumor. Obstruction of urine flow, although an uncommon cause of acute renal failure, is a relatively frequent cause of azotemia. Obstructive renal failure above the bladder must be due to bilateral obstruction; a single, normally functioning kidney shows no impairment of renal function. However, if one kidney has lost its function, stones obstructing the other ureter may cause postrenal acute renal failure.

Prostatic hyperplasia, which interferes with complete emptying of the bladder, is the major cause of urinary obstruction in the elderly man (Fig. 5-6). Increased pressure within the ureters, renal pelvis, and calyces may diminish renal function. Obstructive uropathy is best diagnosed by bladder catheterization and renal x-ray examination. Examination of the urine is not diagnostic. Renal-function studies become altered when obstruction persists and secondary damage to the kidneys occurs. The impaired-function studies then resemble those occurring in intrarenal renal failure.

### LABORATORY FINDINGS

Table 5-1 shows the urinary indices that are commonly found in oliguric renal failure of prerenal and intrarenal origin.[8] Findings of postrenal obstructive renal failure resemble those of intrarenal failure; administration of diuretics or mannitol may result in indices resembling acute tubular necrosis.

Urine volume—<400 ml/day for an average of 10 days, followed by a diuretic or recovery phase in which excretion is usually more than 1000 ml/day. In about 50% of cases of acute renal failure, urine volume is above 600 ml/day. This is termed *nonoliguric* or *high-output* renal failure.

Very rarely, complete anuria occurs; this usually indicates urinary-tract obstruction or bilateral renal cortical necrosis.

Urine—RBC, WBC, protein, and casts; renal tubular casts in ATN and red-cell casts in acute glomerulonephritis

Decreased creatinine clearance is the earliest predictor of postoperative renal failure.[4]

Increased serum creatinine, urea nitrogen, magnesium, phosphorus, uric acid, amylase, lipase

Potassium—in the oliguric phase, serum concentration increases and urine concentration decreases; in the diuretic phase, increased urinary potassium excretion may result in decreased serum potassium.

Decreased serum $CO_2$ content, $p$H (metabolic acidosis), sodium, calcium
Normocytic anemia appears during the second week.

## CHRONIC RENAL FAILURE

Chronic renal failure is the end stage of any severe renal disease (*e.g.*, glomerulonephritis, polycystic disease, pyelonephritis, hereditary nephritis, nephrosclerosis, and amyloidosis). All of the following functions of the kidneys are affected: acid–base and fluid balance, excretion of wastes, maintenance of blood pressure, and production of erythropoietin.

### AZOTEMIA

*Azotemia* refers to the accumulation of nitrogenous waste products in the blood. The BUN concentration in azotemia chiefly reflects the GFR. Although the normal person reabsorbs 50% to 60% of filtered urea, tubular reabsorption of urea diminishes in advanced renal failure. Impaired GFR, rather than tubular absorption, thus accounts for the azotemia of chronic renal failure. Another determinant of urea formation and plasma level is the dietary protein intake. Serum creatinine more accurately reflects the GFR than does the BUN, because it is largely unaffected by exogenous factors such as protein intake. Calculation of creatinine clearance is generally considered the best measurement of functioning nephrons.

Uremia is the clinical symptom complex that occurs in advanced chronic renal failure. Some of the symptoms include weakness, fatigue, confusion, tremors, loss of appetite, nausea, vomiting, bleeding, malnutrition, itching, hypertension, and heart failure.

### ACIDOSIS

Loss of functioning nephrons at first produces no apparent disturbance of acid–base regulation, because the remaining nephrons increase their rates of acid excretion. Bicarbonate reabsorption and distal tubular acid secretion are usually well preserved in renal disease. The primary reason for impaired acid excretion is decreased availability of ammonia and urinary phosphate buffers. The first detectable abnormality of acid excretion is a decline in the rate of urinary ammonium excretion. As renal disease progresses, acid excretion depends almost entirely on excretion of titratable acid, which is the excretion of hydrogen ion along with phosphate buffers. This function remains intact until the GFR falls to 15% to 20% of normal. Below this level, renal acid excretion becomes progressively inadequate, leading to severe chronic metabolic acidosis. Over a long period of time, acidosis contributes to the demineralization of bones.

### SODIUM WASTING AND WATER EXCRETION

Patients with chronic renal failure can neither conserve nor excrete sodium and water normally. The obligatory loss of sodium in chronic renal failure is usually small in relation to dietary intake and is therefore not a clinical problem. Impaired ability to excrete enough sodium is a far more common problem, and one that is aggravated by the high salt content of the usual diet. Patients with advanced chronic renal failure also lose their normal ability to conserve sodium, even under conditions of rigid sodium restriction. This occurs as a consequence of impaired tubular reabsorption of sodium and of the effect of osmotic diuresis, which causes large amounts of sodium to be excreted in the urine.

Patients in chronic renal failure gradually lose the ability to reabsorb water and concentrate their urine. They excrete dilute urine, which approaches the osmolarity of serum. Concentrating ability is severely limited by the time the BUN rises above 50 mg/dl. Impaired water reabsorption results from osmotic diuresis, damaged renal collecting tubules, and impaired medullary reabsorptive mechanisms. Impairment of the ability to dilute urine occurs later, as renal disease progresses.

## CALCIUM AND PHOSPHORUS METABOLISM

As the GFR falls to a creatinine clearance level below 25 ml/min, the serum phosphorus rises for the same reasons that BUN increases. As serum phosphorus rises, serum calcium falls to maintain a stable calcium–phosphorus product. Hypocalcemia occurs also secondary to vitamin-D resistance, which is in part based on failure of the kidney to convert vitamin $D_3$ from its inactive form, $25\text{-}(OH)D_3$, to its active form, $1,25\text{-}(OH)_2D_3$. Hypocalcemia stimulates parathyroid hormone (PTH) secretion. Parathyroid stimulation in chronic renal disease is known as *secondary hyperparathyroidism* (see Chap. 6). PTH partially restores serum ionized calcium and phosphorus levels by causing increased intestinal calcium absorption and bone calcium mobilization and diminished renal tubular phosphate reabsorption. This increases urinary phosphorus and lowers serum phosphorus. However, as GFR decreases further, increasing levels of circulating PTH are required to maintain normal serum calcium and phosphorus levels. Overt hypocalcemia and hyperphosphatemia eventually result when GFR is markedly diminished, and additional secretion of PTH can no longer maintain normal phosphate excretion.

Skeletal demineralization accompanies all cases of renal failure as a consequence of several factors: increased PTH activity, decreased intestinal absorption of calcium, chronic acidosis, and vitamin-D resistance. The bone changes are secondary to renal failure and are termed *renal osteodystrophy*.

## ANEMIA

Normocytic, normochromic anemia is characteristic of azotemia. There is a general depression of erythropoiesis; this is seen as bone-marrow hypoplasia and decreased reticulocyte formation. Impaired renal formation of the RBC-stimulating hormone erythropoietin is considered to be the major cause of anemia in chronic renal failure. There is also diminished marrow responsiveness to the erythropoietin that is formed. Furthermore, there is increased destruction of circulating RBC in patients with uremia. These red cells are abnormal, presumably owing to some factors in uremic plasma. Hemolysis is a less significant factor in contributing to anemia than is decreased RBC formation.

## BLEEDING TENDENCY

Thrombocytopenia occurs in 5% of azotemic patients. Bleeding in chronic renal failure is usually due to defective platelet function, which appears as impaired platelet-factor-3 activation and failure of platelet aggregation in the presence of adenosine diphosphate (ADP).

## HYPERTENSION

Relative renal ischemia with activation of the renin–angiotensin system contributes to the development of hypertension in some patients. Patients in chronic renal failure are unable to adjust the sodium content of body fluids, leading to overexpansion of extracellular fluid volume and to an increase in blood pressure.

## IONIC DISTURBANCES

There may be elevated levels of magnesium owing to impaired renal excretion. Because of secretory efficiency, homeostasis for potassium and satisfactory plasma $K^+$ levels may usually be maintained until late stages of chronic renal failure. The urinary excretion of potassium in chronic renal failure tends to be fixed, and plasma levels reflect only dietary intake less that excreted.

## NEUROLOGIC DYSFUNCTION

Patients with long-standing chronic renal failure often develop dysfunctions of the nervous system, most often involving peripheral nerves. In patients with poor kidney function, drugs that depend on renal excretion for their removal from the body accumulate in body fluids and exert toxic effects on the nervous system.

## LABORATORY FINDINGS

Decreased creatinine clearance

Increased serum BUN, creatinine, phosphorus, magnesium (when GFR <30 ml/min), lipoproteins, and triglycerides (40%–50% of patients)

Decreased serum calcium (due to increased serum phosphorus, decreased calcium absorption, and decreased serum albumin), albumin, and total protein (due to proteinuria)

Increased serum PTH occurs in response to increased serum phosphorus and decreased serum calcium.

Decreased $pH$ and $CO_2$ content (metabolic acidosis) due to failure to excrete acid as $NH_4^+$ and to reabsorb bicarbonate

Decreased $PCO_2$ due to hyperventilation as compensation for metabolic acidosis

Normochromic, normocytic anemia (hematocrit 20%–30%), proportionate to the degree of azotemia

Decreased glucose tolerance due to impaired cellular utilization of glucose

Fixed urine volume (1 liter/day–4 liters/day)

Decreased urine osmolality (250 mOsm/Kg $H_2O$–400 mOsm/Kg $H_2O$); this becomes fixed close to normal plasma level of 280 mOsm/Kg $H_2O$–295 mOsm/Kg $H_2O$

Decreased urine specific gravity, <1.020; as renal impairment becomes more severe, specific gravity approaches 1.010

Increased urine sodium

Decreased urine calcium—occurs before hypocalcemia occurs

# RENAL TUBULAR ACIDOSIS

*Renal tubular acidosis* (RTA) is a term applied to disorders in which the kidneys are unable to excrete $H^+$ normally even though they function adequately in most other respects. This results in renal metabolic acidosis, characterized by a urinary $pH$ that is inappropriately high (alkaline) for the degree of systemic acidosis.

An understanding of renal function in maintaining a normal acid–base balance is essential to comprehending its malfunction, which ultimately results in RTA. Bicarbonate is freely filtered by the glomeruli and is almost totally reabsorbed into the bloodstream through the proximal renal tubules. As bicarbonate is reclaimed, about 97% of the hydrogen ions are excreted in exchange for reabsorbed sodium. In the distal renal tubules new bicarbonate is generated and absorbed into the bloodstream. The newly formed bicarbonate replenishes that which has been depleted as a result of buffering metabolic acids. These acids normally are formed through the oxidation of foods, especially meats. Also, at the site of the distal tubules, the kidneys excrete hydrogen ions along with phosphate buffers and ammonia. A small amount of free hydrogen ion is secreted; this determines the urine $pH$ and enhances the production of ammonia. In states of metabolic acidosis, $NH_3$ synthesis by the distal renal tubular cells increases greatly in order to excrete the excess of hydrogen ions.

RTA results from one of two renal tubular defects: impaired bicarbonate reabsorption by the proximal tubules (proximal RTA) or impaired acid secretion by the distal tubules (distal RTA).

## PROXIMAL RENAL TUBULAR ACIDOSIS

The proximal form of RTA is due to the inability of the proximal tubules to absorb even normal amounts of bicarbonate from the glomerular ultrafiltrate. Consequently, large quantities of bicarbonate are delivered into the distal tubules, overwhelming their reabsorptive capacity. This excess bicarbonate is excreted in the urine, and alkaline urine and hyperchloremic metabolic acidosis result. This is often referred to as *bicarbonate-wasting RTA*. When the plasma bicarbonate falls to very low levels, the distal tubules are able to reabsorb the small amount of bicarbonate that is filtered. The urine then becomes maximally acidified to $pH$ 4.7, indicating that the distal tubular hydrogen-ion secretory mechanism is intact. This feature helps distinguish proximal from distal RTA.

As sodium is lost in the alkaline urine, there is contraction of extracellular fluid volume, which enhances aldosterone secretion by the adrenal gland. This causes potassium excretion and depletion. Demineralization of the skeleton occurs as a consequence of phosphate loss, metabolic acidosis, and secondary hyperparathyroidism. The proximal form of RTA occurs in any of the following conditions:

Fanconi syndrome, a genetically transmitted, complex tubular disorder characterized by glycosuria, aminoaciduria, uricosuria, and phosphaturia
Multiple myeloma
Vitamin-D deficiency
A primary disorder of the proximal tubules
Previous damage of proximal tubules by drugs or heavy metals, as in Wilson's disease

### DISTAL RENAL TUBULAR ACIDOSIS

The distal, or classical, form of RTA is due to impaired secretion of $H^+$ by the distal renal tubules. Another possible mechanism is "back diffusion" of hydrogen ion from the tubular fluid.[11] Consequently, urine is not acidified and remains above $pH$ 6.0, even in the presence of severe systemic acidosis. Bicarbonate conservation and ammonia production are usually normal. The inability to secrete hydrogen ions at a rate equivalent to their rate of formation results in their retention and systemic metabolic acidosis. There is also potassium loss in the urine and mobilization of bone calcium with hypercalciuria. Potassium depletion causes muscle weakness, hyporeflexia, and paralysis. The continued loss of bone calcium results in rickets and osteomalacia. Renal calculi and calcification of renal tissue result from the increased excretion of calcium and phosphate in an alkaline urine. The distal form of RTA associated with normal (or low) plasma potassium occurs in any of the following conditions:[2]

A primary or idiopathic disorder
Secondary to increased serum $\gamma$-globulin, accompanying lupus erythematosus, Sjögren's syndrome, Hodgkin's disease, sarcoidosis
Secondary to altered calcium metabolism
Secondary to interstitial nephropathies caused by obstructive uropathy or sickle-cell disease
Secondary to drugs or toxins

Distal RTA is occasionally associated with increased plasma potassium in the following conditions: obstructive uropathy, sickle-cell disease, amyloidosis, and interstitial nephritis.[2]

## LABORATORY FINDINGS

### Proximal RTA

Decreased blood $pH$, serum bicarbonate (metabolic acidosis)

Alkaline urine in the presence of low serum bicarbonate

Acid urine in the presence of *very* low serum bicarbonate

Increased serum chloride—normal anion gap

Normal or decreased serum potassium, sodium

Increased urine sodium, potassium

Increased urine glucose, phosphorus, amino acids, and uric acid in Fanconi syndrome.

### Distal RTA

Decreased blood $pH$, serum bicarbonate (metabolic acidosis)

Alkaline urine ($pH > 6.0$), regardless of serum bicarbonate level and even with an acid load test (ammonium chloride 100 mg/kg orally)

Increased serum chloride—normal anion gap

Decreased serum potassium, calcium, phosphorus; some cases are associated with hyperkalemia

Increased urine sodium, potassium, calcium, phosphate; the last two account for an increased frequency of calculus formation


## *PYELONEPHRITIS*

*Pyelonephritis* indicates bacterial infection of the kidney that involves the renal pelvis, the renal tubules, and the interstitial tissues between the tubules. This is usually a complication of infection of the lower urinary tract and is most frequently due to *Escherichia coli*. Bacteria from the urethra and bladder usually reach the kidneys through the ureters. Less frequently, bacteria gain access to the kidneys through the bloodstream in the course of septicemia or endocarditis.

Ascending bacterial infection may be secondary to chronic prostatitis or to bladder catheterization. Bacteria introduced into the normal bladder are usually cleared within a few days. The clearance mechanisms are compromised when there is obstruction to urine flow or incomplete bladder emptying. In these situations, bacteria multiply and inflammation of the bladder develops. Inflammation may remain localized in the urinary bladder for years without ascending to the kidney. In some patients, however, bacteria eventually reach the renal pelvis as a result of an abnormal condition in which urine is forced into one or both ureters during urination. This is termed *vesicoureteral reflux*. In the most severe cases of reflux, urine and bacteria may reach the renal pelvis and medulla, where bacterial multiplication occurs. Reflux is frequently seen in children with urinary infections and in adults with bladder tumors, prostatic hyperplasia, or urinary stones.

The normal kidney is resistant to blood-borne infection. However, obstruction to urinary outflow at any site or impaired ureteral peristalsis increases the susceptibility of the kidney to infection. The main cause of this increased susceptibility appears to be increased tissue pressure in the kidney, possibly interfering with the renal microcirculation. In experimental *E. coli* pyelonephritis, the acute infection persists for 1 week to 2 weeks. After six weeks, the kidneys become sterile and the areas of acute inflammation are replaced by scars. *E. coli* antibodies eliminate the bacteria. There is no impairment of renal function.

In the acute phase of infection, urine characteristically contains many leukocytes. The presence of leukocytes in the urine does not differentiate renal infection from bladder infection. However, renal involvement and tubular inflammation are indicated by the presence of leukocyte casts. The WBC are arranged in the shapes of the renal tubules in which they have formed.

In the presence of obstruction, vesicoureteral reflux, or other predisposing conditions, repeated infections occur and the development of chronic pyelonephritis is likely. When chronic pyelonephritis is due to ascending infection, there is damage to the renal pelvis and calyces. The renal medulla is particularly vulnerable to infection because its biochemical environment inactivates leukocytes, antibodies, and complement. Chronic renal infection causes impairment of renal function but does not usually cause renal failure.

## LABORATORY FINDINGS

Quantitative culture of properly collected clean midstream urine:
>100,000 colonies/ml urine indicates infection
10,000 colonies/ml urine–100,000 colonies/ml urine probably indicates infection if only one organism is isolated or is predominant
<10,000 colonies/ml urine usually indicates contamination

It is important to note the following:
1. If a patient is asymptomatic, *two* positive cultures are needed to establish a diagnosis of infection.
2. If cultures are persistently negative in the presence of other evidence of pyelonephritis, three to five first morning urine specimens should be cultured for tubercle bacilli.

Presence of bacteria on Gram's stain of properly collected uncentrifuged urine

Pyuria is of greatest significance when it is associated with bacteriuria. When either urinary WBC or bacteria occur without the other, this is of less significance. WBC and bacteria are often intermittent and are usually absent in chronic pyelonephritis.

WBC casts are diagnostic of renal, rather than bladder, infection.

Proteinuria (>2 g/24 hr)

Decreased urine specific gravity—concentrating ability is impaired relatively early

Decreased creatinine clearance precedes increased BUN or serum creatinine.

Leukocytosis—in acute pyelonephritis

Markedly increased serum C-reactive protein indicates acute infection.

Normocytic anemia—in chronic pyelonephritis

Laboratory findings of associated diseases, such as diabetes mellitus, bladder infection

## *RENAL AND PERINEPHRIC ABSCESSES*

Renal abscesses occur owing to bloodstream infection, renal calculi, chronic ureteral obstruction, or chronic suppurative pyelonephritis (Fig. 5-4). In chil-

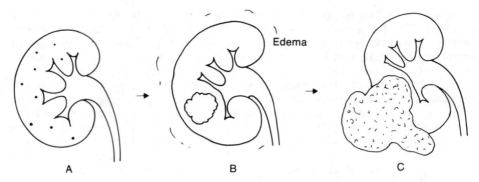

**Fig. 5-4.** Abscesses of the kidney. (*A*) Multiple embolic septicemic abscesses scattered throughout the renal cortex. (*B*) Renal abscess. (*C*) Perinephric abscess. (Blandy J: Lecture Notes on Urology, p 69. Oxford, Blackwell Scientific Publications, 1976)

dren, abscesses may be a complication of urine reflux from the bladder into the ureter. Gram-negative organisms may ascend into the renal collecting tubules. If the diagnosis is not made until late in the course of infection, an abscess could rupture into the pelvic calyceal system or into the perirenal space to form a perinephric abscess (Fig. 5-4C). Perinephric abscess is usually a complication of an advanced, chronic, nonspecific renal infection but may occur secondary to staphylococcal infection of the kidney. Perinephric abscesses become quite large.

### LABORATORY FINDINGS

Leukocytosis (often >30,000/$\mu$l)

Increased sedimentation rate reflects acute inflammation.

Urine—trace of protein, few RBC, many bacteria; culture usually yields *Staphylococcus,* if the infection is of bloodstream origin, or gram-negative organisms, if the infection is of renal origin.

If urinalysis is normal and sterile, acid-fast smear and culture should be done.

Normocytic anemia due to chronic infection

## *RENAL CALCULI*

Renal calculi or stones are collections of salts, deposited around a core of protein or mucoid material, derived from cellular debris or bacteria. Calculi occur when there is increased urinary excretion of salts associated with a change in the $p$H of urine. The $p$H change reduces the solubility of salts, which then precipitate. Most calculi are comprised of calcium oxalate alone or in conjunction with calcium phosphate and calcium carbonate.

Since at least 90% of all renal stones contain calcium as a major constituent, the factors that influence renal calcium excretion might affect calculus formation.

Most patients with calcium stones have no abnormality in either calcium excretion or blood calcium levels.

Three factors interact in the formation of calculi: liberation of mucoprotein from renal connective tissue or inflammatory exudate; increased urinary excretion of calcium and phosphorus; and a systemic factor in the form of dehydration, prolonged bedrest, obstruction of urine excretion, or hypercalcemia.

Factors other than urinary calcium concentration are important in stone formation. There may be factors in normal urine that inhibit crystal formation and growth. Absence or decrease in such factors, which might occur with urinary-tract infections or stasis, allows precipitation of calcium salts, even in the absence of hypercalciuria. Increased urinary oxalate due to increased dietary intake or to endogenous production may also increase stone formation.

Renal stones usually are formed in the renal pelvis. Their presence at that site enhances renal infection. Obstruction of the ureteral lumen results in dilatation of the renal pelvis and calyces. This is known as *hydronephrosis*. Stones may pass down the ureter and may also form in the bladder.

### LABORATORY FINDINGS

Hematuria commonly occurs.

Urinalysis is often normal, but might show pus cells, bacteria, and crystals.

Increased urine calcium (approximately 35% of patients)

Leukocytosis indicates associated infection.


## *RENAL INFARCTION*

A *renal infarct* refers to a well-demarcated, wedge-shaped zone of necrosis of the kidney. Initially the necrotic zone is surrounded by inflammatory cells, which later become replaced by granulation tissue and, ultimately, by a fibrous scar. Microscopically, the infarcted zone is composed of scarred glomeruli, collapsed or absent tubules, and interstitial scars, which show varying degrees of chronic inflammation. Infarcts are frequently multiple. An infarct is usually caused by obstruction of the renal artery or its branches. When the main renal artery is occluded, the entire kidney is affected and becomes functionless and atrophic as it undergoes necrosis and scarring. Arterial obstruction may be due to emboli, which originate from mitral- or aortic-valve infective endocarditis, to an ulcerated aortic atherosclerotic plaque that occludes the origin of the renal artery, or to thrombosis of the renal artery (in polyarteritis or scleroderma).

### LABORATORY FINDINGS

Hematuria, proteinuria, and leukocytosis commonly occur.

Increased SGOT (AST), lactate dehydrogenase (LDH), and C-reactive protein if the infarct is large; LDH isoenzymes show no specific tissue localization

Normal creatine phosphokinase (CPK)

## RENAL-VEIN THROMBOSIS

Thrombotic occlusion of renal veins may result from severe dehydration in infancy, in association with abdominal trauma, secondary to various malignancies, and from various renal diseases. Following venous thrombosis the kidney becomes swollen and engorged with blood. The kidney later undergoes atrophy. Many patients with renal-vein thrombosis develop the nephrotic syndrome. In such cases, renal biopsy shows membranous glomerulonephritis.

Recent evidence indicates that renal-vein thrombosis is a *result* of the hypercoagulability of blood occurring in the nephrotic syndrome, rather than a *cause* of the nephrotic syndrome.[9] Pulmonary embolism or infarction is a frequent complication of renal-vein thrombosis.

### LABORATORY FINDINGS

**Children**

Hematuria

Oliguria

Leukocytosis

Renal failure

**Adults**

Nephrotic syndrome

Increased serum creatinine and BUN

## POLYCYSTIC KIDNEY DISEASE

Polycystic kidney disease is hereditary and commonly affects both kidneys symmetrically. It occurs as a consequence of defects in the development of the collecting and convoluted tubules and in the mechanism of their joining together. Blind convoluted tubules, which are connected to functioning glomeruli, fill with urine and become cystic. As these cysts enlarge, they compress and destroy adjacent kidney tissue and occlude normal tubules. The result is progressive renal functional impairment. The kidneys are studded with variously sized cysts and are larger then normal, often filling much of the abdomen (Fig. 5-5).

This disease in infants is much rarer than in adults, is autosomal recessive, and usually leads to early death. The adult disorder, which is the most common hereditary renal disease, is autosomal dominant and is usually asymptomatic until middle adult life. In association with both forms there might be cysts of the liver, spleen, and pancreas. Cerebral-vessel aneurysms occur with increased frequency in association with polycystic kidney disease. Hypertension is found in about 50% of patients with polycystic renal disease.

Exacerbations of progressive chronic renal failure may be due to any of the following:

1. Salt and water loss leading to dehydration
2. Obstruction of the ureters by cysts or by clots from hemorrhage into cysts
3. Bacterial infection of the cysts
4. Cardiovascular complications such as congestive heart failure or hypertension

### LABORATORY FINDINGS

Increased urine volume commonly occurs.

Hematuria—there are episodes of gross hemorrhage or microscopic bleeding

Proteinuria is progressive.

Pyuria is common, even in the absence of bacteriuria.

Increased BUN and creatinine

Anemia is characteristic, reflecting blood loss or azotemia.

**Laboratory Findings of Complications**
  Pyelonephritis
  Renal calculi

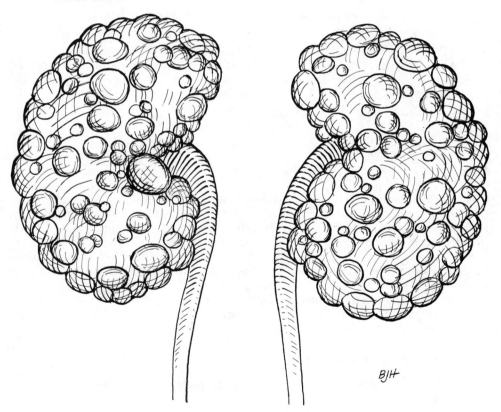

**Fig. 5-5.** Polycystic kidneys.

## *ADENOCARCINOMA OF THE KIDNEY*

Renal carcinoma constitutes 80% of the malignant tumors of the kidney. About one third of patients with renal-cell carcinoma have no complaints directly related to the tumor when it is first detected. About one third of the patients already have metastases when the diagnosis is first made.

Renal carcinoma causes many systemic effects that frequently mimic those of other diseases. The tumor may provoke release of renin from the kidney, resulting in hypertension; it may secrete PTH-like material, resulting in hypercalcemia; or it may form gonadotropins, stimulating the release of gonadal hormones. The tumor has a propensity to invade renal veins and lymphatics and to form tumor emboli. The most common site of metastasis is the lung, with the liver and bone being next in frequency.

### LABORATORY FINDINGS

Hematuria is common.

Anemia is due to impairment of erythropoietin formation by the kidney and to bone-marrow depression.

Increased RBC, hemoglobin, and hematocrit occasionally occur due to erythropoietin formation by the tumor.

Leukemoid reaction (up to 100,000/$\mu$l)

Abnormal liver function tests in the absence of hepatic metastases—increased alkaline phosphatase, prolonged prothrombin time; decreased albumin and increased $\alpha_2$-globulin.

Increased sedimentation rate (up to 150 mm/hr)

## *CYSTITIS*

Cystitis is inflammation of the urinary bladder. The flushing action of urine outflow normally maintains a state of sterility in the bladder. Retention of urine favors bacterial growth. Other factors that play a role in infection are the ability of bacteria to adhere to the bladder mucosa and host resistance. The latter includes development of circulating antibodies, antibacterial substances in the bladder wall and prostatic fluid, and bacterial colonization of the periurethral mucosa.

Prostatitis is the usual source of bladder infection in men. In women, fecal organisms gain access to the vulva and then to the urethra and bladder. *E. coli* and *Streptococcus fecalis* are the major pathogens.

### LABORATORY FINDINGS

Presence of bacteria on Gram's stain of properly collected and uncentrifuged urine

Increased neutrophils in the urine

Quantitative culture of properly collected clean midstream urine:

>100,000 colonies/ml urine indicates infection.

10,000 colonies/ml urine–100,000 colonies/ml urine probably indicates infection if only one organism is isolated or is predominant.

<10,000 colonies/ml urine usually indicates contamination.

It is important to note the following:

1. If a woman has symptoms suggesting bladder infection, the presence of coliform organisms >100 colonies/ml urine in the presence of pyuria is significant. This should not be considered to be contamination.[10]
2. If a patient is asymptomatic, *two* positive cultures are needed to establish diagnosis of infection.
3. If cultures are persistently negative in the presence of other evidence of cystitis, three to five first morning urine specimens should be cultured for tubercle bacilli.

## BENIGN PROSTATIC HYPERPLASIA

The prostate gland reaches its adult weight by the age of 20 years and remains so for 20 years to 30 years; then a second growth phase occurs. Hyperplasia begins in the periurethral region of the gland, causing progressive obstruction of the flow of urine. Incomplete bladder emptying contributes to the development of cystitis. There are also gradual dilatation of the bladder and thickening of the bladder wall. The obstructive mechanism is shown in Figure 5-6. Obstructive symptoms occur in 50% to 75% of men over the age of 50. In the later stages, prostatic enlargement increases back pressure in the kidneys, enhancing the establishment of pyelonephritis.

Prostatic enlargement is an almost universal aging feature in men; it occurs only in men with intact testes. Testosterone from the testes is metabolized in the prostate gland to dihydrotestosterone (DHT). It is postulated that increased amounts of prostatic DHT is causally related to the hyperplasia.

### LABORATORY FINDINGS

Urine—normal or showing changes of infection: proteinuria, pyuria, hematuria, bacteriuria

Increased serum creatinine occurs when urinary-tract obstruction impairs renal function; this is an example of postrenal acute renal failure.

## PROSTATITIS

Acute prostatic infection may be blood-borne or may occur as a result of the ascent of bacteria into the urethra. Most cases of prostatitis are nonbacterial and are of uncertain cause.[7] Some are due to *Chlamydia*, as a complication of non-gonococcal urethritis.[5] Prostatitis is usually complicated by acute cystitis and, often, by acute urinary retention. It may resolve, progress to abscess formation,

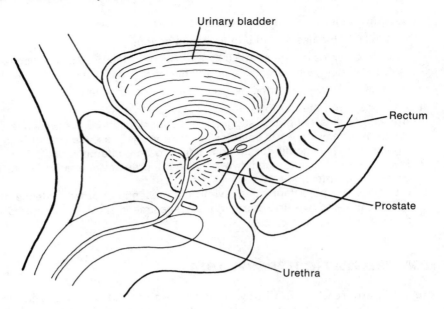

Normal prostate and pelvic organs

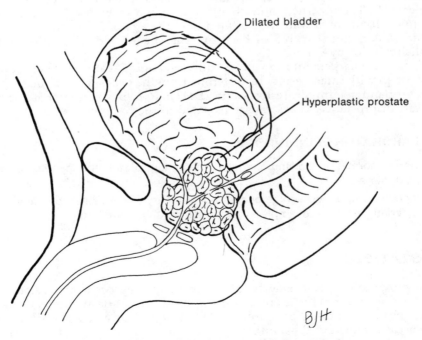

**Fig. 5-6.** Effects of benign prostatic hyperplasia.

or persist as chronic prostatitis. The latter is one of the most common causes of recurrent urinary-tract infection in men. A chronic quiescent prostatic infection may be activated following prostatic massage or bladder catheterization.

## LABORATORY FINDINGS

### Acute Prostatitis

Following prostatic massage, the *last* portion of voided urine shows increased numbers of WBC when compared to the first portion of voided urine.

The *last* portion of voided urine also shows a positive culture and higher colony count when compared to the first portion of voided urine, which is usually sterile.

Culture usually yields *E. coli.* Other less common organisms include *Proteus, Pseudomonas, Klebsiella,* and *Enterobacter.*

### Chronic Prostatitis

Prostatic fluid shows >10 WBC per high-power field
Cultures usually show only 500–1000 bacteria/ml.

## *CARCINOMA OF THE PROSTATE*

The cause of prostatic carcinoma is not known, but it is clear that its growth is increased by androgens and decreased by estrogens or castration.[12] It is usually associated with benign prostatic hyperplasia but does not develop from it. The initial lesion is usually a firm area on the posterolateral surface of the gland; this gradually spreads to involve the hyperplastic prostatic tissue. The seminal vesicles then become involved. Later, the tumor extends through the urethral mucosa or bladder wall. The cancer spreads through the lymphatics to the pelvic lymph nodes or through the veins to the bones of the pelvis, spine, and thighs. This tumor stimulates bone formation at sites of bony metastasis.

The adult prostate is the major site of elaboration of acid phosphatase. The enzyme concentration is 1000 times higher in the prostate than in other tissues. In advanced prostatic cancer, particularly that which has metastasized to bone, 75% of patients have markedly increased amounts of this enzyme in the blood.

## LABORATORY FINDINGS

Increased serum acid phosphatase indicates local extension or distant metastases of the tumor. Elevated levels show a marked fall within 3 days to 4 days after castration or within 2 weeks after estrogen therapy has begun. Normal levels may occur with prostatic cancer.

Increased serum alkaline phosphatase reflects new bone formation, which occurs with bone metastases. The enzyme increases when there is a favorable response to therapy, reaches a peak in 3 months, and then declines. Recurrence of bone metastases causes the enzyme to increase again.

Anemia, normocytic—due to infection, hemorrhage, or bone-marrow replacement by tumor

Increased bone-marrow acid phosphatase occurs earlier than does increased serum acid phosphatase.

## VAGINITIS

Specific causes of vaginal inflammation include *Trichomonas vaginalis, Gardnerella vaginalis,* and *Candida albicans.* (For other female genital infections see Chap. 11.) *T. vaginalis* is a sexually transmitted protozoan. Diabetes, antibiotic use, and pregnancy predispose a woman to vaginal infections with the fungus *C. albicans. G. vaginalis* is thought to be the cause of nonspecific vaginitis, but this is controversial. The occurrence of vaginitis during childhood and after the menopause is due to the fact that at these times the vaginal mucosa is thin and lacks normal resistance to infection.

### LABORATORY FINDINGS

Gram's stain and culture might show *G. vaginalis, Neisseria gonorrhoeae, C. albicans*

Wet mount or Gram's stain might show masses of gram-negative rods clustered about vaginal epithelial cells. These so-called clue cells are suggestive of *G. vaginalis* infection.

Saline suspension or Pap smear might show *T. vaginalis.*

## ECTOPIC PREGNANCY

An ectopic pregnancy is one that occurs outside the uterine cavity (Fig. 5-7). Its most frequent site is within the fallopian tube. This is usually due to partial tubal obstruction resulting from previous infection of the tube.

A fertilized egg may implant itself on the tubal mucosa. The implantation is followed by an erosive action of trophoblastic tissues, which are the embryonal portion of the placenta. These tissues penetrate into or through the tubal wall, and into the peritoneal cavity.

A tubal pregnancy may terminate in one of the following ways:

*Tubal rupture*—the tube becomes enlarged and distended with blood and trophoblastic tissues. It then erodes, and massive bleeding into the peritoneal cavity occurs.

*Tubal abortion*—the ovum may move out of the end of the tube and succumb with only minimal bleeding.

*Secondary abdominal pregnancy*—the tubal placental tissue may grow through the tubal wall, or out of the end of the tube, and become secondarily implanted on the peritoneal surface, the omentum, the mesentery, or other intraperitoneal organs. A full-term abdominal pregnancy may result.

*Cessation of ovum viability*

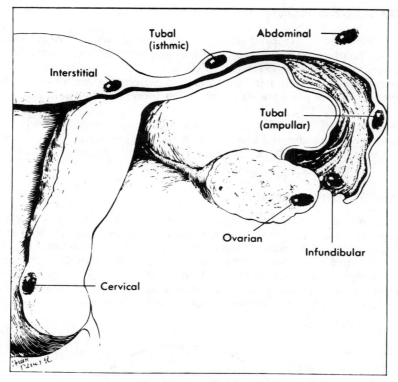

**Fig. 5-7.** Sites of ectopic pregnancies. (McLennan CE, Sandberg EC: Synopsis of Obstetrics, 9th ed, p 236. St Louis, CV Mosby, 1974)

## LABORATORY FINDINGS

Pregnancy tests—latex and hemagglutination-inhibition tests are positive in only 50% of these patients. Radioimmunoassay tests on serum are required to detect the very low levels of human chorionic gonadotropin (HCG) which occur in ectopic pregnancy.[3] Decreasing levels of HCG indicate loss of viability of an ectopic pregnancy.

### Ruptured Tubal Pregnancy

Leukocytosis, which usually returns to normal in 20 hours; 50% of patients have normal WBC, 75% have WBC $< 15,000/\mu$l

Anemia may or may not be present; progressive anemia indicates continued bleeding.

Increased serum amylase

Increased sedimentation rate

## *HYDATIDIFORM MOLE*

Hydatidiform mole is a trophoblastic disease of pregnancy in which embryonic portions of the placenta become edematous and overdistended with fluid. They form translucent grapelike vesicles, which fill the entire uterine cavity (Fig. 5-8).

The mole is considered to be either a degenerative process, a tumor, or a malformation of the placenta. It occurs with increased frequency in older patients.

There are other trophoblastic diseases. Chorioadenoma destruens is a mole that superficially invades the uterine wall. Choriocarcinoma is an invasive malignant tumor of trophoblastic elements that usually metastasizes widely.

### LABORATORY FINDINGS

Increased serum HCG—normally, from the 7th to the 10th week of the average pregnancy, there is a sharp rise in HCG; this occurs especially with multiple pregnancies and is similar to the amount seen with hydatidiform mole. After the 10th to 12th week of a normal pregnancy there is a fall in HCG. In the presence of hydatidiform mole, HCG continues to rise. After removal of the mole, the HCG levels should normally become negative within 60 days. If an elevated titer persists or continues to increase, then an invasive mole or choriocarcinoma probably exists.

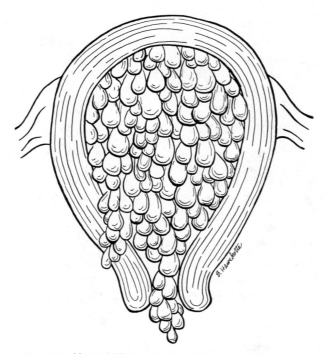

**Fig. 5-8.** Hydatidiform mole in bisected uterus.

Increased urine HCG, often markedly elevated, parallels serum levels. Quantitative titers are important for diagnosis and for following the course of the disease and response to treatment.

Laboratory findings of disseminated intravascular coagulation (see Chap. 8), which may occur with hydatidiform mole.

## REFERENCES

1. Arbeit LA, Weinstein SW: Acute tubular necrosis: Pathophysiology and management. Med Clin North Am 65:147–163, 1981
2. Batlle D, Kurtzman NA: Distal renal tubular acidosis: Pathogenesis and classification. Am J Kid Dis 1:328–344, 1982
3. Berry CM, Thompson JD, Hatcher R: The radioreceptor assay for hCG in ectopic pregnancy. Obstet Gynecol 54:43–46, 1979
4. Brown R, Babcock R, Talbert J et al: Renal function in critically ill postoperative patients: Sequential assessment of creatinine, osmolar, and free water clearance. Crit Care Med 8:68–72, 1980
5. Felman YM, Nikitas JA: Nongonococcal urethritis. JAMA 245:381–386, 1981
6. Levinsky NG: Pathophysiology of acute renal failure. N Engl J Med 296:1453–1458, 1977
7. Meares EM: Prostatitis. Annu Rev Med 30:279–288, 1979
8. Miller TR, Anderson RJ, Linas SL et al: Urinary diagnostic indices in acute renal failure, a prospective study. Ann Intern Med 89:47–50, 1978
9. Sherman RA, Dodelson R, Gary NE, Eisinger RP: Membranous nephropathy. J Med Soc NJ 77:649–652, 1980
10. Stamm WE, Counts GW, Running KR et al: Diagnosis of coliform infection in acutely dysuric women. N Engl J Med 307:463–468, 1982
11. Stinebaugh BJ, Schloeder FX, Tam SC et al: Pathogenesis of distal renal tubular acidosis. Kidney Int 19:1–7, 1981
12. von Eschenbach AC: Cancer of the prostate. Curr Probl Cancer 5:1–54, 1981

## BIBLIOGRAPHY

Early LE, Gottschalk CW (eds): Strauss and Welt's Diseases of the Kidney, 3rd ed. Boston, Little, Brown, 1979
Harrington AR, Zimmerman SW: Renal Pathophysiology. New York, John Wiley & Sons, 1982
Knox FG (ed): Textbook of Renal Pathophysiology. Hagerstown, Harper & Row, 1978
Leaf A, Cotran R: Renal Pathophysiology, 2nd ed. New York, Oxford University Press, 1980
Smith DR: General Urology, 9th ed. Los Altos, Lange Medical Publications, 1978
Weller JM (ed): Fundamentals of Nephrology. Hagerstown, Harper & Row, 1979

# 6

# *ENDOCRINE DISEASES*

## PITUITARY TUMORS

Most pituitary tumors are benign tumors, or *adenomas.* Endocrine symptoms in patients with pituitary tumors reflect either hypofunction due to destruction of normal pituitary tissue (see Anterior Pituitary Insufficiency) or hyperfunction due to increased hormone formation by the tumor. Using currently available radioimmunoassays for anterior pituitary hormones, studies have found 70% to 80% of pituitary adenomas to be functioning tumors, with the majority secreting prolactin (PRL). This hormone normally induces the formation and secretion of breast milk. Other functioning pituitary tumors form adrenocorticotropic hormone (ACTH) (see Cushing's Syndrome) or growth hormone (GH) (see Acromegaly).

The most common pituitary tumor is the prolactinoma. PRL-secreting tumors in women are responsible for amenorrhea–galactorrhea. Women with these tumors usually have irregular menses or cessation of menstruation (*amenorrhea*). The most likely explanation for the ovarian hypofunction that accompanies increased PRL formation is interference with hypothalamic secretion of luteinizing hormone-releasing hormone (LH-RH). *Galactorrhea* indicates spontaneous flow of breast milk that either does not occur in relation to pregnancy or else persists for more than 6 months postpartum. Normal or abnormal lactation begins when the breasts, which have been stimulated by long exposure to high levels of PRL, estrogen, and progesterone, experience the sudden withdrawal of the latter two hormones.

PRL-secreting tumors in men are not clinically manifested as early as are those in women. Testosterone levels are uniformly depressed; this is secondary to impaired LH-RH secretion by the hypothalamus.

## LABORATORY FINDINGS

Increased plasma PRL (>300 ng/ml)—this finding is more diagnostic than are tests designed to stimulate or suppress PRL secretion

Diminished PRL increase following administration of thyrotropin-releasing hormone (TRH) or phenothiazines, such as chlorpromazine or perphenazine

## *ANTERIOR PITUITARY INSUFFICIENCY*

The clinical picture in anterior pituitary insufficiency varies greatly depending on the patient's age at onset, on whether there is the presence of a tumor that compresses the optic nerves and impairs vision, and on which anterior pituitary hormones are affected. GH is usually the first hormone affected. With progressive insufficiency there are decreases in gonadotropins, thyroid-stimulating hormone (TSH), and finally ACTH. A pituitary tumor is the most common cause of primary hypopituitarism. Although hypopituitarism is commonly chronic, it might occur suddenly following postpartum pituitary necrosis or hemorrhage into a pituitary tumor. Clinical hypopituitarism does not occur until about 70% to 75% of the gland is destroyed.

Secondary hypopituitarism may be caused by numerous central nervous system (CNS) disorders, all of which have in common the disruption of delivery of releasing factors or inhibiting factors from the hypothalamus to the pituitary.

Pituitary insufficiency results in secondary insufficiency of the target endocrine organs: thyroid, adrenal cortex, testis, and ovary. This insufficiency is characterized biochemically by decreased "-tropic" hormones. In *primary* failure of the thyroid, adrenal cortex, or gonads, the pituitary "-tropic" hormones are characteristically increased (see Hypothyroidism, Addison's Disease, Klinefelter's Syndrome, Turner's Syndrome).

## GONADOTROPIC HORMONES

The gonadotropic hormones include follicle-stimulating hormone (FSH) and luteinizing hormone (LH).

The gonadotropic hormones are stimulated by gonadotropin-releasing hormone (Gn-RH, LH-RH) produced by the hypothalamus.

FSH causes follicle development in the ovary and production of an androgen-binding protein in the testis. In the presence of FSH, LH develops and matures ovarian follicle and thecal tissue to secrete estrogens, stimulates ovulation, and develops functioning corpus luteum which produces progesterone. In the man, LH stimulates Leydig cells to form androgens, particularly testosterone. LH is known in men as interstitial cell-stimulating hormone. The androgen-binding protein brings testosterone into the testicular tubules, where it enhances sperm maturation.

If gonadotropin production fails before sexual maturity, puberty does not take place and secondary sex characteristics remain infantile. When gonadotropin deficiency develops in adult life, there is gradual loss of the secondary sex characteristics. LH deficiency also impedes ovulation, resulting in amenorrhea or infertility. LH deficiency is frequently seen with small, benign, PRL-producing pituitary tumors.

Estrogens either stimulate or suppress LH, depending on their degree and duration of increase. Progesterone and testosterone usually decrease LH levels. FSH is suppressed by a hormone known as *inhibin,* which is produced both by the ovaries and testes.

## THYROID-STIMULATING HORMONE

Although TSH deficiency may produce all of the characteristic signs of hypothyroidism, secondary hypothyroidism is usually less severe than is the primary form; it is also far less frequent. TSH is stimulated by TRH, produced by the hypothalamus, and is inhibited by triiodothyronine ($T_3$) and thyroxine ($T_4$) produced by the thyroid. Somatostatin produced by the hypothalamus also inhibits TSH secretion.

## ADRENOCORTICOTROPIC HORMONE

Adrenal cortical insufficiency secondary to diminished ACTH is characterized by decreased concentration of cortisol but not of aldosterone. The latter adrenal cortical hormone is largely, but not entirely, independent of ACTH control. ACTH is stimulated by stress; this results in production of corticotropin releasing factor (CRF) by the hypothalamus. ACTH is inhibited by cortisol, produced by the adrenal cortex. ACTH is normally secreted at its highest levels in the early morning and at its lowest levels at night. Cortisol secretion exhibits similar diurnal rhythmicity in response to ACTH stimulation.

## GROWTH HORMONE

GH deficiency in children may account for growth failure. These patients are extremely sensitive to insulin and often have episodes of spontaneous fasting hypoglycemia. GH is inhibited by somatostatin and stimulated by GH releasing hormone (GH-RH), both of which are produced in the hypothalamus. GH secretion is normally stimulated by hypoglycemia, protein ingestion, exercise, stress, and deep sleep. Glucose administration suppresses secretion of GH.

## LABORATORY FINDINGS

One or more of the pituitary hormones will be either decreased or in the low-normal range with an attendant decrease in target hormones. The pituitary hormones do not increase appropriately following stimulation.

Decreased GH, which does not respond to stimulation by at least two of the following: hypoglycemia, arginine, L-dopa

Decreased FSH → decreased estrogens and progesterone

Decreased LH (ICSH) → decreased estrogens and progesterone or testosterone

Decreased FSH and LH do not respond to stimulation by Gn-RH or clomiphene citrate.

Decreased TSH → decreased free $T_4$ index

Decreased TSH does not respond to stimulation by TRH

Decreased ACTH → decreased cortisol

Decreased ACTH does not respond to stimulation by metyrapone

## *ACROMEGALY*

Increased formation of GH by a benign pituitary tumor or *adenoma,* results in gigantism if increased hormone formation precedes complete skeletal maturation. The hormone causes proportional growth in the lengths and widths of all bones. If excess GH secretion by a pituitary tumor *follows* skeletal maturation, acromegaly (Greek, meaning *great extremities*) results. In acromegaly, there is accentuation of bone width, great enlargement of the hands and feet, lengthening of the lower jaw, broadening of the bridge of the nose, and increased soft-tissue growth. Overgrowth of bone around the joints may eventually result in severe joint dysfunction. Enlargement and hyperfunction of other endocrine glands are common in acromegaly.

Although the precise mechanism of stimulation of growth through GH is not completely understood, it is clear that GH does not work directly at the cellular level, but rather stimulates formation of mediating or intermediary hormones, called *somatomedins.* These directly stimulate deoxyribonucleic acid (DNA), ribonucleic acid (RNA), protein synthesis, mitosis, and collagen formation. Cartilage cells are the probable target of somatomedin control of skeletal growth. The source and identity of the somatomedins have not been fully determined.

A pituitary tumor responsible for acromegaly might also induce signs of deficiency of gonadotropins, TSH, and ACTH.

## LABORATORY FINDINGS

### Diagnostic Studies

Increased serum GH, which is not suppressed by oral administration of glucose; there is suppression of GH by glucose in normal persons.

GH is increased in response to TRH administration; there is no such increase in normal persons.

### Other Laboratory Findings

Increased serum phosphorus due to increased renal tubular phosphate reabsorption

Increased serum alkaline phosphatase reflects increased bone formation.

Increased serum and urine calcium reflect increased intestinal absorption of calcium.

Increased serum and urine creatine and creatinine reflect an increased rate of tissue synthesis.

Diabetes mellitus occurs in 10% of patients and there is impaired glucose tolerance in 50% of patients; these occur as a result of the antagonistic effect of GH on insulin.

## DIABETES INSIPIDUS

Central diabetes insipidus results from a deficiency of the hormone vasopressin (antidiuretic hormone [ADH]), which is stored in the posterior lobe of the pituitary gland. Deficiency of ADH may be either complete or incomplete. Most cases are of unknown origin, although many are due to hereditary, traumatic, inflammatory, degenerative, malignant, or granulomatous disorders. Lesions involve the hypothalamus, the pituitary gland, or the nerve pathways joining them.[10]

ADH is required to maintain the normal osmotic pressure of the plasma. Dehydration, which increases plasma osmolality by as little as 2%, stimulates osmoreceptors in the anterior hypothalamus. This causes the posterior lobe of the pituitary gland to release ADH into the general circulation. The hormone acts on the distal renal tubules and collecting ducts to increase reabsorption of water and to stimulate the thirst mechanism.

Hormone deficiency results in the formation of large volumes of urine of low specific gravity. These findings also occur in a renal disorder in which the kidneys cannot respond to ADH; this is termed *renal diabetes insipidus.* Psychogenic polydipsia, also known as compulsive water drinking, may produce the same clinical findings. Differentiation of these conditions may be accomplished by overnight fluid restriction, infusion of hypertonic saline, and, if indicated, observation of response to ADH injection.

### LABORATORY FINDINGS

Increased urine volume (4 liters/24 hr–15 liters/24 hr)

Decreased urine specific gravity ( < 1.004)—not appreciably increased when fluids are withheld

Decreased urine osmolality (<200 mOsm/Kg $H_2O$) in the presence of high-normal or elevated plasma osmolality

### Diagnostic Studies

Overnight water deprivation causes an increase in serum osmolality, but urine osmolality is less than 400 mOsm/Kg $H_2O$, and is usually less than that of serum. Patients also show weight loss due to continued renal loss of water despite water deprivation.

If the diagnosis is uncertain after overnight water deprivation, a hypertonic saline infusion test should be performed. Failure to demonstrate a rise in urine osmolality and a decrease in urine volume indicates diabetes insipidus.

If concentrated urine is not produced following the infusion of hypertonic saline, aqueous ADH may then be given to determine whether the diabetes insipidus is of renal or pituitary origin. Following ADH injection, pituitary diabetes insipidus shows increased urine osmolality and decreased urine output; renal diabetes insipidus shows no change in urine osmolality or urine output.

## SYNDROME OF INAPPROPRIATE SECRETION OF ANTIDIURETIC HORMONE

The syndrome of inappropriate secretion of ADH (SIADH) is secondary to a variety of pulmonary and CNS disorders and secondary to certain tumors, especially small-cell (oat cell) carcinoma of the lung. These tumors produce an ADH-like substance. Hormone secretion is without the normal physiologic stimulus of dehydration; hence, it is "inappropriate." The consequences of this disorder are fluid retention and subsequent dilution and decrease of serum sodium. The patient with SIADH is somewhat overhydrated.

### LABORATORY FINDINGS

Decreased serum sodium due to dilution by retained fluid

Decreased serum osmolality (<285 mOsm/Kg $H_2O$) due to fluid retention

Increased urine osmolality (300 mOsm/Kg $H_2O$–400 mOsm/Kg $H_2O$)—reflects decreased fluid excretion

Increased ratio of urine osmolality to serum osmolality

Normal urine sodium and creatinine clearance

## HYPERTHYROIDISM

Hyperthyroidism is also known as *thyrotoxicosis*. This condition results in the increased formation and release of thyroid hormones and from the effects these hormones have on body tissues. The effects result from a generalized increase in cellular metabolism. The most frequent clinical symptoms include heat intolerance, increased sweating, weight loss, increased appetite, nervousness, palpitations, fatigue, and weakness. The most frequent clinical signs include atrial fibrillation, tachycardia, hyperactivity and thyroid enlargement or goiter. Hyperthyroidism is due to excessive release of thyroid hormone from a toxic diffuse goiter (Graves' disease) or a toxic nodular goiter (Plummer's disease).

Graves' disease is the most common cause of thyrotoxicosis. Approximately 50% of patients have clinically evident infiltrative ophthalmopathy, which is also known as *exophthalmos*. This is manifested as protrusion of one or both eyes associated with an accumulation of mucopolysaccharides and lymphocytes in the tissues behind the eyes. Treatment of hyperthyroidism does not seem to have an appreciable influence on exophthalmos, which may occasionally be so severe as to threaten loss of vision due to corneal damage resulting from an inability to close the eyelid or due to optic-nerve damage.

A patient with Graves' disease usually has thyroid-stimulating immuno-globulins in his serum. Long-acting thyroid stimulator (LATS) was the first ab-normal thyroid stimulator discovered. Its name is derived from the fact that its thyroid-stimulating actions in mice or guinea pigs were more prolonged than were those of TSH. More recently, additional thyroid-stimulating immuno-globulins have been described. LATS is an autoantibody that operates at the cellular level similarly to TSH. It binds to the thyroid receptor for TSH, stimulat-ing iodine uptake, adenylate-cyclase activation, and formation of adenosine 3' : 5'-cyclic phosphate (cyclic AMP) (Fig. 6-1). The latter is the first intracellular

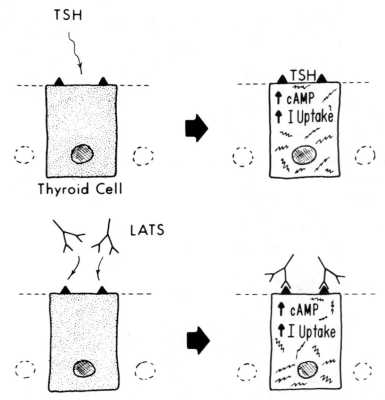

**Fig. 6-1.** The action of LATS on the thyroid mimics that of TSH, stimulating iodine uptake and activating cyclic AMP (cAMP). (Thaler MS, Klausner RD, Cohen HJ: Medi-cal Immunology, p 405. Philadelphia, JB Lippincott, 1977)

messenger through which peptide hormone action is expressed. Unlike TSH, LATS is an immunoglobulin produced by the patient's lymphocytes and is not subject to suppression by hormones produced by the thyroid gland.

Toxic nodular goiter is a nodular enlargement of the thyroid gland with some, but not all, of the nodules being functionally hyperactive. It is regarded as a late complication of long-standing nontoxic nodular goiter and is associated with neither exophthalmos nor elevated levels of LATS. It is accompanied by increased levels of free thyroid hormones, $T_4$, and $T_3$.

In hyperthyroidism, the secretion rates of $T_4$ and $T_3$ is increased, usually resulting in increased serum concentrations of both hormones. The increases in $T_3$ production and serum concentration are characteristically greater than are those in $T_4$. $T_3$ is the major physiologically active hormone at the cellular level; $T_4$ is predominantly a prohormone. Rarely, hyperthyroidism may be associated with elevation of only free $T_3$ ($T_3$ toxicosis) or of only free $T_4$ ($T_4$ toxicosis).

## LABORATORY FINDINGS

### Diagnostic Studies

Increased serum $T_4$—this may be normal

Increased resin $T_3$ uptake—this measures the availability of unbound binding sites for $T_4$ and $T_3$ on $T_4$-binding proteins; this may be normal even more often than is $T_4$.

Increased free $T_4$ index—this is the product of $T_4 \times$ resin $T_3$ uptake; this usually parallels absolute free $T_4$ concentration.

Increased serum $T_3$—measurement of this hormone is indicated when the free $T_4$ index is normal or borderline and clinical suspicion of hyperthyroidism is high.

Increased free $T_3$ index—this is the product of $T_3 \times$ resin $T_3$ uptake; this usually parallels absolute free $T_3$ concentration.

Minimal or absent increase in TSH following IV administration of TRH—this reflects pituitary suppression by increased $T_4$ and $T_3$ and indicates thyroid autonomy. *Autonomy* means that thyroid function is independent of pituitary regulation, but does not necessarily imply clinical thyrotoxicosis.

Presence of thyroid-stimulating immunoglobulins such as LATS in patients with Graves' disease

### Other Laboratory Findings

Increased serum glucose due to increased intestinal absorption and gluconeogenesis

Decreased serum cholesterol and triglycerides due to increased utilization

## HYPOTHYROIDISM

Inadequate peripheral tissue levels of thyroid hormone result in hypothyroidism. Most cases are primary and are due to deficiencies in the thyroid gland. Most cases of primary hypothyroidism are of unknown origin. Hypothyroidism may follow Hashimoto's disease or radioactive iodine treatment for hyperthyroidism. Uncommonly, the condition might be secondary to deficient TSH production by the pituitary gland.

A congenital form of primary hypothyroidism exists. If this is undiagnosed and untreated, cretinism results. *Cretinism* has been defined as permanent neurologic and skeletal retardation resulting from an inadequate supply of thyroid hormone during fetal and neonatal life. Newborn screening programs for the diagnosis of hypothyroidism include assays of T$_4$ and TSH. The reported incidence of neonatal hypothyroidism in North America is 1 : 5900 live births.

The most frequent clinical symptoms in hypothyroidism include cold intolerance, dry skin, weight gain, hoarseness, and fatigue. The most frequent clinical signs of severe hypothyroidism include coarse dry skin and hair, slow reflex relaxation, pallor, and periorbital edema.

Throughout all of the organ systems, one common result of hypothyroidism is excessive interstitial accumulation of glycosaminoglycan. This highly hydrophilic material causes the mucinous edema known as *myxedema,* which accounts for many of the clinical manifestations of hypothyroidism.

## LABORATORY FINDINGS

### Diagnostic Studies

Decreased serum T$_4$, resin T$_3$ uptake, and free T$_4$ index—the degree of depression of these indices depends on the extent of destruction of the thyroid gland.

Increased serum TSH—this is the single most important diagnostic laboratory test for primary hypothyroidism. This might be elevated, even with a normal free T$_4$ index. TSH is low or undetectable in cases of secondary hypothyroidism.

### Other Laboratory Findings

Increased serum cholesterol and triglycerides reflect decreased utilization.

Increased serum creatine phosphokinase (CPK), lactate dehydrogenase (LDH), and serum glutamic-oxaloacetic transaminase (SGOT)—myxedema of skeletal muscles causes leakage of these enzymes through the muscle membranes into capillaries

Flat glucose tolerance curve due to decreased gastric emptying and diminished cellular utilization of glucose

Anemia, usually normocytic, due to decreased erythropoietin production, decreased tissue oxygen needs, or impaired marrow function. Microcytic anemia might follow increased menstrual blood loss. The occasional occurrence of macrocytic anemia is due to vitamin-B$_{12}$ or folate deficiency.

Achlorhydria and parietal cell antibodies occur in up to 40% of patients.

## HASHIMOTO'S DISEASE

Hashimoto's disease is also known as *struma lymphomatosa, lymphocytic thyroiditis,* and *chronic autoimmune thyroiditis.* It is probably the most common cause of hypothyroidism in the United States. Diffuse thyroid enlargement is the most frequent physical finding in this disorder. Almost all patients have elevated serum levels of antibodies against thyroglobulin or against microsomal cytoplasmic antigen. The antibody titers do not correlate with the severity of the disease, and it has not been definitely established whether the circulating antibody is the cause or the result of thyroid destruction. The thyroid gland shows destroyed thyroid follicles and many lymphocytes and plasma cells, the appearance of which suggests an autoimmune mechanism. It has been postulated that antigen–antibody complexes are deposited in the thyroid, activating killer lymphocytes, which destroy thyroid tissue.

Hashimoto's disease occurs in association with, or as an end stage of, Graves' disease. It is also associated with other autoimmune disorders such as pernicious anemia, idiopathic adrenal insufficiency, hypoparathyroidism, diabetes mellitus, and primary gonadal failure.

### LABORATORY FINDINGS

Increased serum antithyroglobulin and antimicrosomal antibodies. Microsomal antibody titers correlate with the degree of lymphocytic infiltrate in the thyroid gland. Thyroglobulin antibodies correlate with the degree of thyroid fibrosis and occur in the chronic stage of the disorder. Children often do not have elevated antibody titers.

Increased TSH characteristically reflects primary hypothyroidism; this occurs before the free $T_4$ index decreases.

Free $T_4$ index is normal early in the disease but decreases as the disease progresses and more of the thyroid gland is destroyed.

## SUBACUTE THYROIDITIS

Subacute thyroiditis is also called *granulomatous, nonsuppurative,* or *giant cell thyroiditis*. This condition is the most common cause of thyroid pain and tenderness. The disorder is thought to be of viral origin. Mumps, influenza, and adenovirus have been associated with this disease. Pathologically, the gland shows destruction of thyroid follicles, mononuclear and polymorphonuclear infiltrates, fibrosis, and characteristically multinucleated giant cells.

The capacity to form thyroid hormone is blocked and there is unregulated and excessive breakdown of thyroglobulin, resulting in the increased release of $T_3$ and $T_4$. Clinical manifestations of hyperthyroidism occur in approximately 50% of patients, although biochemical hyperthyroidism occurs transiently in almost all patients. After six months, virtually all patients are clinically normal.

### LABORATORY FINDINGS

Increased sedimentation rate is a characteristic finding.

Free $T_4$ index and free $T_3$ index are usually elevated but may be normal early in the course of the disease; they are often decreased later in the disease; they are normal after six months.

Increased antithyroglobulin antibodies—slight elevation, which falls to normal with recovery

Mild normocytic anemia

## *CARCINOMA OF THE THYROID*

An increased incidence of thyroid cancer is associated with prior external radiation of the thyroid. The time required for the development of clinically evident thyroid carcinoma after external radiation ranges from 3.5 to 35 years or longer. There is no clear relation between the radiation dose and the interval between exposure and detection of the tumor.

The most common form of thyroid cancer is papillary carcinoma, which has a relatively benign course. This comprises 60% of thyroid malignancies. It is not unusual for affected patients to live 20 years to 30 years with known metastatic disease. Follicular carcinomas are less common, occur at a somewhat older age, and have a higher degree of malignancy. These constitute 20% of cases.

Medullary carcinomas make up 5% to 10% of thyroid cancers. These tumors arise from parafollicular cells, or C cells, which are situated between the thyroid follicles and produce calcitonin. The best-known pharmacologic effect of calcitonin is to lower plasma calcium and inorganic phosphorus by acting on the bones and kidneys.[1] This hormone is antagonistic to parathyroid hormone. In approximately 15% of patients with medullary carcinoma of the thyroid, the disease is familial and is transmitted as an autosomal dominant trait. The familial form usually occurs as part of the syndrome of multiple endocrine neoplasia, which is characterized by the combination of medullary thyroid carcinoma, bilateral adrenal pheochromocytomas, and parathyroid adenomas.

Anaplastic, or undifferentiated, carcinomas make up 10% to 20% of thyroid cancers and are the most malignant. They cannot be monitored by laboratory tests.

### LABORATORY FINDINGS

Biopsy of the thyroid gland is required for definitive diagnosis.

Increased serum calcitonin—characteristic finding in medullary carcinoma. An increased level may occur only following stimulation by calcium or pentagastrin infusion. These stimulation tests should be performed on relatives of patients with medullary carcinoma to facilitate early recognition of the disease at a stage when it might be curable.

Increased serum thyroglobulin—this occurs in many patients with untreated papillary and follicular carcinomas; it might also be elevated in Graves' disease and in subacute thyroiditis. The major use of this assay is in the follow-up of patients with thyroglobulin-secreting thyroid carcinoma. Very low or undetectable postoperative thyroglobulin levels indicate complete removal of the tumor. Persistence of elevated thyroglobulin indicates that residual thyroid carcinoma probably remains. Thyroglobulin is also elevated when metastases develop.

# CUSHING'S SYNDROME

*Cushing's syndrome* refers to the effects on the body of an excess of cortisol produced by the adrenal cortex. Cortisol regulates gluconeogenesis and the loss of nitrogen and potassium from tissues, decreases tissue utilization of carbohydrates, increases insulin resistance and circulating neutrophils, and decreases circulating eosinophils and lymphocytes. The major clinical features of Cushing's syndrome, in order of frequency of occurrence, are obesity, facial flushing, increased body hair, menstrual disorders, hypertension, muscular weakness, back pain, and reddish purple skin streaks. Protein depletion is manifested as thin skin, poor wound healing, and a decrease in bone mineral and muscle mass.

Cushing's syndrome may result from adrenal stimulation by ACTH of pituitary origin or from extrapituitary tumors. The former is known as *Cushing's disease* and the latter as *ectopic ACTH syndrome*. Cushing's disease accounts for approximately 70% of patients with Cushing's syndrome. Most of these patients have benign pituitary adenomas as the source of ACTH production, although pituitary histology may, rarely, be normal. The ectopic ACTH syndrome accounts for approximately 15% of patients with Cushing's syndrome. Undifferentiated oat cell carcinoma of the lung is the most frequent source of ectopic nonpituitary ACTH formation. Thus, the vast majority of cases of Cushing's syndrome are ACTH dependent and show enlargement or hyperplasia of both adrenal glands. In Cushing's disease, the benign pituitary tumors release ACTH irregularly rather than in the normal diurnal cycle of high morning levels and low evening levels. As a consequence, irregular, usually elevated levels of plasma cortisol occur. Furthermore, because the feedback inhibition of ACTH by cortisol is defective, the elevated cortisol secretion does not suppress ACTH secretion. Patients with ectopic ACTH syndrome usually have a greater degree of ACTH and cortisol hypersecretion than is seen in Cushing's disease.

Primary adrenocortical tumors are ACTH independent and cause approximately 15% of cases of Cushing's syndrome. Half of these tumors are benign adenomas and half are malignant carcinomas. Cortisol produced by adrenal tumors suppresses pituitary ACTH release. This is in striking contrast to ACTH-dependent Cushing's syndrome, in which there is persistent elevation of ACTH. Adrenal tumors, which hypersecrete cortisol, cause shrinkage or atrophy of the adrenal cortices not involved by the tumor.

## LABORATORY FINDINGS

### Diagnostic Studies

*Low-Dose Dexamethasone Test*
In normal persons, dexamethasone inhibits pituitary ACTH release and consequently suppresses adrenal cortisol secretion. Patients with Cushing's syndrome, in whom feedback control is abnormal, do not usually show cortisol suppression with low doses of dexamethasone.

Following a low dose of dexamethasone given over two days, these patients show no suppression of the 24-hour urinary excretion of 17-hydroxycorticosteroids (17-OHCS) and urinary free cortisol. For outpatient

**Table 6-1.** Dexamethasone Differentiation of Cushing's Syndrome

| DISORDER | PLASMA ACTH | SUPPRESSION OF URINARY STEROIDS |
|---|---|---|
| Cushing's disease | Normal or slightly elevated | To <50% of baseline values |
| Ectopic ACTH syndrome | Markedly elevated | None |
| Adrenal tumor | Low or undetectable | None |

screening, a single bedtime low dose of dexamethasone will not suppress plasma cortisol drawn the next morning.

*High-Dose Dexamethasone test*
This test is performed following an abnormal low-dose dexamethasone test to establish the origin of the hypercortisolism.

A high dose of dexamethasone is given over a period of 48 hours, or as a single bedtime dose. A basal blood sample is obtained for ACTH. Twenty-four-hour urine samples are collected before and after dexamethasone for measurement of urinary free cortisol and 17-OHCS to determine whether there is cortisol suppression.

Table 6-1 indicates the differential laboratory findings.

**Other Laboratory Findings**

Slightly increased hemoglobin and hematocrit

Decreased total lymphocyte, monocyte, and eosinophil counts—these cells move out of the circulation into the bone marrow, spleen, and lymph nodes.

Decreased serum potassium occurs in ectopic ACTH syndrome and adrenocortical carcinoma with markedly elevated cortisol levels; potassium loss is due to both increased glomerular filtration rate (GFR) and increased protein catabolism with loss of intracellular potassium.

Increased blood $p$H and bicarbonate (metabolic alkalosis) accompanies hypopotassemia.

Increased serum and urine glucose and decreased glucose tolerance—cortisol is a glucocorticoid that increases hepatic glycogen and glucose production and decreases glucose uptake and utilization in peripheral tissues.

Increased urine calcium, in approximately 40% of patients—glucocorticoids decrease renal reabsorption of calcium.

# ADRENOCORTICAL INSUFFICIENCY

Adrenocortical insufficiency is a rare disorder. Primary adrenocortical insufficiency is known as *Addison's disease.* Secondary adrenocortical insufficiency is usually due to prolonged therapeutic administration of glucocorticoids, such as cortisone or prednisone. Glucocorticoid therapy suppresses pituitary ACTH production and thereby results in secondary adrenocortical insufficiency. Less commonly, this disorder is due to decreased ACTH formation caused by a pituitary tumor.

Almost 95% of the adrenal glands must be destroyed to produce symptoms and signs of insufficiency. The major clinical features of adrenocortical insufficiency include weakness and fatigue, weight loss, loss of appetite, increased skin pigmentation, hypotension, and gastrointestinal (GI) symptoms. Pigmentation reflects the effect of excess ACTH, which is a finding in primary insufficiency. The other features reflect cortisol deficiency. Mineralocorticoid deficiency is indicated by fluid and electrolyte imbalance.

Primary adrenocortical insufficiency is idiopathic in more than 80% of cases. It is believed to be due to an autoimmune process, because adrenal antibodies are found in approximately 60% of these patients. About 50% of patients with idiopathic adrenocortical insufficiency have one or more of the following associated disorders: primary ovarian failure, diabetes mellitus, hypothyroidism, absence of skin pigmentation, thyrotoxicosis, hypoparathyroidism, and pernicious anemia. Tuberculosis currently accounts for fewer cases of Addison's disease than it did formerly.

In secondary adrenal insufficiency due to pituitary tumor, ACTH deficiency is almost always accompanied by deficiencies of GH and gonadotropins. The predominant effect of ACTH deficiency is decreased cortisol secretion. Hyperpigmentation, dehydration, and electrolyte abnormalities, which occur in primary adrenal insufficiency, do not occur.

## LABORATORY FINDINGS

### Diagnostic Studies

*Rapid ACTH Stimulation Test Using Cosyntropin (synthetic ACTH)*
A lack of increase in plasma cortisol following cosyntropin injection indicates adrenocortical insufficiency.

*Differentiation of Primary From Secondary Adrenocortical Insufficiency*
Increased plasma ACTH indicates primary insufficiency.

Normal or low plasma ACTH indicates secondary insufficiency.

### Other Laboratory Findings

*Primary Adrenocortical Insufficiency*
Presence of adrenal antibodies occurs in 50% to 70% of patients with nontuberculous Addison's disease.

Effects of mineralocorticoid deficiency:
Decreased serum sodium due to loss in urine; this finding might be obscured by associated dehydration

Increased serum potassium

Increased blood urea nitrogen (BUN) and creatinine due to decreased blood volume and dehydration

Effects of glucocorticoid deficiency:
Normocytic, normochromic anemia—this finding might be obscured by associated dehydration

Decreased neutrophils, increased lymphocytes, increased eosinophils

*Secondary Adrenocortical Insufficiency*
Adrenal effects are only those of glucocorticoid deficiency (listed above), because the mineralocorticoid, aldosterone, is not affected by diminished ACTH secretion.

Decreased GH, gonadotropins, and possibly TSH reflect pituitary insufficiency.


# ALDOSTERONISM

Aldosterone is a hormone of the adrenal cortex that primarily causes sodium and water to be reabsorbed in exchange for potassium and hydrogen ions at the distal renal tubules. The chief controlling mechanism of aldosterone production is the renin–angiotensin system, which is stimulated by low serum sodium or by a fall in intravascular fluid volume and renal blood pressure. These stimuli cause increased production of renin by the juxtaglomerular cells of the kidney. The enzyme renin activates angiotensinogen to angiotensin I, which is in turn converted to angiotensin II, which stimulates aldosterone secretion by the adrenal cortex and also increases blood pressure. Increases in plasma potassium stimulate aldosterone production independently of sodium and angiotensin.

Increased serum levels of aldosterone occur following stimulation by the renin–angiotensin system, by increased plasma potassium, or by dehydration. Conditions producing secondary aldosteronism occur with diuretic abuse, congestive heart failure with sodium and fluid retention, cirrhosis with ascites, nephrosis, toxemia of pregnancy, accelerated hypertension, and unilateral renal artery disease.

Primary aldosteronism is due to an aldosterone-producing benign tumor of the adrenal cortex in about 85% of cases. It may, occasionally, be due to bilateral adrenocortical hyperplasia or, very rarely, to carcinoma of the adrenal cortex. Patients with primary aldosteronism characteristically are hypertensive and have hypokalemia. The hypokalemia is associated with alkalosis, muscular weakness, and electrocardiogram (ECG) abnormalities.


## LABORATORY FINDINGS

### Diagnostic Studies

Increased urinary and plasma aldosterone—these cannot be reduced with high-sodium diet, with saline infusion, or with administration of fludrocortisone acetate.

Increased plasma aldosterone : plasma renin activity ratio (>400) occurs in primary aldosteronism.[5] This ratio does not seem to be influenced by variations of sodium intake or diuretic administration. The ratio seems to separate patients with aldosterone-producing adenomas from other hypertensive patients.

Decreased plasma renin indicates primary aldosteronism. Renin is not increased following salt restriction, diuretics, and upright posture. These mechanisms decrease plasma volume and stimulate the renin–angiotensin system.

Normal or increased plasma renin indicates secondary aldosteronism.

**Other Laboratory Findings**

Increased urine potassium (> 30 mEq/24 hr)—this degree of urine potassium loss reflecting the aldosterone effect is inappropriately excessive in the presence of hypokalemia.

Decreased plasma potassium—20% of patients may have normal plasma potassium, between 3.5 mEq/liter and 4.0 mEq/liter. In these patients, hypokalemia may be demonstrated by increasing sodium intake. This will cause a significant fall in plasma potassium and an increase in urine potassium in all patients with aldosteronism.

Increased serum $p$H and $CO_2$ content (metabolic alkalosis) accompany potassium depletion and urinary hydrogen-ion loss.

# PHEOCHROMOCYTOMA

Pheochromocytoma is a rare tumor of the sympathetic nervous system.[12, 14] Approximately 90% arise in the adrenal medullae; the remainder occur in association with sympathetic ganglia. The tumors produce increased amounts mostly of norepinephrine but also of epinephrine. These hormones are termed *catecholamines*. Metabolites of catecholamines excreted in urine are *metanephrines*. In 50% to 70% of familial cases and 10% to 20% of sporadic cases, the tumor is bilateral. About 5% to 10% of pheochromocytomas are malignant. Excessive release of catecholamines into the bloodstream commonly produces sustained or intermittent hypertension, severe headache, excessive perspiration, palpitations, pallor, nervousness or anxiety, and tremor. Hypotension commonly occurs after an attack. This tumor is responsible for less than 0.5% of all cases of hypertension. Complications include heart failure, myocardial infarction, stroke, and aneurysm.

There is an associated familial occurrence of pheochromocytoma and neurofibromatosis; this combination is known as multiple endocrine adenomatosis type IIb. Neurofibromatosis is a familial condition characterized by developmental changes in the nervous system, muscles, bones, and skin and marked by the formation of multiple benign nerve tumors covering much of the skin surface. Another familial syndrome associated with pheochromocytoma includes medullary carcinoma of the thyroid gland and parathyroid adenoma. This combination of tumors is referred to as multiple endocrine adenomatosis type IIa.

## LABORATORY FINDINGS

**Diagnostic Studies**

Increased 24-hour urine metanephrines—this is the best single screening test; metanephrines might be elevated even between hypertensive attacks.

Increased plasma norepinephrine (noradrenalin)—this is not suppressed by clonidine hydrochloride.[2] This is the best definitive test and should be done regardless of urinary metanephrine excretion if the entire clinical picture is strongly suggestive of pheochromocytoma.

Increased urine metanephrine–creatinine ratio (> 2.2 mcg/mg)

### Other Laboratory Findings

Increased serum and urine glucose due to catecholamine-induced suppression of insulin secretion and acceleration of glucose production

## KLINEFELTER'S SYNDROME

Klinefelter's syndrome is the most common form of male hypogonadism and is due to a chromosome abnormality that results in primary testicular failure. The syndrome is characterized by small and firm testes, absence of sperm formation, and gynecomastia (enlargement of the male breasts). Classically, this syndrome is due to the presence of an extra X chromosome, resulting in an XXY sex chromosome constitution, producing a 47XXY karyotype. The normal male karyotype is 46XY. In variants of Klinefelter's syndrome, any of a number of abnormal chromosome patterns may be present.

Although these persons have the physical features of men, the presence of an XX chromosome pair results in a Barr body, which may be seen microscopically in most cells of the body. A Barr body is a nuclear chromatin mass, on the inner membrane of the nucleus, that represents an inactivated X choromsome. It is found in the cells of normal females; when found in males it indicates the presence of an extra X chromosome, as in Klinefelter's syndrome. Scrapings of cells from the inner lining of the oral cavity provide a convenient means of examining cells for Barr bodies.

### LABORATORY FINDINGS

Barr bodies are present in >20% of oral-cavity cells

Decreased serum free testosterone—does not increase following stimulation by human chorionic gonadotropin (HCG)

Increased serum and urine FSH and LH—this finding characterizes primary hypogonadism and differentiates it from secondary hypogonadism

Absence of sperm in seminal fluid

Testicular biopsy shows atrophy with hyalinized tubules and absence of spermatogenesis

Karyotype is usually 47XXY.

## SECONDARY TESTICULAR FAILURE

Secondary hypogonadism indicates testicular failure secondary to either pituitary failure, excessive prolactin production, or failure of the hypothalamus to produce Gn-RH. This is a less common cause of male hypogonadism than is Klinefelter's syndrome.

Increased levels of GH or prolactin indicate an underlying pituitary tumor as the cause of secondary hypogonadism. A pituitary tumor may cause secondary testicular failure without evidence of pituitary hormone formation.

## LABORATORY FINDINGS

Decreased or low-normal serum and urine FSH and LH—Failure of increase following stimulation by clomiphene citrate, along with a strong increase following Gn-RH stimulation, suggests a hypothalamic lesion. Failure of increase following stimulation by Gn-RH suggests a pituitary lesion.

Decreased serum free testosterone, which increases following administration of HCG

Absence of sperm in seminal fluid

Testicular biopsy shows atrophy and failure of spermatogenesis.

Possible increase in GH or prolactin

## *TESTICULAR TUMORS*

Although testicular neoplasms are uncommon, their peak occurrence in the third and fourth decades makes them one of the most common malignancies in this age group. About 5% of men with testicular tumors have histories of an undescended testis.

Most testicular tumors originate from the germinal cells of the seminiferous tubules, which are the site of sperm formation. The most common testicular tumor is the seminoma, which only rarely forms hormones. Other testicular tumors are hormonally active and produce HCG, which is found in the urine in large quantities. This is the same hormone that is produced by the normal placenta. Certain other testicular tumors, derived from fetal yolk-sac cells, produce a substance called $\alpha_1$-*fetoprotein*. This substance is produced by normal embryonic tissues during fetal development but is not normally found after birth. Inactive fetal genes might be reactivated during the process of malignant transformation.

Monitoring the levels of HCG or $\alpha_1$-fetoprotein is useful in following the effects of treatment and detecting tumor recurrence. The hormonal tumor markers are not helpful in the early detection of testicular malignancy. The preoperative hormone level is not related to prognosis.

Interstitial Leydig cell tumors of the testis are rare and usually benign. Androgen-producing Leydig cell tumors cause pseudoprecocity in the prepubertal boy. Enlargement of the breasts, termed *gynecomastia*, occasionally occurs in a man as a consequence of estrogen formation by some testicular and adrenal tumors.

## LABORATORY FINDINGS

Increased urine HCG—this is formed by tumors having chorionic tissue, such as choriocarcinoma and embryonal carcinoma. The HCG assay should be $\beta$-subunit specific to avoid a false-positive result due to cross-reaction with LH.

Increased serum $\alpha_1$-fetoprotein occurs with embryonal carcinomas and yolk-sac tumors.[4]

## TURNER'S SYNDROME

Turner's syndrome, or ovarian dysgenesis, is the most commonly encountered form of primary ovarian hypogonadism. As in Klinefelter's syndrome, this is due to defective chromosomal constitution. About 80% of patients have only one X chromosome, rather than two, and thus are designated 45XO in their sex-chromosome makeup.

The ovaries fail to develop and, as a consequence, these women remain sexually infantile, although their internal and external genitalia are female. These patients have other associated abnormalities, the most common of which are short stature, webbing of the neck, and a wide chest with broadly spaced nipples.

### LABORATORY FINDINGS

Absence of Barr bodies (approximately 80% of patients)—reflects the presence of only one X chromosome

Decreased serum and urine estrogens, which do not increase following administration of HCG

Increased FSH—this is elevated in early childhood and again prepubertally, but may be normal in mid-childhood

Increased LH—this usually does not increase until puberty

Karyotype shows 45XO in typical cases; other chromosomal abnormalities also occur.

## POLYCYSTIC OVARY SYNDROME (STEIN-LEVENTHAL SYNDROME)

Stein-Leventhal syndrome comprises some or all of the following features: bilateral polycystic ovaries, amenorrhea, oligomenorrhea, infertility, increased body and facial hair, obesity, and acne.[16]

Patients have decreased levels of sex-hormone-binding globulin; this results in increased circulating free testosterone. The excess androgens are primarily of ovarian origin, but might partially arise from the adrenal gland. The androgen excess accounts for elevated estrogen levels as a result of tissue conversion of the former to the latter. Hirsutism is a consequence of elevation of circulating androgenic hormones and their precursors.

A major characteristic of Stein-Leventhal syndrome is chronic anovulation. The constant secretion of excessive amounts of androgen and its conversion to estrogen constitute the basis for chronic anovulation. Persistently elevated estrogen levels augment pituitary sensitivity to LH-RH of hypothalamic origin. This stimulates greater pituitary secretion of LH than of FSH. The excess of LH and lack of the normal midcycle LH surge cause loss of normal ovarian cycles and result in chronic anovulation.[16]

The increased LH–FSH ratio stimulates ovarian androgen formation and

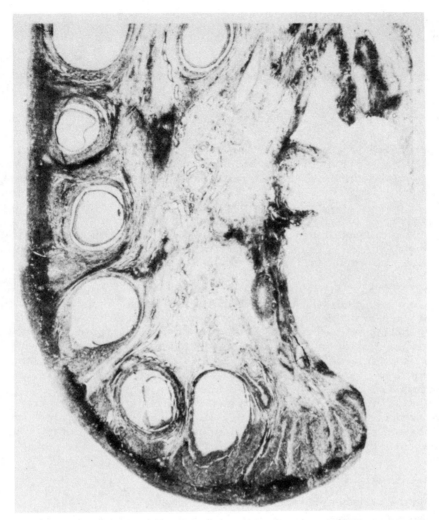

**Fig. 6-2.** Multiple cysts in the cortex of the ovary in Stein-Leventhal syndrome. The lack of corpora lutea reflects the failure of ovulation. (Novak ER, Woodruff JD: Gynecologic and Obstetric Pathology, 7th ed, p 364. Philadelphia, WB Saunders, 1974)

suppresses ovarian estrogen formation. Chronic LH stimulation and excessive androgen production cause ovarian enlargement, thickening of ovarian capsules, and impaired follicle maturation. These result in degeneration of ovarian follicles and consequent characteristically increased follicular cyst formation and absence of corpora lutea, which are normally seen only following ovulation (Fig. 6-2).

### LABORATORY FINDINGS

Increased LH–FSH ratio is a characteristic finding.

Increased serum free testosterone

Increased serum androstenedione, which is a testosterone precursor

## SECONDARY OVARIAN FAILURE

Ovarian failure may be secondary to organic or functional disturbances of the pituitary gland or hypothalamus or to any condition associated with excessive androgen production. Absence of menstruation, or *amenorrhea*, indicates ovarian failure.

Amenorrhea may be the first indication of a slowly growing pituitary tumor, occurring years before it is otherwise clinically evident. Sometimes the suspicion of a pituitary tumor is increased because of clinical signs of acromegaly, Cushing's syndrome, or inappropriate lactation due to pituitary formation of GH, ACTH, or prolactin, respectively.

Sheehan's syndrome is one cause of permanent failure of pituitary formation of FSH and LH. In this disorder, varying degrees of postpartum pituitary failure are seen. The syndrome is thought to be the result of temporary postpartum hypotension which causes pituitary necrosis, hemorrhage, or infarction.

In the majority of patients with pituitary gonadotropin deficiency and amenorrhea there is no evidence of organic hypothalamic or pituitary disease, and it is presumed that there is a functional defect resulting in failure of gonadotropin secretion. An acquired form of amenorrhea is seen in anorexia nervosa, in which amenorrhea is associated with weight loss.

Almost any disease that disturbs metabolism or nutrition may be associated with secondary amenorrhea through depression of ovarian function via hypothalamic–pituitary controls. Emotional and psychic stimuli may have a similar effect in some women.

### LABORATORY FINDINGS

Normal or decreased serum and urinary FSH and LH

Normal or decreased serum and urinary estrogens—these will increase following administration of gonadotropins.

## OVARIAN TUMORS

The vast majority of ovarian tumors is nonfunctional (*i.e.*, the tumors produce no hormones and consequently are not detectable through clinical or laboratory hormonal effects).

Estrogen-producing tumors include granulosa cell tumor and thecoma. Clinical evidence of these tumors is seen as precocious puberty, if they occur in childhood, or as resumption of menstruation, if they occur after menopause. Clinical features are not readily evident during the reproductive years.

Androgen-producing tumors include arrhenoblastomas, hilar cell tumors, and adrenal rest tumors. Patients with such tumors present with amenorrhea and virilization. Adrenal rest tumors may also produce cortisol and present as Cushing's syndrome.

## LABORATORY FINDINGS

### Feminizing Ovarian Tumors

Increased serum and urinary estrogens

Decreased urinary FSH as a result of suppression by increased ovarian estrogens

Lack of serum progesterone and urinary pregnanediol

### Masculinizing Ovarian Tumors

Markedly increased serum free testosterone

Decreased urinary FSH as a result of suppression by increased ovarian testosterone

Increased cortisol and other laboratory findings of Cushing's syndrome in adrenal rest tumors

Increased 17-ketosteroids (17-KS) produced by adrenal rest tumors

Pap smear shows decreased estrogen effect

# DIABETES MELLITUS

Diabetes mellitus is a disorder manifested by an increase in blood sugar due to relative or absolute insulin deficiency.

Diabetes is now categorized as insulin-dependent or insulin-independent rather than as juvenile-onset or adult-onset.[15] Insulin-dependent diabetes is associated with certain genetically determined histocompatibility antigens. It appears that environment determines whether this form of diabetes will become clinically evident in the genetically susceptible person. One such environmental factor is a viral infection that, either directly or through an autoimmune response, leads to injury and death of pancreatic $\beta$ cells. Failure of insulin formation and secretion is the primary pathogenetic factor in insulin-dependent diabetes. Glucagon excess may exaggerate the effects of insulin lack in such patients.

In insulin-independent diabetes, which accounts for 85% to 90% of diabetes, insulin deficiency does not occur. Affected patients appear to have insulin resistance.[13] Insulin resistance occurs both in the liver and in the peripheral tissues, principally the muscle. Hepatic resistance is present in the form of inappropriately high glucose production in the fasting state and deficient glucose uptake following glucose ingestion. Peripheral resistance becomes manifest as reduced glucose uptake, mostly by muscle, after exposure to insulin and reduced clearance of plasma glucose in the fasting state. Insulin resistance is intensified by obesity, which is present in 80% of diabetics. Obesity appears to enhance a genetic susceptibility to diabetes. Obese patients have increased demand for insulin secretion from genetically impaired $\beta$ cells. Obesity is associated with a decreased number of insulin receptors, alterations in glucose transport, and alterations in intracellular glucose metabolism.[13]

Insulin is the body's major storage hormone, and insulin deficiency results in a diminished ability of the body to increase its storage reservoir of fuels because of inadequate metabolism of ingested foodstuffs. Ingested glucose is not stored but appears as hyperglycemia. Ingested protein is not stored but appears as hyperaminoacidemia. Hypersecretion of glucagon in response to protein ingestion also causes hyperglycemia. Ingested fat is not stored but appears as hypertriglyceridemia. When there is a major deficiency of insulin, not only is fuel accumulation after eating hampered, but there is also excessive mobilization of stored body fuels in the fasting state. In diabetic ketoacidosis, there is overproduction of glucose and ketones from amino acids and fatty acids and a marked acceleration of fat and protein breakdown.

The complications of diabetes may be divided into the following:

1. Those associated with insulin therapy
2. Those associated with pregnancy
3. Diabetes-induced acidosis or coma
4. Vascular and neuropathic complications

### COMPLICATIONS OF INSULIN THERAPY

The most frequent complication of insulin therapy is hypoglycemia, which may produce convulsions or coma. If hypoglycemia is prolonged, there may be permanent brain damage. Local temporary allergic reactions to insulin injections may occur. Occasionally, atrophy of subcutaneous fat occurs at the site of insulin injections. With the advent of purer insulin preparations, this has occurred less frequently.

### DIABETES AND PREGNANCY

When very carefully controlled, diabetes during pregnancy has no adverse effect on mother or fetus. With poor diabetes control, however, diabetic retinopathy in the mother is accelerated during pregnancy. Babies of diabetic mothers are usually born heavier than normal but, despite their weight, are like premature babies in that they are more subject than normal to respiratory distress syndrome, hypoglycemia, and hypocalcemia.

### DIABETIC ACIDOSIS AND COMA

Diabetic coma is associated with severe ketoacidosis or with hyperglycemia and dehydration. The relative lack of insulin leads to overproduction of glucose from endogenous precursors such as amino acids. This causes hyperglycemia, which increases plasma osmolarity and tends to draw fluid out of cells and into the extracellular space, resulting in cellular dehydration. Hyperglycemia results in glycosuria, producing an osmotic diuresis and further aggravating dehydration and loss of electrolytes. Insulin deficiency contributes to renal sodium loss. Lack of insulin and acidosis result in the transfer of potassium out of cells and into the plasma; it is then rapidly excreted in the urine. Accelerated gluconeogenesis results in conversion of amino acids to sugar and urea. Urea has an osmotic effect, which leads to tissue and urinary fluid loss, further accentuating dehydration. In fully developed diabetic ketoacidosis, therefore, all body compartments are dehydrated and there are absolute deficiencies of water, sodium, potassium, magnesium, chloride, and bicarbonate.

Insulin lack results in augmented breakdown of fat and mobilization of free fatty acids. Within the liver, free fatty acids are readily converted to acetoacetic acid and $\beta$-hydroxybutyric acid. The increased ketones released by the liver cannot normally be metabolized by muscle tissues and tend to accumulate in the blood. The presence of large amounts of ketone bodies, which are moderately strong acids, causes an increase in the hydrogen-ion concentration of body fluids. As a result there is a fall in serum bicarbonate, producing metabolic acidosis. The lowered $p$H stimulates the central respiratory center to increase ventilation.

In hyperosmolar nonketotic coma, there are extreme degrees of hyperglycemia ($>$600 mg/dl), dehydration, and azotemia, but there is no ketosis. The patient's serum is hyperosmolar, exceeding 350 mOsm-Kg $H_2O$, and in extreme cases approaches 500 mOsm/Kg $H_2O$. (Normal serum osmolarity is 275 mOsm-Kg $H_2O$ to 295 mOsm/Kg $H_2O$.) The pathogenesis of this condition is thought to be due to the presence of an amount of insulin sufficient to inhibit fatty-acid mobilization but insufficient to prevent hyperglycemia, osmotic diuresis, and potassium loss. Many patients have a concurrent illness, such as renal insufficiency, pneumonia, GI hemorrhage, or gram-negative sepsis. The associated illness either initiates or accentuates the sequence of events.

## VASCULAR AND NEUROPATHIC COMPLICATIONS

Vascular and neuropathic complications appear with increasing frequency the longer the duration of the disease. The two major theories for the pathogenesis of diabetic microvascular and neuropathic complications are those based on metabolic and genetic factors. Probably both factors play a role.

### Large Vessels

For unknown reasons the diabetic is more likely to develop atherosclerosis than is the nondiabetic. Atherosclerosis may result in partial or complete blockage of arteries, leading to increased occurrence of myocardial infarction, cerebrovascular accidents, or gangrene of the lower extremities. Many factors have been implicated to explain increased atherosclerosis in diabetes. There is recent evidence suggesting that hyperinsulinemia may be one such important factor.

### Small Vessels

Capillary basement-membrane thickening or microangiopathy occurs throughout the body, including skin and muscle, but is of greatest clinical significance in the retina and glomerulus.

In the retina, damaged capillaries cause microaneurysms, hemorrhages, and exudates, which are the consequence of fluid that has leaked out of capillaries. Scarring associated with hemorrhage leads to retinal detachment. For unknown reasons, retinal capillaries tend to proliferate. The diabetic also has increased frequency of cataract formation. All of these effects combine to make diabetes the leading cause of blindness in this country today.

Diabetic renal disease is manifested primarily by thickening of the glomerular capillary basement membranes. This leads to increased glomerular capillary permeability and occlusion of capillary lumina, resulting in diminished glomerular filtration. The result is varying degrees of proteinuria and azotemia. Diabetics' increased susceptibility to infection results in interstitial nephritis and tubular damage.

### Neuropathy

The most common neuropathy is sensory neuropathy of the feet, in which there is numbness, tingling, burning, and sharp shooting pains. The pathogenesis of this disorder is not understood. Lack of sensation in the soles of the feet, coupled with poor circulation, commonly leads to ulcerations that become infected and lead to gangrene. Diabetic mononeuropathies are probably the result of nerve infarction.

## LABORATORY FINDINGS

### Diagnostic Studies

Fasting venous plasma glucose >140 mg/dl on more than one occasion.

Oral glucose tolerance test utilizing 75-g carbohydrate solution—2 hr, and one other sample, plasma glucose above 200 mg/dl[9]

### Other Laboratory Findings

Increased urine glucose when blood glucose is above the renal threshold

Increased urine volume and osmolality—glucose in the urine acts as an osmotic diuretic

Decreased serum phosphorus—insulin causes phosphate to enter cells; there is also increased phosphate loss in urine

Decreased serum sodium—this is inversely related to increased blood sugar; osmotic diuresis accounts for increased sodium loss in the urine.

### Laboratory Findings in Ketoacidosis

Increased plasma glucose

Plasma acetone is usually present; increased $\beta$-hydroxybutyrate.

Increased BUN and creatinine—prerenal azotemia reflects dehydration and fall in blood pressure

Increased urine glucose, ketones, protein, and casts

Decreased blood $p$H, $CO_2$ content (metabolic acidosis)—reflects increased formation of ketoacids and diminished bicarbonate consequent to buffering of acids; increased anion gap

Decreased $PCO_2$ reflects increased ventilation as compensation for metabolic acidosis.

Increased serum potassium—acidosis causes potassium to shift from within the cells into the extracellular space. Potassium may be normal or low, particularly after therapy has been started.

Leukocytosis may be >20,000/$\mu$l, even without infection.

# HYPOGLYCEMIA

Hypoglycemia is a reduction in plasma glucose to less than 45 mg/dl with development of symptoms that generally are relieved with glucose or eating. Symptoms of hypoglycemia are perspiration, palpitation, tremor, tingling, numbness or burning, hunger, and irritability. These symptoms result from hypoglycemic stimulation of the sympathoadrenal system, which in turn results in an increased secretion of epinephrine and norepinephrine. Hypoglycemia also stimulates secretion of GH, cortisol and glucagon. Epinephrine and glucagon are essential for restoration of the plasma glucose level to normal. This is accomplished by increased hepatic glucose production. Hepatic stores of glycogen can meet the body's needs for no more than about 24 hours. During fasts longer than 24 hours, the blood glucose level is normally maintained by an increased rate of gluconeogenesis, which is glucose formation from noncarbohydrate sources.

### ORGANIC PRIMARY HYPOGLYCEMIA

Hypoglycemia occurs *during fasting* in this group of conditions.

### Insulin-Producing Islet Cell Tumors (Insulinomas)

Insulinomas usually occur in the pancreas, and 90% are benign. They are an unusual cause of hypoglycemia, but when present they have a pattern of gradually increasing fasting hypoglycemia. It is currently felt that the underlying defect is an inability of the tumor cells to store insulin; this results in increased levels of plasma insulin.

### Extrapancreatic Tumors That Produce Hypoglycemia

Uncommon extrapancreatic tumors produce hypoglycemia by secreting an insulinlike material, utilizing glucose at an accelerated rate, or inhibiting the ability of the liver to release glucose.

### Deficiency of Factors That Normally Counter Insulin Effects

A deficiency of GH, cortisol, or $T_4$ increases a patient's sensitivity to insulin and decreases his capacity to correct hypoglycemia. Patients with deficiencies of these hormones often have fasting hypoglycemia, which is accompanied by an appropriate reduction in plasma insulin.

### Hepatic Disorders

Patients with severe hepatic necrosis might manifest fasting hypoglycemia because the liver can neither store glycogen nor provide glucose through gluconeogenesis.

In von Gierke's disease (see Chap. 10), glycogen accumulates in various tissues, particularly the liver. Glycogen accumulates because the patient lacks enzymes necessary to metabolize glycogen to form glucose. This results in fasting hypoglycemia.

## ORGANIC SECONDARY HYPOGLYCEMIA

Hypoglycemia may be secondary to administration of insulin, sulfonylureas, or alcohol. Insulin-induced and alcohol-induced hypoglycemia are the two most common types of hypoglycemia encountered in adults. Alcoholic hypoglycemia is the result of depleted liver glycogen and impaired gluconeogenesis.

## POSTPRANDIAL OR REACTIVE HYPOGLYCEMIA

Reactive hypoglycemia is characterized by the development of symptoms within a few hours *after eating.* Fasting does not provoke this type of hypoglycemia. Many theories of pathophysiology have been proposed. The precise mechanism to explain this condition has not been determined.

The most common form of this condition is idiopathic, or functional, postprandial hypoglycemia. This frequently occurs in association with manifestations of anxiety or other psychoneuroses. Postprandial hypoglycemia also occurs following subtotal gastrectomy. This is considered to be due to rapid passage of ingested glucose into the duodenum, from which it is quickly absorbed, leading to early hyperglycemia and excessive insulin secretion. Postprandial hypoglycemia might also be an early manifestation of insulin-dependent diabetes mellitus. Patients have normal fasting glucose levels. However, with glucose tolerance tests, they show an exaggerated early rise in plasma glucose due to inadequate insulin release and late hyperinsulinemia as a response to hyperglycemia early in the test. The delayed insulin response accounts for the marked fall in blood sugar.

## LABORATORY FINDINGS

### Insulin-Producing Islet Cell Tumor

Symptoms of hypoglycemia occur *while fasting* and are accompanied by plasma glucose <45 mg/dl and an inappropriately high plasma insulin level (>10 $\mu$U/ml). In about 50% of patients, overnight fasting produces the characteristic findings. Some patients require as much as a 72-hour fast, followed by exercise, to demonstrate hypoglycemia and hyperinsulinemia and establish the diagnosis.

### Postprandial (Reactive) Hypoglycemia

Plasma glucose below 45 mg/dl and appropriate symptoms occur 2–4 hours after eating but *not during fasting.* The glucose frequently returns to normal spontaneously. The 5-hour glucose tolerance test is an artificial situation and is not recommended for establishing the diagnosis. A standard meal may be used in an attempt to produce postprandial hypoglycemia. Blood sugar should be drawn *at the time symptoms occur.* It is not necessary to measure serum insulin levels.

#### Other Laboratory Findings

Laboratory findings of Cushing's syndrome, hypothyroidism, hypopituitarism, hepatic failure, von Gierke's disease—if hypoglycemia is secondary to any of these disorders

## ZOLLINGER-ELLISON SYNDROME

The Zollinger-Ellison (Z-E) syndrome is characterized by intractable ulcerations of the duodenum and jejunum, diarrhea, steatorrhea, and non-$\beta$-cell tumors of the pancreatic islets. The cells constituting these tumors produce increased levels of gastrin. The tumors are called gastrinomas.

Gastrin is normally produced by mucosal cells in the gastric antrum, the distal non–acid-secreting segment of the stomach. The hormone is physiologically stimulated by a meal. Upon release, the hormone is absorbed into the bloodstream and carried to the fundic cells of the stomach, stimulating them to release hydrochloric acid. Control of gastrin secretion is normally mediated by a negative feedback mechanism in which acid bathing the antrum acts directly on the gastrin-producing cells to inhibit further release of the hormone. Gastrin produced by gastrinomas is not inhibited by gastric acid in the normal fashion. Persistently increased gastrin formation stimulates secretion of large volumes of highly acid gastric secretions, causing peptic ulceration.

The syndrome may be associated with adenomas of the parathyroid, adrenal, or pituitary glands. This is known as *multiple endocrine adenomatosis* type I.

### LABORATORY FINDINGS

#### Diagnostic Studies

Increased fasting serum gastrin (>500 pg/ml)—borderline levels (250 pg/ml– 500 pg/ml) will be markedly increased following stimulation by IV secretin

#### Other Laboratory Findings

Increased volume of highly acid gastric juice; baseline acidity is >60% of the maximally stimulated level. A recent report revealed that gastric analysis does not improve on the diagnostic ability of the fasting serum gastrin test.[8]

Increased stool lipids—duodenal hyperacidity inactivates pancreatic enzymes and causes maldigestion and malabsorption of lipids and consequent diarrhea and steatorrhea

Decreased serum potassium secondary to severe diarrhea, which often accompanies this syndrome

Decreased serum albumin—possibly due to protein malabsorption or protein-losing enteropathy

## HYPERPARATHYROIDISM

In primary hyperparathyroidism, the normal feedback control of parathyroid hormone (PTH) secretion is lost and excessive hormone production continues despite elevated plasma calcium levels.

Hyperparathyroidism is usually due to a benign tumor or adenoma of one or more parathyroid glands. Approximately 15% of cases are due to diffuse enlargement or hyperplasia of all four parathyroid glands. Rarely, hyperparathyroidism is caused by parathyroid carcinoma.

PTH acts on bones to increase calcium resorption, stimulates the kidney to produce 1,25-dihydroxyvitamin $D_3$, acts on the intestinal tract through increased 1,25-dihydroxyvitamin $D_3$ to increase absorption of calcium, and acts on the kidneys to increase tubular absorption of ionized calcium and to decrease proximal renal tubular reabsorption of phosphate. The net result of these actions is to elevate serum calcium, decrease serum phosphate, and increase urinary calcium and phosphate.

Most cases of hyperparathyroidism are asymptomatic and are detected by finding hypercalcemia on a "routine" or screening chemistry profile. When present, the symptoms and signs of the disease are primarily due to hypercalcemia, which results from the formation of excess PTH. The symptoms and signs are quite varied. Renal calculi and bone disease are considered to be specific complications of hyperparathyroidism. Hypertension, peptic ulcer, and fatigue, although disease-related, are nonspecific findings.

Hypercalciuria appears to be the most important risk factor predisposing the patient to stone formation in primary hyperparathyroidism. Increased calcium excretion results from increased intestinal absorption of calcium as a consequence of increased serum levels of 1,25-dihydroxyvitamin $D_3$. In the past, approximately 50% of patients with primary hyperparathyroidism have had renal calculi. In a recent series, only 21% of patients had renal calculi.[7]

Hypercalcemia may also be responsible for calcification of kidney tissue and for interference with the ability of the kidneys to concentrate urine. This might result in polyuria and polydipsia (increased thirst).

Bone involvement in primary hyperparathyroidism consists of varying degrees of skeletal mineral resorption with variable clinical, radiologic, and histologic findings. The severity of bone disease depends on the aggressiveness of the basic disease and the systemic mechanisms that restore the bone minerals.

Secondary hyperparathyroidism is the normal adaptive response of parathyroid hyperplasia and increased PTH production, which occurs secondary to hypocalcemia. The most common cause is uremia and the second most common cause is GI malabsorption of calcium and vitamin D. Secondary parathyroid hyperplasia does not lead to hypercalcemia because the feedback control mechanism functions normally in regulating PTH secretion to restore the lowered serum calcium to only normal levels.

Tertiary hyperparathyroidism is defined as the state of unregulated, overcompensated parathyroid hyperfunction occurring after long-standing secondary hyperparathyroidism. This results in marked elevation of serum calcium and phosphorus, alkaline phosphatase, and BUN. By far the most common cause is uremia.

The following sequence of events is responsible for secondary hyperparathyroidism that could eventually result in tertiary hyperparathyroidism: With loss of renal function, the ability of the kidney to excrete phosphate diminishes and hyperphosphatemia occurs. This causes a lowering of serum calcium, apparently by driving calcium into the bone and other tissues. This could result in calcification of soft tissues. In an effort to keep the serum calcium normal, the parathyroid glands are stimulated. As renal function decreases further, there is diminished conversion of 25-hydroxyvitamin $D_3$ to 1,25-dihydroxyvitamin $D_3$. This results in impaired intestinal absorption of calcium. Softening of bones due to failure of calcification occurs and the parathyroid glands are further stimulated. (See Osteomalacia, Chap. 10.) As a consequence of continued parathyroid stimulation, there is increased PTH secretion and hypercalcemia. Metabolic bone disease secondary to renal failure is termed *renal osteodystrophy*.

There are several syndromes in which hyperparathyroidism is associated with other diseases. In multiple endocrine adenomatosis type I, hyperparathyroidism coexists with adenomas of the pituitary and pancreatic islets and often is associated with severe peptic ulceration and, sometimes, with adrenal tumors. In multiple endocrine adenomatosis type II, hyperparathyroidism is associated with pheochromocytoma, a tumor of the adrenal medulla, and with medullary thyroid carcinoma.

## LABORATORY FINDINGS

### Diagnostic Studies

Increased serum calcium (11 mg/dl–13 mg/dl) is the single most important test in the diagnosis of primary hyperparathyroidism. It should be elevated on at least three occasions. Levels >13 mg/dl suggest nonparathyroid causes of hypercalcemia (*e.g.*, malignant tumors, multiple myeloma, and hypervitaminosis D).

Decreased serum phosphate (<3.8 mg/dl). This is lower in hyperparathyroidism than in nonparathyroid hypercalcemia.

Increased serum chloride—levels above 103 mEq/liter strongly suggest hyperparathyroidism in the absence of thyrotoxicosis; levels below 103 mEq/liter suggest nonparathyroid hypercalcemia in the absence of diuretic administration or vomiting.

Normal hematocrit is characteristic of primary hyperparathyroidism; hematocrit <37% is often found in nonparathyroid hypercalcemia because this is most frequently associated with malignant tumors.

Lafferty uses the above parameters in the following discriminant formula, constructed so that a positive score indicates hyperparathyroid hypercalcemia and a negative score suggests nonparathyroid hypercalcemia:[7]

$$0.22 \text{ HCT} + 0.76 \text{ Cl} - 1.5 \text{ Ca}_{ex} - 1.9 \text{ P} - 7.44*†$$

### Other Laboratory Findings

Increased urine phosphate due to decreased renal tubular reabsorption

Increased urine calcium due to increased intestinal absorption, increased renal tubular reabsorption, and increased mobilization from bone

* HCT = hematocrit
  Cl = chloride
  $Ca_{ex}$ = the difference between the total serum calcium and the upper limits of normal in a given laboratory
  P = phosphorus
† The formula is not useful in separating hyperparathyroid patients from normal patients. Patients who are vomiting or using diuretics might be misclassified using this formula.

Increased urine volume due to increased urinary phosphate and calcium

Decreased and fixed urine specific gravity—result of hypercalcemic interference with renal concentrating ability

Decreased serum $p$H and bicarbonate (metabolic acidosis) due to renal loss of bicarbonate

Increased serum PTH, which must be correlated with serum calcium:
  High serum calcium—primary hyperparathyroidism
  Low serum calcium—secondary hyperparathyroidism, as in chronic renal disease
  In patients with hypercalcemia due to malignant disease, PTH values are generally lower than those seen with hyperparathyroidism, but *with significant overlap*.

Radioimmunoassay of PTH might help in the patient with borderline elevation of serum calcium, unresolved metabolic bone disease, or recurrent calcium stone formation, but is not usually needed to diagnose hyperparathyroidism.

A major cause of variability in PTH determinations is that the available immunoassays measure different portions of the PTH. Some assays measure carboxy-terminal fragments and intact PTH, whereas others measure the amino-terminal portion of the PTH molecule. The latter is the biologically active region of the molecule. In a study of 29 patients with hypercalcemia, Raisz *et al* had serum PTH assays done by four commercial laboratories and observed, " . . . we found considerable variation in the frequency of elevated values [of PTH] in hyperparathyroidism and the degree to which the assay discriminated between primary hyperparathyroidism and hypercalcemia of malignancy . . . it is still necessary to use multiple tests in the differential diagnosis of hypercalcemia."[11]

## HYPOPARATHYROIDISM

Hypoparathyroidism is an uncommon clinical disorder.[3] Damage or accidental removal of the parathyroid glands following surgical excision of the thyroid gland is the most common cause of hypoparathyroidism. Idiopathic hypoparathyroidism, in which there is severe damage to all four parathyroid glands, is possibly due to an autoimmune mechanism. Parathyroid antibodies may be demonstrated in about one third of cases. Idiopathic hypoparathyroidism occasionally occurs in association with a syndrome of adrenal insufficiency, diabetes mellitus, hypothyroidism, and ovarian failure.

Hypoparathyroidism results from deficiency, ineffectiveness, or resistance of PTH with resultant inability to stimulate target tissues. Consequently, there is impaired renal phosphate excretion and renal calcium reabsorption and decreased renal production of 1,25-dihydroxyvitamin $D_3$. This affects calcium and skeletal metabolism.

Pseudohypoparathyroidism, also known as *Albright's hereditary osteodystrophy,* is a rare, usually familial, disorder. In this condition, the parathyroid glands are normal but there appears to be resistance of bones and renal tubules to the actions of PTH. The findings are hypocalcemia, hyperphosphatemia, increased PTH, developmental skeletal abnormalities, mental retardation, and soft-tissue calcifications.

The symptoms and signs of hypoparathyroidism are largely attributable to hypocalcemia. Diminished calcium-ion concentration in extracellular fluid increases the excitability of motor-nerve fibers and lowers the threshold of peripheral sensory-nerve receptors to excitation. These effects of hypocalcemia are antagonized by magnesium and enhanced by potassium. With severe hypocalcemia, spontaneous nerve activity occurs, giving rise to tingling and numbness of the hands, feet, and mouth and tongue area; convulsions; and spasm of smooth and skeletal muscles. This complex is called *tetany*. Other symptoms of hypoparathyroidism include emotional lability, anxiety, depression, delirium, and mental retardation.

## LABORATORY FINDINGS

Increased serum phosphorus, which reflects increased renal reabsorption of phosphorus

Decreased serum calcium—decreased PTH and 1,25-dihydroxyvitamin $D_3$ result in decreased calcium entry into the blood from bones, GI tract, and renal tubules

Decreased urine calcium and phosphorus

Decreased or undetectable serum parathyroid hormone; increased PTH occurs in pseudohypoparathyroidism

Increased serum $p$H, bicarbonate (metabolic alkalosis)—due to renal retention of bicarbonate

## *PRECOCIOUS PUBERTY*

*Precocious puberty* indicates sexual development before the age of 10 in boys and before the age of 8 in girls. This is due to early secretion of increased gonadotropins by the pituitary. It is manifested by spermatogenesis in boys and onset of menses in girls. True precocious puberty might be secondary to lesions in the brain involving the posterior hypothalamus. Other hypothalamic functions may also be disturbed, resulting in diabetes insipidus, obesity, emotional lability, somnolence, or unstable temperature control.

*Pseudoprecocious puberty* refers to the early development of secondary sexual characteristics without spermatogenesis or menarche and is independent of gonadotropin secretion. Approximately 60% of affected boys have significant organic disease of the brain, adrenals, or gonads, whereas only 20% of girls have similar findings. Pseudoprecocious puberty is usually due to congenital adrenal hyperplasia, in the boy, or to hormonally active testicular or ovarian tumors.

## LABORATORY FINDINGS

Increased pituitary gonadotropins in true precocious puberty

Decreased or low-normal pituitary gonadotropins in pseudoprecocious puberty

**Girls**

Estrogen effect seen on Pap smear

Increased estrogens due to granulosa cell tumor of the ovary

**Boys**

Increased HCG in choriocarcinoma of the testis

Increased urinary pregnanetriol or serum 17-hydroxyprogesterone in congenital adrenal hyperplasia

Increased serum free testosterone in interstitial cell tumor of the testis

## ECTOPIC HORMONE PRODUCTION

*Ectopic hormone production* refers to hormone production by a neoplasm of an organ that is not generally accepted as the site of production of the hormone in question.[6] Currently, nearly 40 different neuroendocrine cell systems have been identified; these are widely dispersed throughout the body. They are found in such sites as the carotid body and other chemoreceptors, the thyroid gland, thymus, lung, GI tract, pancreas, and adrenals. Each of these cell systems may undergo physiologic hyperplasia or may form benign or malignant tumors, which secrete various hormones. The clinical syndromes produced are indistinguishable from disorders of the endocrine glands normally producing those hormones. Ectopic hormone secretion is usually, but not always, autonomous (*i.e.*, the ectopic hormone is not suppressed by mechanisms that suppress the normally produced hormone).

### LABORATORY FINDINGS

The most commonly produced hormones that are formed at ectopic sites are listed below. For the laboratory findings see the disorder indicated.

ACTH—small-cell (oat cell) carcinoma of lung, epithelial thymoma, pancreatic islet-cell tumor, medullary carcinoma of thyroid, bronchial carcinoid tumor (see Cushing's Syndrome)

ADH (vasopressin)—small-cell (oat cell) carcinoma of lung (see Syndrome of Inappropriate ADH Secretion)

PTH—squamous cell carcinoma of lung, adenocarcinoma of kidney (see Hyperparathyroidism)

Non–islet-cell tumors producing hypoglycemia—fibrosarcoma, liposarcoma, mesothelioma, leiomyosarcoma, hepatoma, adrenocortical carcinoma (see Hypoglycemia)

Erythropoietin—cerebellar hemangioblastoma, uterine fibromas, liver carcinoma (see Secondary Erythrocytosis, Chap. 8)

HCG—carcinoma of lung, kidney, liver, adrenal gland

Calcitonin—small cell (oat cell) carcinoma of the lung, breast cancer (see Carcinoma of the Thyroid)

# REFERENCES

1. Austin LA, Heath H: Calcitonin. N Engl J Med 304:269–278, 1981
2. Bravo EL, Tarazi RC, Fouad FM et al: Clonidine-suppression test. N Engl J Med 305:623–626, 1981
3. Breslau NA, Pak CYC: Hypoparathyroidism. Metabolism 28:1261–1276, 1979
4. Catalona WJ: Tumor markers in testicular cancer. Urol Clin North Am 6:613–628, 1979
5. Hiramatusu K, Yamada T, Yukimura Y et al: A screening test to identify aldosterone-producing adenoma by measuring plasma renin activity. Arch Intern Med 141:1589–1593, 1981
6. Imura H: Ectopic hormone syndromes. Clin Endocrinol Metab 9:235–260, 1980
7. Lafferty FW: Primary hyperparathyroidism. Arch Intern Med 141:1761–1766, 1981
8. Malgelada JR, Davis CS, O'Fallon WM et al: Laboratory diagnosis of gastrinoma. Mayo Clin Proc 57:211–218, 1982
9. National Diabetes Data Group: Classification and diagnosis of diabetes mellitus and other categories of glucose intolerance. Diabetes 28:1039–1057, 1979
10. Oberfield SE: Diabetes insipidus and other disorders of water balance. Pediatr Ann 9:384–389, 1980
11. Raisz LG, Yajnik CH, Bockman RS et al: Comparison of commercially available parathyroid immunoassays in the differential diagnosis of hypercalcemia due to primary hyperparathyroidism or malignancy. Ann Intern Med 91:739–740, 1979
12. Ram CVS, Engleman K: Pheochromocytoma, recognition and management. Curr Probl Cardiol 4:1–37, 1979
13. Salans LB: Diabetes mellitus, a disease that is coming into focus. JAMA 247:590–594, 1982
14. Sever PS, Roberts JC, Snell ME: Phaeochromocytoma. Clin Endocrinol Metab 9:543–568, 1980
15. Williams TF: Diabetes mellitus. Clin Endocrinol Metab 10:179–194, 1981
16. Yen SSC: The polycystic ovary syndrome. Clin Endocrinol 12:177–207, 1980

# BIBLIOGRAPHY

Felig P, Baxter JD, Broadus AE et al: Endocrinology and Metabolism. New York, McGraw-Hill, 1981
Ryan WG: Endocrine Disorders: A Pathophysiologic Approach, 2nd ed. Chicago, Year Book Medical Publishers, 1980
Watts NB, Keffer JH: Practical Endocrine Diagnosis, 3rd ed. Philadelphia, Lea & Febiger, 1982
Williams RH: Textbook of Endocrinology, 6th ed. Philadelphia, WB Saunders, 1981

# 7

# *NEUROLOGIC DISEASES*

## *MENINGITIS*

Meningitis is inflammation of the meningeal coverings of the brain and spinal cord. It may be due to a great variety of pathogenic organisms including bacteria, mycobacteria, rickettsiae, fungi, and viruses.

The most common route by which microorganisms reach the central nervous system (CNS) is the bloodstream. Primary sources of infection include adjacent infected foci, penetrating cranial injuries, the lungs, the heart valves, the placenta, and the birth canal. In most patients the precise route by which bacteria infect the meninges cannot be determined.

It has been postulated that the entry of blood-borne bacteria into the subarachnoid space is facilitated by damage to the barrier that normally separates the vascular circulation from the cerebrospinal circulation. This damage may follow trauma, circulating endotoxin, or an antecedent viral infection of the meninges. Once organisms enter the subarachnoid space, they grow in the cerebrospinal fluid (CSF). The circulation of the CSF aids in rapid dissemination of the infecting organisms throughout the subarachnoid space. Dural sinus thrombophlebitis may be a complication of meningitis (see Dural Sinus Thrombophlebitis). A superficial brain inflammation, *encephalitis*, usually accompanies purulent meningitis.

The most common meningeal pathogens, accounting for 80% to 90% of cases, are type B *Hemophilus influenzae, Neisseria meningitidis,* and *Streptococcus pneumoniae.* Meningococci and *H. influenzae* are frequently found in the nasopharynx of a carrier. The meningococcal carrier state may last for a few days or months; it enhances the immunity of the host. The factors that predispose such carriers to bloodstream invasion include lack of adequate levels of immunity, prior viral respiratory-tract infection, and pneumococcal pneumonia. Meningococcal antibodies are present in most adult serum, and they play a role in preventing disease. The newborn very rarely contracts meningococcal meningitis but, with loss of maternal antibodies, susceptibility appears. The risk of this disease is greatest between the ages of 6 months and 24 months. Meningococci in the bloodstream damage blood-vessel walls producing petechiae and, occasionally, intravascular coagulopathy. In meningococcemia, foci of infection develop in the skin, joints, lungs, ears, and adrenal glands.

Meningitis due to type B *H. influenzae* occurs most frequently between 2 months and 7 years of age. Few people in this age group have *Hemophilus* antibodies; most are, therefore, susceptible to infection with this organism. Infection usually begins as nasopharyngitis, probably initiated by a viral respiratory-tract infection.

The incidence of meningitis is increased in the very young and in the elderly. In these patients, the disease process tends to increase in severity. Factors that have been implicated as predisposing neonates to meningitis include premature rupture of the fetal membranes, prolonged labor, maternal infection during the last week of pregnancy, and infection with Group B streptococci from the birth canal. *Escherichia coli* meningitis in the newborn may be due to impaired antibody formation in the first few months of life or to increased gastrointestinal (GI) permeability to *E. coli.* Premature infants placed in a humidified environment might develop septicemia and meningitis owing to organisms such as *Pseudomonas aeruginosa* and *Serratia marcescens,* which proliferate in a moist atmosphere.

Leukemia, lymphoma, multiple myeloma, and Hodgkin's disease have all been associated with increased CNS infections. These infections occur as a consequence of decreased production of normal immunoglobulins, delayed and defective antibody response to bacteria, production of abnormal immunoglobulins, decreased macrophage activity, and depression of cellular immunity. CNS infection also occurs with increased incidence and severity in immunosuppressed and debilitated patients, in alcoholics, and in patients with diabetes mellitus or renal failure. The patient whose reticuloendothelial system has been suppressed by disease or medication is likely to be infected with such organisms as *Corynebacterium diphtheriae, Listeria monocytogenes, Pseudomonas aeruginosa, Serratia marcescens,* and *Staphylococcus aureus.* In addition, CNS infection in this setting is more frequent with such uncommon organisms as *Nocardia, Aspergillus, Candida, Cryptococcus, Mucor,* cytomegalovirus, and herpesvirus.

Tuberculous meningitis is not commonly seen today because there is a general decrease in systemic tuberculosis. Meningeal involvement is secondary to bloodstream spread from a pulmonary tuberculous infection. It may also occasionally occur as a complication of miliary or widespread tuberculosis with extensive mycobacterial seeding of the meninges. Meningeal foci rupture and discharge organisms into the subarachnoid space and spinal fluid (see Tuberculosis, Chap. 2).

*Cryptococcus neoformans* is the most frequent fungal CNS infection. Primary infection begins in the respiratory tract and may spread to the brain through the bloodstream. In addition to the meninges, the cerebral cortex may also be involved. Cryptococcal meningitis is frequently found in association with chronic debilitating diseases such as diabetes mellitus and Hodgkin's disease (see Cryptococcosis, Chap. 2).

## LABORATORY FINDINGS

The diagnosis of CNS infection is made primarily by documentation of changes within the CSF obtained by lumbar puncture (Fig. 7-1).[9] A deep yellow color of spinal fluid is derived primarily from bilirubin pigment. In the absence of hemorrhage, this is most frequently associated with elevated protein concentration and may be seen when the CSF circulation has been impaired. Increased CSF protein generally accompanies an increase in white blood cells (WBC) and is the result of injury to the meninges by an inflammatory process and subsequent passive diffusion of albumin into the CSF from serum. As few as 200 WBC/$\mu$l to 300 WBC/$\mu$l impart haziness to CSF; 500 WBC/$\mu$l give the CSF an opalescent appearance; and 700 WBC/$\mu$l to 800 WBC/$\mu$l cause a turbid appearance. Fluid containing thousands of cells will look like pus. Polymorphonuclear leukocytes predominate in bacterial infections, whereas

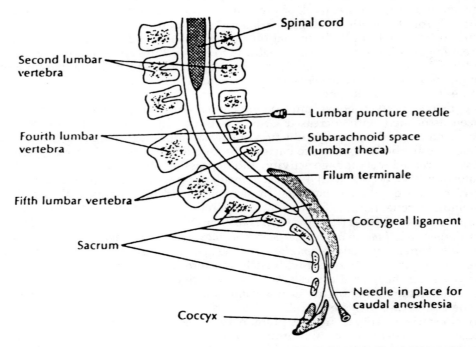

**Fig. 7-1.** Lumbar puncture, showing the needle inserted through the third lumbar intervertebral space, caudal to the termination of the spinal cord. (Albernaz JG: Nervous system. In Didio LJA: Synopsis of Anatomy, p 383. St Louis, CV Mosby, 1970)

lymphocytes predominate in tuberculous and nonbacterial infections. A lack of cells does not invariably exclude the possibility of bacterial meningitis but this certainly is a rare occurrence. Various stains (Gram's, immunofluorescent, acid-fast, auramine–rhodamine, india ink) and cultures on several media should be done on CSF to identify the pathogenic organism. There is a decrease in CSF glucose in bacterial, tuberculous, mycotic, and carcinomatous meningitis. Decreased CSF glucose is the result of increased glucose utilization by rapidly growing microorganisms, phagocytosis of bacteria by WBC, and impaired glucose transport into the CSF from the bloodstream across the inflammatory exudate.

## Acute Bacterial Meningitis

*CSF*
CSF appears opalescent to purulent, slightly yellow, and might have a coarse clot.

Protein 50 mg/dl–1500 mg/dl (usually 100 mg/dl–500 mg/dl)

Glucose 0 mg/dl–40 mg/dl; <31% of the blood glucose concentration[12]

WBC 100 $\mu$l to >50,000/$\mu$l (usually 4,000/$\mu$l–10,000/$\mu$l), 85%–95% neutrophils; as the disease progresses there is a gradual increase in lymphocytes and large mononuclear cells. Cell counts above 50,000/$\mu$l raise the possibility that a brain abscess has ruptured into the subarachnoid space. (see Brain Abscess)

One or more bacterial organisms are usually seen on a gram-stained smear and recovered on culture—usually *Hemophilus influenzae, Neisseria meningitidis, Streptococcus pneumoniae*; in newborns, *Escherichia coli* and group B streptococci are frequently recovered. Prior antibiotic treatment decreases the frequency of positive cultures.

Through counterimmunoelectrophoresis and latex agglutination, soluble bacterial capsular antigens in CSF may be detected. These tests are of great help for rapid diagnosis and also for diagnosis after treatment has been started and the smears and cultures are negative. They are used to test for the antigens of meningococcus, pneumococcus, *H. influenzae,* and group B streptococci.

Increased CSF lactate dehydrogenase (LDH), especially $LDH_4$ and $LDH_5$, which are derived from granulocytes

*Other Laboratory Findings*
Blood cultures are positive in 40%–60% of patients with bacterial meningitis.

Nasopharyngeal cultures often yield pathogenic *H. influenzae* or *N. meningitidis.*

Leukocytosis with a shift to the left

Markedly increased serum C-reactive protein

## Tuberculous Meningitis

CSF appears opalescent, slightly yellow; a delicate clot may be seen

Protein 45 mg/dl–500 mg/dl (usually 100 mg/dl–200 mg/dl)

Glucose 10 mg/dl–40 mg/dl; not usually as low as in bacterial meningitis

WBC 25/$\mu$l–500/$\mu$l, chiefly lymphocytes; neutrophils may equal lymphocytes early in the infection

Organisms may be seen on an acid-fast- or auramine–rhodamine-stained smear of the fibrin clot or pellicle and recovered on culture.

Decreased serum sodium—this might be due to inappropriate secretion of antidiuretic hormone

**Cryptococcal Meningitis**

CSF appears normal.

Protein 20 mg/dl–50 mg/dl

Glucose reduced in more than half of the cases

WBC 0/$\mu$l–800/$\mu$l (average 50/$\mu$l), chiefly lymphocytes

Identification of organisms on india ink or Nigrosin wet-mount preparation and isolation of *Cryptococcus* on culture

Latex agglutination test of CSF and serum detects cryptococcal capsular antigen. This is more sensitive than the use of india ink.

Indirect immunofluorescence and tube agglutination tests for cryptococcal antibodies; these usually become positive after the latex agglutination test becomes negative

# VIRAL INFECTIONS

Viruses gain entrance to the body through several pathways. The most common viruses—mumps, measles, and varicella—enter the body through the respiratory passages. Polioviruses and other enteroviruses enter by the oral route; herpes simplex virus enters through oral or genital routes. Rabies is acquired as a result of animal bites, and arbovirus infections are the result of mosquito bites. The fetus may be infected *in utero* by rubella virus or cytomegalovirus.

Following entry into the body viruses multiply, usually giving rise to primary viremia and systemic dissemination. Further replication results in continued or secondary viremia, during which phase the virus often involves the CNS. Viremia usually terminates coincidentally with the appearance in the circulation of interferon and the specific viral antibody. Virus infections of the brain produce two distinct syndromes: aseptic meningitis and encephalitis. In aseptic meningitis, the inflammatory process is confined to the meninges. In viral encephalitis, viruses invade and destroy nerve cells in the brain. Viral inclusion bodies are seen within the involved cells. Inflammation and thrombosis of small vessels contribute to widespread destruction of cerebral tissue. There is often also swelling and inflammation of the spinal cord.

## ASEPTIC MENINGITIS

The term *aseptic meningitis* is used for any suspected CNS viral inflammation in which there is a predominance of lymphocytes in the CSF. A specific cause cannot be established in one third or more of cases of presumed viral origin. Aseptic meningitis occurs more frequently than does bacterial meningitis. The most common causes of viral meningitis are the enteroviruses, which include echoviruses, coxsackieviruses, and the polioviruses. Enteroviruses initially replicate in the intestinal epithelium, enter the bloodstream, and then involve the meninges, where further replication occurs. Lifelong immunity follows infection by a particular enterovirus serotype, but there is no protective immunity to infection with other serotypes. Other viruses that cause aseptic meningitis are mumps virus, herpes simplex virus, and lymphocytic choriomeningitis virus. Clinical and laboratory findings similar to those seen in aseptic meningitis occur with leukemic and lymphomatous meningeal infiltration or carcinomatous metastases to the meninges.

## LABORATORY FINDINGS

### CSF

Clear, turbid, or xanthochromic

Protein 20 mg/dl–200 mg/dl (usually 80 mg/dl–100 mg/dl)

Glucose normal

WBC <500/$\mu$l; chiefly neutrophils on the first day, then lymphocytes predominate; >1000 lymphocytes/$\mu$l usually occurs in lymphocytic choriomeningitis and may also occur with mumps and echovirus infections

Negative bacterial smears and cultures

Virus isolation

### Blood

Neutralization viral serologic tests show a fourfold rise in titer from acute to convalescent sera; the latter should be drawn 10 days to 2 weeks after the onset of illness.

Indirect immunofluorescent test for lymphocytic choriomeningitis may become positive 3 days after the onset of symptoms. Titers increase rapidly and decline slowly over several months.

### ACUTE ENCEPHALITIS

Encephalitis is a nonsuppurative inflammation of the substance of the brain. Susceptible neurons are directly invaded by virus and the cells are destroyed. Because the meninges are inflamed in most forms of encephalitis, the term *meningoencephalitis* is often used. When the spinal cord is also involved, this is termed *encephalomyelitis*.

### Arboviruses

Arboviruses are arthropod-borne viruses. Viruses that cause acute encephalitis and are transmitted by mosquitoes include eastern equine encephalomyelitis virus, western equine encephalomyelitis virus, St. Louis encephalitis virus, and California encephalitis virus. Arboviruses are inoculated directly into the bloodstream by infected mosquitoes. The viruses multiply within the blood-vessel lining cells within two to four days. They then reach the CNS, where further replication and encephalitis occur.

## LABORATORY FINDINGS

### CSF

*Early* (first 2–3 days):  Cell count <100/µl, mostly neutrophils
Protein and glucose normal

*Later* (after 3rd day):  Cell count 50 µl–500/µl, mostly lymphocytes
Protein up to 100 mg/dl
Glucose normal
Bacterial culture negative

### Blood

Viral serologic tests show fourfold increase in titer from acute to convalescent sera.

Hemagglutination inhibition and neutralization antibodies are detected within 1 week after onset of symptoms and persist for at least 8 years.
Complement-fixation antibodies first appear 2 to 3 weeks after onset and persist for 1 to 3 years (Fig. 7-2).

Isolation of virus from blood and CSF of patients during the acute disease is unusual.

## Herpes Simplex Virus

Herpes simplex virus may cause severe acute encephalitis, usually terminating in death. Type 1 herpes simplex virus is the single most important cause of fatal nonepidemic encephalitis in the United States. In herpes infection, the virus remains latent in nerve cells for long periods until immunity declines or some other factor activates an acute neurologic infection. Reactivated virus reaches the brain through the trigeminal or olfactory nerves (see Chap. 11).

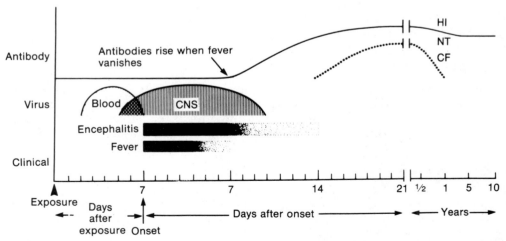

**Fig. 7-2.** Pathogenesis of arbovirus infection: Time course of clinical features, virus detection, and antibodies. (CNS, central nervous system; HI, hemagglutination inhibition; NT, neutralizing antibody; CF, complement fixation test.) (McLean DM: Virology in Health Care, p 167. Baltimore, Williams & Wilkins, 1980)

## LABORATORY FINDINGS

### CSF

Spinal fluid findings are similar to those described above for the arbovirus encephalitides.

Fourfold rise in herpes antibodies in 80%–85% of proven infections;[16] specificity ranges from 81% to 88%. Ratio of herpes simplex virus antibodies in serum to the same antibodies in CSF is <20 by the 5th or 6th day of the disease.

### Brain Biopsy

Herpesvirus may be cultured or identified by immunofluorescence, immunoperoxidase, or electron-microscopy techniques in 76% of cases.[16]

Culture of brain biopsy material is the most sensitive and specific diagnostic test.

## Herpes Zoster

Herpes zoster, also known as *shingles,* is a disease characterized by blisters and severe nerve pain in skin areas supplied by peripheral sensory nerves arising in infected dorsal root ganglia. It is caused by the varicella-zoster virus, which also causes chickenpox (see Chap. 11). In herpes zoster, the virus may infect spinal or cranial sensory ganglia, the posterior gray matter of the spinal cord, and adjacent meninges. Neurologic involvement may be in the clinical form of viral encephalomyelitis, aseptic meningitis, or postinfectious polyneuropathy. The latter is the most common form.

The pathogenesis is presumed to be as follows: After a primary infection with the varicella-zoster virus, seen as chickenpox, the virus makes its way from the initial skin lesions, along sensory nerves, to the sensory ganglia. The virus remains latent in the ganglionic nerve cells until it is activated. Activation occurs with decreased resistance and may accompany aging, tuberculosis, cancer, lymphomas, or treatment with immunosuppressive drugs or radiation. At the time of reactivation, the virus produces inflammation and necrosis of the sensory ganglia and then progresses down the nerve, causing severe nerve symptoms. The virus multiplies in the skin cells and causes skin blisters along the distribution of the affected nerve. If the inflammation spreads into the spinal cord and motor nerves, paralysis results.

## LABORATORY FINDINGS

### CSF

Cell count up to 300 lymphocytes/$\mu$l

Protein 20 mg/dl–110 mg/dl

### Skin Biopsy

Intranuclear inclusions in skin cells or in multinucleated giant cells

Immunofluorescent identification of the virus

## Poliomyelitis

Poliomyelitis is caused by the poliovirus, which enters the body orally, multiplies in the pharynx and intestine, and has a viremic stage but usually does not

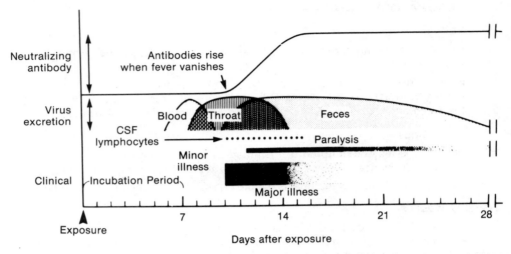

**Fig. 7-3.** Pathogenesis of poliomyelitis: Time course of clinical features, virus detection, and antibodies. (McLean DM: Virology in Health Care, p 68. Baltimore, Williams & Wilkins, 1980)

invade the CNS. When the virus does invade the CNS, aseptic meningitis occurs as a mild, nonparalytic disease. Rarely, encephalomyelitis occurs as a severe, paralytic disease. The virus affects primarily lower motor neurons in the anterior horn of the spinal cord and brain stem. Other neural structures affected include neurons of the cerebellum, basal ganglia, and the cerebral cortex. Pathogenesis is depicted in Figure 7-3.

## LABORATORY FINDINGS

### CSF

Cell count 25/$\mu$l–500/$\mu$l; at first, mostly neutrophils; after several days, lymphocytes predominate

Protein normal at first; 50 mg/dl–200 mg/dl within 2 weeks; normal by 6th week

Glucose normal

### Blood

Leukocytosis (<15,000/$\mu$l) within 1st week

Viral serologic tests show a fourfold increase in the titer of neutralizing antibody from acute to convalescent sera.

## Slow Virus Infections

Slow virus infections of the brain simulate degenerative neurologic diseases. In these disorders, the infecting viral agent continues to multiply within the host, producing progressive disability over a period of many months or years. Slow viral infections include subacute sclerosing panencephalitis, which is due to measles virus; progressive rubella panencephalitis, and progressive multifocal leukoencephalopathy, which is due to papovavirus. The latter disorder is usually encountered in association with chronic lymphocytic leukemia, Hodgkin's disease, lymphosarcoma, or sarcoidosis. The impaired immunologic status in these disorders contributes to activation of the papovavirus infection. The pathogenesis of these diseases is not yet understood. Death occurs within months to years.

## LABORATORY FINDINGS

### CSF

Increased $\gamma$-globulin, especially IgG

Slight increase in lymphocytes

Moderate increase in protein

Increased measles antibody titer in subacute sclerosing panencephalitis

Increased rubella antibody titer in progressive rubella panencephalitis

Normal CSF in progressive multifocal leukoencephalopathy

### Serum

Increased measles antibody titer in subacute sclerosing panencephalitis

Increased rubella antibody titer in progressive rubella panencephalitis

### Brain Biopsy

Brain biopsy is required for a definitive diagnosis of progressive multifocal leukoencephalopathy.

## *NEUROSYPHILIS*

Syphilis is caused by *Treponema pallidum* and is contracted by sexual contact (see also Chaps. 1 and 11). Following the initial infection, the organisms gain access to the CNS, presumably through perineural and perivascular spaces.[10,14] This usually occurs within 3 months to 18 months. Meningitis and inflammation of the meningeal blood vessels constitute the initial stage of neurologic involvement.

The late or chronic stages of CNS syphilis include meningovascular syphilis, general paresis, tabes dorsalis, optic atrophy, and meningomyelitis. Meningovascular syphilis is usually seen 6 years to 7 years after the initial infection. In this stage there are inflammation and thrombosis of cerebral vessels with resulting infarctions in the brain.

Paretic neurosyphilis involves the frontal and temporal lobes of the brain and is seen clinically as progressive mental and physical deterioration with dementia, impaired speech, tremors, seizures, and delusions. It is also known as *general paresis of the insane.* This occurs 15 years to 20 years after the original infection. Paresis is a subacute encephalitis with thickening of the meninges, atrophy of the brain, and diffuse vasculitis. Spirochetes in the brain substance may be demonstrated by special staining techniques.

Tabetic neurosyphilis is characterized clinically by lightninglike pains, unstable walking, loss of sensation in the feet, numbness and tingling in many body areas, and urinary incontinence. Tabetic crises consist of sudden attacks of abdominal pain, nausea, and vomiting. All of these symptoms reflect syphilitic involvement of dorsal root ganglia, sensory-nerve roots, and sensory columns of the spinal cord.

Syphilitic optic atrophy appears as progressive blindness. Meningomyelitis becomes manifest in sensory- and motor-nerve disorders of the spinal cord.

## LABORATORY FINDINGS

### Serologic Tests for Syphilis[10,14]

Positive serum FTA-ABS test (95%) and VDRL test (75%)—negative VDRL usually occurs in late neurosyphilis

Positive CSF VDRL test (25%–82%)—this is highly specific for neurosyphilis but not very sensitive. Positive CSF VDRL test with a positive serum FTA-ABS is diagnostic of neurosyphilis. There are no standard procedures for the FTA-ABS test on spinal fluid.

### CSF[10,14]

Normal findings (30%)

*Active disease*

WBC 200/$\mu$l–300/$\mu$l, mostly lymphocytes

Protein 40 mg/dl–200 mg/dl

Increased $\gamma$-globulin.

Normal glucose

## *EPIDURAL ABSCESS*

An epidural abscess is a collection of pus outside the dura, which is the firm outer meningeal covering of the brain (Fig. 7-4). This localized infection more frequently involves the epidural space of the spine than it does that of the skull. In spinal epidural abscess the source is often infected hair follicles of the back, bacteremia, or osteomyelitis of adjacent vertebrae. Epidural pus may extend widely and cause compression of the spinal cord and veins of the cord. The meningeal vessels become infected and occluded by thrombi, further injuring the spinal cord.

## LABORATORY FINDINGS

Leukocytosis

Culture of abscess—the most common organism is *Staphylococcus aureus;* other organisms include streptococci, gram-negative bacilli, anaerobes

### CSF

WBC 20/$\mu$l–100/$\mu$l

Protein 100 mg/dl–400 mg/dl

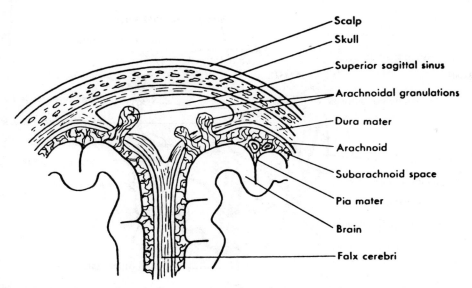

**Fig. 7-4.** Frontal section through the medial portion of the head illustrates the meningeal coverings of the brain. (Albernaz JG: Nervous System. In Dido LJA: Synopsis of Anatomy, p 379. St Louis, CV Mosby, 1970)

Glucose normal

Cultures normal

### Laboratory Findings of Underlying Conditions

Vertebral osteomyelitis (see Chap. 9)

Bacteremia due to dental, respiratory, or skin infections or abscesses at other sites

Diabetes mellitus (see Chap. 6)

## SUBDURAL EMPYEMA

A subdural empyema is a collection of pus beneath the dura and outside the arachnoid meninges (see Fig. 7-4). This usually results from the direct extension of infected nasal sinuses or, less often, from a middle-ear infection. It may also occur following penetrating wounds of the skull or osteomyelitis of the skull or as a complication of meningitis or brain abscess. Infection spreads through infected bone or infected dural venous sinuses (Fig. 7-5). This accounts for the development of an empyema at a distance away from the original focus of infection.

### LABORATORY FINDINGS

Leukocytosis 20,000/$\mu$l–40,000/$\mu$l

Cultures of empyema—in about half the cases, no organisms can be cultured or seen on Gram's stain. Nonhemolytic streptococci are the most common

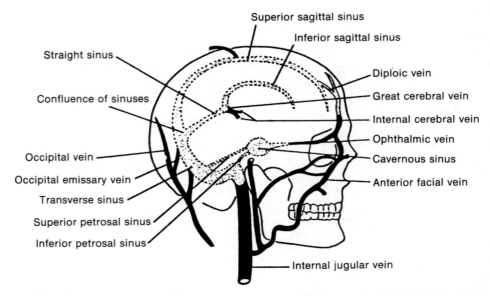

**Fig. 7-5.** The dural venous sinuses, the internal jugular vein, and some diploic and emissary veins. (Albernaz JG: Nervous System. In Didio LJA: Synopsis of Anatomy, p 393. St Louis, CV Mosby, 1970)

organisms when the preceding condition is sinusitis. *Staphylococcus aureus* or gram-negative organisms are usually recovered following trauma or surgery.

**CSF**

WBC 50/$\mu$l–1000/$\mu$l; 20%–80% neutrophils

Protein 75 mg/dl–300 mg/dl

Normal glucose

Cultures negative

## BRAIN ABSCESS

A brain abscess is a collection of pus within the substance of the brain. Most abscesses arise from sinusitis, mastoiditis, or middle-ear infections. About one third of brain abscesses are from blood-borne infections elsewhere in the body. These are commonly secondary to suppurative processes in the lungs, such as bronchiectasis, lung abscess, or pleural empyema. Less frequently, brain abscess follows acute infective endocarditis. About 20% of cases have no clearly identifiable sources. A small proportion of brain abscesses follows skull fracture in which infection is introduced from the outside.

### LABORATORY FINDINGS

Leukocytes are normal or increased up to 15,000/$\mu$l.

Increased sedimentation rate

If the subarachnoid space becomes involved by extension of the abscess to the surface of the brain or to the ventricles, then the CSF findings will be those of bacterial meningitis with grossly purulent spinal fluid and WBC >50,000/μl

In recent years, cultures of brain abscesses have shown increased isolation of obligate anaerobes, especially *Bacteroides* species. Anaerobic streptococci are also frequently isolated.[2] These organisms usually originate in the lung. Enteric organisms are almost always associated with ear infections, and staphylococcal abscess commonly follows penetrating head trauma or bacteremia.

### CSF (when meninges are not involved)

WBC 20/μl–300/μl; 10%–80% neutrophils

Protein <100 mg/dl

Glucose normal

Culture negative

### Laboratory Findings of Underlying Diseases

Lung abscess, pleural empyema, bronchiectasis (see Chap. 2) infective endocarditis (see Chap 1)

## DURAL SINUS THROMBOPHLEBITIS

Venous drainage of the brain occurs through the cerebral veins, which flow into several large channels known as *dural sinuses*. The sinuses drain into the jugular veins (Fig. 7-5). Dural sinuses may become occluded when there is infection in the epidural or subdural spaces, meningitis, brain abscess, skull injury, clot formation (in polycythemia vera or sickle cell anemia), or tumor emboli. Severe dehydration also may lead to dural sinus thrombosis.

Occlusion of cerebral veins results in increased intracranial pressure, headache, seizures, fever, and toxemia. Infected emboli may be released from the veins into the bloodstream, causing pulmonary sepsis and petechiae in the skin and mucous membranes.

Thrombosis of the transverse or lateral sinus is usually secondary to chronic infection of the middle ear and mastoid air cells. Cavernous sinus thrombosis is usually secondary to acute suppurative processes in the orbit, nasal sinuses, or upper half of the face. The superior sagittal or longitudinal sinus is less commonly the site of an infective thrombosis than are the other venous sinuses.

### LABORATORY FINDINGS

Leukocytosis

Positive blood culture in about 50% of cases

CSF—usually normal, but may show 10 WBC/μl–4000 WBC/μl and slightly increased protein

## REYE'S SYNDROME

Reye's syndrome is an acute neurologic disorder of childhood. It is of unknown cause and is accompanied by fatty degeneration of the liver and kidneys.[3]

Reye's syndrome is usually preceded by influenza or varicella virus infections, although no virus has been identified as a cause of this rapidly progressive and often fatal disease.

The brain becomes markedly swollen owing to extracellular edema. Cerebral symptoms may be due in part to profound hypoglycemia, marked hyperammonemia, and an increase in circulating short-chain fatty acids. These metabolic disturbances reflect severe liver impairment. The liver is the site of marked lipid deposits but there is no sign of inflammation or liver cell necrosis. Fatty deposits in the kidneys may result in azotemia.

The mechanisms of this disorder are not clear, but most evidence suggests that it results from widespread injury to hepatic and neuronal mitochondria. Hepatocellular damage results in disruption of fatty-acid and carbohydrate metabolism.

### LABORATORY FINDINGS

Markedly increased serum ammonia; increased serum glutamic-oxaloacetic transaminase (SGOT) (AST [aspartate aminotransferase]), serum glutamic-pyruvic transaminase (SGPT) (ALT [alanine aminotransferase]), amino acids, fatty acids, and LDH reflect hepatic injury

Increased blood urea nitrogen (BUN) and creatinine reflect renal injury.

Increased lactic acid, decreased bicarbonate, decreased $pH$ (metabolic acidosis) due to impaired oxidative metabolism

Later there is often decreased $PCO_2$ and increased $pH$ (respiratory alkalosis)—increased ammonia leads to hyperventilation

Decreased blood glucose, sodium, potassium

Prolonged prothrombin time reflects severe hepatic damage.

Normal serum bilirubin

Increased serum creatine phosphokinase (CPK), especially MM* (muscle) fraction, occurs in severely affected children. Progressive increase indicates a poor prognosis.

CSF glucose is decreased in proportion with the decreased blood glucose level.

## *MULTIPLE SCLEROSIS*

Multiple sclerosis is the most common of the demyelinating diseases. These are diseases characterized by a loss of myelin from the CNS. Complete loss of the lipid myelin sheath that surrounds nerve fibers interferes with their ability to conduct nerve impulses. Multiple sclerosis is manifested clinically by a great variety of features, which include motor weakness, tingling of the extremities, impaired vision and speech, tremors, irregular gait, bladder dysfunction, and altered emotional responses. In addition to its widespread involvement of the

---

* See definition on page 12 in Chapter 1.

brain and spinal cord, the disorder is characterized clinically by periods of remission and relapse.

There are discrete, irregularly shaped demyelinated lesions scattered throughout the CNS. The lesions are called *plaques* and they appear at different times during the course of the disease.

Although the gross and microscopic pathology help to explain some of the clinical features of multiple sclerosis, the pathogenesis of the disease remains obscure. Several theories that have been put forth have both experimental support and evidence that challenges them. The most promising theory at present is the suggestion than an initial viral insult is followed by a secondary mechanism, which is probably immunologic. A suggested sequence of events is initiated by the action of a slow virus on myelin basic protein. The protein acts as an antigen, stimulating production of antibody; this appears in the CSF as IgG. Myelin breakdown is detected as myelin basic protein in the spinal fluid and as myelin antibodies in the serum. The plaquelike zones of demyelination found in the brain and spinal cord are considered to be the scars that remain as the end stage of the disease.

## LABORATORY FINDINGS[4,8]

$$\text{Increased CSF IgG index } (>0.65) = \frac{\text{CSF IgG/CSF albumin}}{\text{Serum IgG/Serum albumin}}$$

The IgG index is reported to have a higher degree of sensitivity and specificity than have other laboratory tests for multiple sclerosis when cerebral infections and immunologic diseases are eliminated.[5]

Increased CSF IgG and IgG/total protein ratio (about 67% of patients)

Multiple discrete (oligoclonal) bands of CSF $\gamma$-globulins are seen when using high-resolution agarose gel electrophoresis (85%–95% of patients)

Slight increase in CSF mononuclear cells ($>50/\mu l$)—in 25% of patients during an acute episode; this reflects activity of the disease

Slight increase in CSF protein ($<100$ mg/dl)—in 25% of patients

Presence of myelin basic protein in CSF reflects fragments of myelin sheaths in the spinal fluid, indicating recent demyelination or acute disease activity

## *EPILEPSY*

*Epilepsy* has been defined as a disorder of the nervous system characterized by sudden recurrent attacks, usually with alteration of consciousness, with or without convulsive movements.

Seizures are episodic, abrupt, excessively rapid, and generally short-lived electrical discharges of cerebral neurons. The primary epileptic discharge results from instability or irritability of a group of neurons. A seizure usually begins with a local neuronal electrical discharge, which induces CNS dysfunction either at that site or at a distant site by spreading along nerve pathways.

Neuronal discharges may be monitored by means of an electroencephalogram (EEG); this is analogous to the use of an electrocardiogram (ECG) to monitor the electrical discharges from the heart. EEG patterns seen in idiopathic epilepsy are similar to those that may be seen in seizures caused by a brain tumor, anoxia, hypoglycemia, disturbances of blood electrolyte composition, convulsant drugs, or electric shock. This suggests that a common pathophysiology underlies many different seizure states.

In childhood, about 50% of convulsions are of unknown etiology. The remainder are secondary to fever or birth injury to the brain. Many adult patients with recurrent convulsive seizures have no demonstrable causes for their disorders. The diseases and conditions that are frequently accompanied by seizures include developmental and congenital defects, birth injuries, anoxia in infancy and childhood, acute infectious diseases of childhood, meningitis, encephalitis, cerebral trauma, tumors, abscesses, granulomas, parasitic cysts, CNS degenerative diseases, uremia, alcohol or drug withdrawal, cerebral edema, cerebrovascular lesions, polycythemia, asphyxia, carbon-monoxide poisoning, anaphylaxis, Raynaud's disease (a vascular occlusive disorder), Stokes-Adams syndrome (slow heart rate, fainting, cerebrovascular arteriosclerosis), tetany (hypocalcemia), insulin shock (hypoglycemia), hyperventilation (respiratory alkalosis), and ingestion of convulsant drugs.

## LABORATORY FINDINGS

Idiopathic epilepsy and many cases of seizures of known origin—no abnormal laboratory findings

Serum anticonvulsant levels are often necessary for optimal management of epileptic seizures and for the diagnosis of recurrent seizures.

Common antiepileptic drugs, which may require blood-level monitoring, include phenobarbital, phenytoin, carbamazepine, primidone, ethosuximide, methsuximide, diazepam, valproic acid, and clonazepam.

### Conditions That Cause Seizures and Have Associated Laboratory Abnormalities

Hypoglycemia (see Chap. 6)

Meningitis*

Encephalitis*

Cerebral infarction*

Cerebral hemorrhage*

Brain tumor*

Multiple sclerosis*

Sickle cell anemia (see Chap. 8)

Leukemia (see Chap. 8)

Phenylketonuria (see Chap. 10)

Von Gierke's disease (see Chap. 10)

Porphyria (see Chap. 10)

* Discussed in this chapter

# CEREBRAL INFARCTION

A cerebral infarction is an area of necrosis of brain tissue. It occurs as a consequence of oxygen or glucose deprivation. Cerebral infarction is commonly referred to as a *stroke*. When hypoxia lasts for less than a minute, no permanent damage results. The exact period of time of cerebral anoxia needed for neuronal necrosis to result has not been precisely established, but it is between 2 minutes and 5 minutes. After brain cells undergo necrosis, the supporting glial cells swell until they compress capillaries, preventing the return of blood to the ischemic area; the result is an infarct.

The causes of cerebral infarction are classified on the basis of whether there is normal or reduced cerebral blood flow. Infarction in the presence of normal blood flow results from pulmonary or anemic hypoxia or from hypoglycemia. Reduced cerebral blood flow is generalized or focal. Generalized reduction of cerebral blood flow may be the result of decreased cardiac output, hypertension, or extensive small-vessel occlusions.

By far the most common cause of focal cerebral infarction in adults is arterial thrombosis associated with arteriosclerotic disease of the intra- and extracranial vessels (see Atherosclerosis, Chap. 1). These vascular changes may be seen as early as the second or third decade of life. The vascular degenerative process is similar to that seen elsewhere in the vascular system. The severity of the process is greater and its development earlier in patients with diabetes mellitus or hypertension. Consequently there is a higher than normal incidence of cerebral infarction in patients with these disorders.

Cerebral embolism is a complication of heart disease. Its most frequent cause is an irregular heart rate and an irregular force known as *chronic atrial fibrillation*. The source of an embolus is usually a thrombus, or clot, attached to the inner lining of the left atrium. The thrombus usually develops as a result of impaired atrial blood flow secondary to a narrowed mitral valve that has been damaged in rheumatic heart disease. An embolus breaks off from the clot, enters the circulation, and blocks one of the small cerebral blood vessels. Another source of an embolus may be a thrombus formed on the damaged heart lining overlying the site of a myocardial infarct.

Sometimes hemorrhage occurs in an area of cerebral infarction. This reflects leakage of blood through the damaged vessels into surrounding tissues. About 65% of infarcts following cerebral embolism are hemorrhagic.[1] Emboli tend to lyse or fragment and the collateral circulation restores blood flow into the infarcted area. This results in hemorrhage into a zone of infarction and accounts for the presence of blood in the CSF.

## LABORATORY FINDINGS

### Cerebral Thrombosis

CSF usually entirely normal

CSF protein might be increased up to 50 mg/dl–80 mg/dl

CSF WBC might be increased up to 50/$\mu$l during first 48 hours; rarely there is a transient increase to 400/$\mu$l–2,000/$\mu$l about the third day.

Increased serum CPK (50% of patients)—appears after 2 days, peaks at 3 days, returns to normal by 14 days

Increased serum SGOT (AST) (50% of patients)—appears after 7 days

**Cerebral Embolism**

Usually the same as in cerebral thrombosis

Up to 65% of patients show slight xanthochromia—reflects the occurrence of hemorrhagic infarction

Rarely, a patient with a hemorrhagic infarct might show up to 10,000 RBC/$\mu$l.

## CEREBRAL HEMORRHAGE

*Cerebral hemorrhage* refers to bleeding into the meningeal spaces or into the brain itself (Fig. 7-6). Hemorrhage into the subdural or extradural spaces occurs

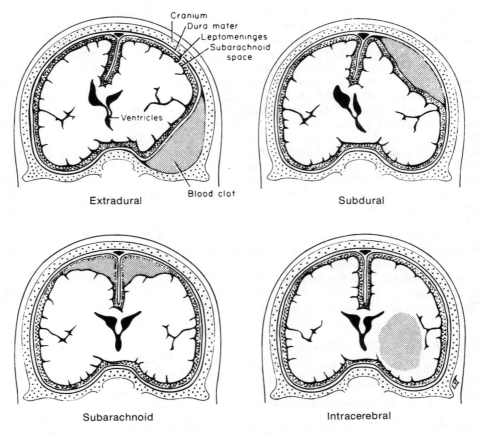

**Fig. 7-6.** Sites of cerebral hemorrhages. (Gilbert EE, Huntington RW: An Introduction to Pathology, p 325. New York, Oxford University Press, 1978)

almost exclusively as a result of trauma. Extradural hemorrhage develops between the dura and the skull and occurs in 0.4% to 3.0% of head injuries. It usually follows laceration of a meningeal artery by a skull fracture. Subdural hematoma is a collection of blood between the dura and the brain; it follows traumatic rupture of meningeal veins. In these hemorrhages, blood does not usually enter the spinal fluid circulation and it consequently is not detected on examination of the CSF.

Hemorrhage into the subarachnoid space is usually a consequence of head trauma or rupture of a saccular aneurysm. These aneurysms most commonly involve an artery of the circle of Willis at the base of the brain. Saccular or congenital aneurysms are presumed to result from developmental defects in the arterial wall. They are not consequences of atherosclerosis. Because of their appearance, they are often referred to as *berry aneurysms.* The aneurysms occur with increased frequency in association with segmental narrowing or coarctation of the aorta and with polycystic kidneys. In subarachnoid hemorrhage, the blood gains access to the cerebrospinal circulation. Within a few hours of the hemorrhage, a large amount of hemoglobin is released into the spinal fluid because of disruption of RBC. Bilirubin, which is a breakdown product of hemoglobin, appears in the CSF about 12 hours after a bleeding episode. Hemoglobin and bilirubin are irritating to the meninges and produce a transient outpouring of polymorphonuclear leukocytes.

Intracerebral hemorrhage is bleeding into the substance of the brain. This usually results from a rupture of a small penetrating artery or arteriole secondary to hypertension. Patients with long-standing hypertension develop degenerative changes in the muscle and elastic tissue of the blood-vessel walls. Hemorrhage is usually preceded by seizures, increased intracranial pressure, and a complex of transient neurologic symptoms termed *hypertensive encephalopathy.* Other causes of intracerebral hemorrhage include ruptured congenital aneurysm, vascular malformation, and bleeding disorders. Blood escaping into brain tissue destroys the area where the bleeding arises and acts as a rapidly expanding mass lesion, which displaces and compresses adjacent brain tissue. Blood seeps into the ventricles in more than 80% of patients, producing bloody CSF.[1] There are no CSF findings if blood does not enter the ventricles or the subarachnoid space. Blood in the ventricular system rapidly leads to coma and death. This is due to pressure transmitted to the brain stem.

## LABORATORY FINDINGS

### Epidural and Subdural Hemorrhage

Usually no CSF findings unless blood enters the subarachnoid space

### Subarachnoid Hemorrhage

Occult blood may be present in CSF within 8 hours after symptoms.

Hemoglobin may persist in CSF for 8 days.

Xanthochromia, due primarily to bilirubin, appears after 8 hr–12 hr and persists for 20 days–30 days.

Gross blood is present in CSF in 85% of patients; blood usually does not clot and is uniform in all tubes; blood clears by the 10th day in 40% of patients.

WBC–RBC ratio in bloody spinal fluid is usually the same as in peripheral blood. However, it may be higher than in peripheral blood because of an accompanying inflammatory reaction in the meninges.

Increased CSF protein (up to 1000 mg/dl)

Transient albuminuria and glycosuria

Leukocytosis of 15,000/$\mu$l–18,000/$\mu$l

Increased sedimentation rate

### Intracerebral Hemorrhage

Laboratory findings are similar to those in subarachnoid hemorrhage only if and when blood enters the ventricles or subarachnoid space.

## BRAIN TUMORS

Primary brain tumors arise from the meninges or from the glial cells, which comprise the supportive tissues of the brain substance. These latter tumors are called *gliomas* and are usually malignant. The most common meningeal tumors are meningiomas, which are benign and which produce clinical effects by pressing against the brain or cranial nerves.

About 20% of brain tumors are metastatic (*i.e.,* they originate at another site). The most frequent sites of origin are the lungs and the breasts.

Only those tumors that penetrate into the subarachnoid space or into the ventricles will be in contact with the CSF and produce CSF changes.

Brain tumors may involve the hypothalamus. This region is the source of hormones that influence the production and release of other hormones from the pituitary gland. Hypothalamic hormones that affect anterior pituitary hormones include corticotropin releasing factor, gonadotropin releasing hormone, thyrotropin releasing hormone, prolactin inhibiting hormone, growth hormone releasing factor, and growth hormone inhibiting factor (somatostatin). The hypothalamus also controls the production of vasopressin (antidiuretic hormone) by the posterior pituitary gland. Brain-tumor involvement of the hypothalamus may result in precocious puberty, hypogonadism, hypothyroidism, dwarfism, diabetes insipidus, hypernatremia, increased or decreased appetite, or disturbed body-temperature control (see Chap. 6).

### LABORATORY FINDINGS

#### CSF

The following findings occur only when products of tumor necrosis or malignant cells gain access to the CSF through the subarachnoid space or ventricles:

Appearance—usually clear, occasionally xanthochromic

WBC up to 150/$\mu$l (25% of patients)

Increased protein, up to 500 mg/dl

Tumor cells may be present on cytologic examination.

Glucose may be decreased if tumor cells are present.

**Altered Hypothalamic Hormones (see Chap. 6)**

Anterior pituitary insufficiency

Diabetes insipidus

Hypothyroidism

Secondary testicular failure

Secondary ovarian failure

Precocious puberty

**Laboratory Findings of the Primary Tumor (when the brain tumor is metastatic)**

Bronchogenic carcinoma (see Chap. 2)

Leukemia (see Chap. 8)

Malignant lymphoma (see Chap. 8)

## SPINAL-CORD TUMORS

Most spinal-cord tumors arise outside of the cord itself and involve the dural covering of the cord. Tumors outside the dura include lymphomas and metastatic carcinomas. Tumors beneath the dura include meningiomas and nerve-sheath tumors, known as *neurilemomas* or *schwannomas.* Tumors of the substance of the spinal cord itself account for only 5% of all spinal-cord tumors. Most spinal-cord tumors are benign and occur with about one fifth of the frequency of brain tumors.

As the cord enlarges because of a tumor growing within it or is compressed by a tumor from without, the subarachnoid space around the cord is obliterated. The CSF below this site is no longer in continuity with the circulating spinal fluid above the lesion. As a consequence of the obstruction, resorption of water from the CSF produces spinal fluid of high protein content. The increased protein imparts a yellowish color to the CSF. The yellow discoloration is termed *xanthochromia.*

### LABORATORY FINDINGS

#### CSF

Protein 50 mg/dl–3500 mg/dl (85% of patients); when protein is high, CSF usually clots because of the presence of increased fibrinogen

Xanthochromia (40% of patients)

WBC 25/$\mu$l–100/$\mu$l (15% of patients)

Glucose normal

## GUILLAIN-BARRÉ SYNDROME

Guillain-Barré syndrome is also known as *acute idiopathic polyneuritis* or *postinfectious polyneuritis.* It is an acute, rapidly progressive form of polyneuropathy, characterized by muscle weakness and slight distal sensory loss, which usually begins 1 week to 3 weeks after a mild respiratory or GI infection. There are widespread inflammation and demyelination throughout the cranial nerves, the ventral and dorsal nerve roots, the dorsal root ganglia, and the entire lengths of the peripheral nerves.

Most evidence suggests that the clinical manifestations of this disorder are the result of a cell-mediated immunologic reaction directed toward peripheral nerves. The antigen in this reaction is a basic protein found only in peripheral nerve myelin. (Myelin is the lipid–protein sheath surrounding nerves.) The consequence of this immunologic reaction is a myelin-sheath breakdown, which results in impaired nerve function. Further effects of the autoimmune process might be disruption of the nerve axon and atrophy of the muscle that has been innervated by the damaged nerves.

### LABORATORY FINDINGS

Early leukocytosis

**CSF**\*

Increased protein (50 mg/dl–100 mg/dl)—this reflects the widespread inflammation of the nerve roots; the protein increase usually begins after the 10th day of the neurologic illness and peaks at 4 wk–6 wk; the increase parallels the clinical severity

Normal cell count (90% of patients); slightly increased mononuclear cells (10% of patients)


## *ALCOHOLIC MUSCLE DISEASE*

Chronic alcoholism may be associated with severe pain, tenderness, and swelling of one or more muscles.[11] The symptoms usually follow a persistently excessive intake of alcohol. Acute alcoholic myopathy is usually self-limited and relatively benign. On occasion, however, severe muscle necrosis gives rise to myoglobinuria and fatal acute tubular necrosis of the kidneys.

Many alcoholics seen with acute alcoholic intoxication or withdrawal syndrome have no muscle symptoms but demonstrate elevation of the muscle enzymes, CPK and aldolase. Biopsies often show evidence of fragmentation, edema, necrosis, and inflammation of muscle tissues.

### LABORATORY FINDINGS

Increased serum CPK; MM† (muscle) band seen on electrophoresis

Increased serum aldolase

Myoglobinuria and acute renal failure might occur.

---

\* The combination of increased CSF protein with the usually normal CSF cellularity is referred to as *albuminocytologic dissociation.*
† See definition on page 12 in Chapter 1.

Frequent macrocytosis and decreased RBC folate result from increased alcoholic intake

Increased γ-glutamyl transpeptidase indicates increased alcoholic intake.

## MYASTHENIA GRAVIS

Myasthenia gravis in an autoimmune disease of voluntary muscles manifested by muscle weakness and fatigability.[13] In this disease, there are circulating antibodies to the acetylcholine receptors located on muscle fibers. The antibodies deplete acetylcholine receptors, interfering with the normal transmission of nerve impulses to the affected muscles; motor function is thereby impaired. The process that initiates the antibody formation is unknown.

Disorders of the thymus gland often occur in association with myasthenia gravis. The relationship has not been clearly established. There might be a thymic polypeptide factor that acts to inhibit neuromuscular transmission at the myoneural junction. The thymus might also be an active site of production of antibodies to acetylcholine receptors. About 80% of patients with myasthenia gravis have thymic enlargement characterized by germinal centers with increased B cells in the central region of the thymus gland. This may indicate thymic inflammation. Approximately 15% of patients with myasthenia gravis have tumors of the thymus gland.

Thyroid disorders are found in 5% of patients. Other autoimmune disorders such as systemic lupus erythematosus, rheumatoid arthritis, and polymyositis may occasionally be seen in association with myasthenia gravis.

### LABORATORY FINDINGS

Presence of serum antibodies to acetylcholine receptors (87%–93% of patients)—this is the best diagnostic test; the antibody titer does not correspond with the severity of the disease or with the response to therapy

Normal CPK, aldolase, SGOT (AST) and LDH

## MUSCULAR DYSTROPHIES

A myopathy is a muscular disorder characterized by weakness or some other symptom of muscle dysfunction that is not due to emotional or neurogenic cause. A dystrophy is a subgroup of myopathy with three characteristics: heritable transmission, progressive weakness, and histologic evidence of muscle degeneration with no evidence of abnormally stored material or structural abnormality of the fibers. Muscular dystrophies are uncommon disorders, usually classified on the basis of genetic pattern and the clinical features of involved muscle groups, age of onset, and rate of progression.

Increasing biochemical and ultrastructural evidence implicates the muscle surface membrane as the site of the fundamental disorder. There is evidence of dysfunction of enzymes that are an integral part of the muscle membrane. Enzymes leak into the bloodstream from defective or damaged muscle fibers.

## LABORATORY FINDINGS

Increased serum CPK, aldolase, SGOT (AST), and LDH reflect skeletal-muscle breakdown and the release of enzymes from muscle into serum. The serum level reflects the severity of muscle damage. CPK isoenzymes include both MM* and MB.* There is increased MB* isoenzyme in diseased skeletal muscle. The increased LDH isoenzyme is usually $LDH_5$.

A recent detailed study demonstrated the following findings in Duchenne's muscular dystrophy:[6]

Early: Moderate increase in $LDH_4$, marked increase in $LDH_5$
Progressing: Moderate increases in $LDH_4$ and $LDH_5$
Late: Moderate increases in $LDH_3$ and $LDH_4$; normal $LDH_5$

This may be interpreted as indicating a gradual disappearance of degenerating mature muscle fibers ($LDH_5$) and an increased synthesis of immature muscle fibers ($LDH_1$–$LDH_3$) as regeneration occurred.


## *FAMILIAL PERIODIC PARALYSIS*

Periodic paralysis is characterized by recurrent attacks of flaccid weakness, usually associated with abnormally high or low concentrations of serum potassium.[7] Familial cases appear to have an autosomal dominant inheritance. There are two variants of this disorder—one in which the serum potassium is low and one in which the serum potassium is high. It is presumed that these changes are secondary to shifts of potassium into and out of the muscles, respectively. In the hyperkalemic type, there are alterations in the muscle electrical potential indicating depletion of muscular potassium. One theory suggests that in the hypokalemic type fluid and electrolytes enter muscles and inhibit the contractility of muscle cells or prevent transmission of nerve impulses.[7]


### LABORATORY FINDINGS

Decreased serum potassium (2.5 mEq/l–3.5 mEq/l)—hypokalemic type

Increased serum potassium (5.0 mEq/l–7.0 mEq/l)—hyperkalemic type

Serum potassium is usually normal between attacks.

Increased CPK during acute attacks


## *REFERENCES*

1. Adams RD, Vander Eecken HM: Vascular diseases of the brain. Annu Rev Med 4:213–252, 1953
2. Alderson D, Strong AJ, Ingham HR et al: Fifteen year review of the mortality of brain abscess. Neurosurgery 8:1–6, 1981
3. Consensus Conference, Office for Medical Applications of Research, National Institutes of Health: Diagnosis and treatment of Reye's syndrome. JAMA 246:2441–2444, 1981
4. Hart RG, Sherman DG: The diagnosis of multiple sclerosis. JAMA 247:498–503, 1982

* See definitions on page 12 in Chapter 1.

5. Hershey LA, Trotter JL: The use and abuse of the cerebrospinal fluid IgG profile in the adult: A practical evaluation. Ann Neurol 8:426–434, 1980
6. Ibrahim GA, Zweber BA, Awad EA: Muscle and serum enzymes and isoenzymes in muscular dystrophies. Arch Phys Med Rehabil 62:265–269, 1981
7. Johnsen T: Familial periodic paralysis with hypokalemia. Dan Med Bull 28:1–27, 1981
8. Johnson KP: Cerebrospinal fluid and blood assays of diagnostic usefulness in multiple sclerosis. Neurology 30:106–109, 1980
9. Karandanis D, Shulman JA: Recent survey of infectious meningitis in adults: A review of laboratory findings in bacterial, tuberculous and aseptic meningitis. South Med J 69:449–457, 1976
10. Luxon LM: Neurosyphilis. Int J Dermatol 19:310–317, 1980
11. Myerson RM, Lafair JS: Alcoholic muscle disease. Med Clin North Am 54:723–730, 1970
12. Powers WS: Cerebrospinal fluid to serum glucose ratios in diabetes mellitus and bacterial meningitis. Am J Med 71:217–220, 1981
13. Scadding GK, Havard CW: Pathogenesis and treatment of myasthenia gravis. Br Med J 283:1008–1012, 1981
14. Simon RP: Neurosyphilis: An update. West J Med 134:87–91, 1981
15. Underman AE, Overturf GD, Leedom JM: Bacterial meningitis—1978. DM 24:1–63, 1978
16. Whitley R: Diagnosis and treatment of herpes simplex encephalitis. Annu Rev Med 32:335–340, 1981

## BIBLIOGRAPHY

**Adams RD, Victor M:** Principles of Neurology, 2nd ed. New York, McGraw-Hill, 1981
**Eliasson SG, Prensky AL, Hardin WB:** Neurological Pathophysiology, 2nd ed. New York, Oxford University Press, 1978
**Gilroy J, Meyer JS:** Medical Neurology, 3rd ed. New York, Macmillan, 1979
**Merritt HH:** A Textbook of Neurology, 6th ed. Philadelphia, Lea & Febiger, 1979

# 8
# *HEMATOLOGIC DISEASES*

## IRON DEFICIENCY ANEMIA

Iron deficiency in adults always arises because of an inability of the diet and intestinal absorption of iron to keep pace with increased requirements imposed either by increased red cell mass or by blood loss. Anemia results when the iron stores of the body have been depleted and there is insufficient iron available for adequate hemoglobin production.

Dietary iron deficiency most frequently occurs in milk-fed infants who are given no iron supplementation. During pregnancy, the mother's red cell mass expands by 20%, the fetus requires iron for blood-cell formation, there is blood loss at delivery, and iron stores are depleted with lactation. Consequently, unless the pregnant woman's iron intake is supplemented, 85% to 100% will become iron deficient.

Iron absorption may be deficient following subtotal gastrectomy. This is a consequence of the rapid passage of food into the jejunum, bypassing the iron-absorptive sites in the duodenum. Intestinal malabsorption of iron is an uncommon cause of iron deficiency. As long as the duodenal surface is well preserved, sufficient amounts of iron may be absorbed to meet requirements.

Blood loss is the most important factor in the development of iron deficiency in the adult. This most frequently occurs with peptic ulcers, which are the most common cause of iron deficiency in men. Reflux esophagitis, hemorrhagic gastritis, and gastrointestinal (GI) cancer are other frequent causes of bleeding from the GI tract. Another cause is bleeding varices, which are large veins developing at the lower end of the esophagus and the upper stomach in the presence of cirrhosis (see Chap. 4). Chronic users of aspirin also have increased GI bleeding owing to superficial gastric erosions. Other causes of intestinal blood loss are regional ileitis, ulcerative colitis, diverticulitis, and hemorrhoids. Chronic intermittent bleeding also occurs following subtotal gastrectomy. Increased menstrual blood loss is the most frequent cause of iron deficiency in premenopausal women. Urinary blood loss may occur with renal or bladder tumors or stones. Chronic intravascular hemolysis results in urinary loss of hemosiderin, ferritin, and hemoglobin; this may result in iron deficiency anemia. Patients undergoing renal hemodialysis lose blood in the dialyzing fluid and may become iron deficient.

Iron deficiency impairs cellular function in many tissues. The rapidly proliferating cells of the upper part of the alimentary tract seem particularly susceptible to the effects of iron deficiency. There may be thinning of the mucosal layer from the mouth to the small intestine. Gastric achlorhydria often occurs as a consequence.

## LABORATORY FINDINGS

### Peripheral Blood

Normal or decreased reticulocytes reflect impaired marrow response to anemia in absence of iron.

*Sequential Stages in the Development of Iron Deficiency*
Normal indices, no anemia, and depleted iron stores, indicated by decreased serum ferritin and marrow hemosiderin—early iron deficiency

Normocytic, normochromic anemia follows complete depletion of iron stores; variable anisocytosis and poikilocytosis

Microcytic, hypochromic anemia indicates late iron deficiency.

### Bone Marrow

Decreased or absent stainable iron (hemosiderin) is the earliest indicator of iron depletion; it precedes anemia. Stainable marrow iron indicates storage iron.

Variable cellularity—there is a poor correlation between the severity of anemia and the degree of erythroid hyperplasia.

Decreased sideroblasts, which are iron-containing normoblasts

### Other Laboratory Findings*

Decreased serum ferritin—this is the earliest indicator of iron depletion, usually corresponding to marrow iron stores. This might be normal in the presence of accompanying chronic disease, liver disease, or malignant neoplasm.[11]

Increased iron binding capacity—this occurs only after storage iron is completely depleted. The iron binding capacity is a measure of serum transferrin.

Decreased serum iron and transferrin saturation (<16% early, <10% late)

Increased free erythrocyte protoporphyrin—this provides the same information as transferrin saturation but is a slower and more stable indicator of iron storage.

### Laboratory Findings of Underlying Disease

See diseases and conditions discussed above.

## MEGALOBLASTIC ANEMIAS AND VITAMIN B$_{12}$ DEFICIENCY

Vitamin B$_{12}$ and folic acid have essential roles in deoxyribonucleic acid (DNA) synthesis. Deficiencies of either or both of these coenzymes lead to disturbances in cell division. This affects bone marrow cells and other proliferating cells, such as those lining the GI tract. Defective DNA synthesis blocks or delays cell division. The resulting state of unbalanced cellular growth causes a predisposition to premature cell death or abnormal cell division and asynchronous nuclear-cytoplasmic maturation. Due to abnormal DNA synthesis, the cell nucleus takes longer to mature than does the cytoplasm. Normal ribonucleic acid (RNA) metabolism allows for normal cytoplasmic maturation. The resulting cells, therefore, have more mature-appearing cytoplasm than nuclei. Delayed cell division results in the affected cells' being much larger in size than are normal cells. Hence, they are termed *megaloblasts* (*megalo* meaning *large*). Megaloblasts are considered to be functionally and morphologically abnormal normoblasts. These abnormal cells occur with deficiencies of both vitamin B$_{12}$ and folic acid.

Megaloblastic anemia is characterized functionally by a striking degree of destruction of developing red blood cells (RBC) within the bone marrow. This destruction is termed *ineffective erythropoiesis*. Circulating RBC are also defective, as evidenced by a shortened life span and a moderate degree of hemolysis. Iron is ineffectively utilized by developing RBC. Abundant plasma iron moves rapidly into the marrow, becoming accumulated in storage cells, rather than

* These all *precede* microcytosis and anemia, and are listed in order of occurrence.

being utilized for hemoglobin formation. After a period of retention, it is gradually released and stored in the liver. Defective DNA synthesis also causes ineffective formation and maturation of leukocytes and platelets.

### PERNICIOUS ANEMIA

Pernicious anemia is a consequence of impaired absorption of vitamin B$_{12}$. It is not due to dietary deficiency. The absorption of vitamin B$_{12}$ is dependent on a mechanism that is unique among the essential nutrients. The parietal cells of the stomach produce hydrochloric acid and a glycoprotein known as *intrinsic factor*. After vitamin B$_{12}$ has been ingested and has been released from complexes in ingested foods, intrinsic factor tightly and specifically binds it. B$_{12}$ is protected by intrinsic factor from destruction by digestive enzymes. Specific receptors on the surface of the microvilli of the terminal ileum take up the intrinsic factor–vitamin B$_{12}$ complex. Vitamin B$_{12}$ is absorbed at this site and enters the circulation. It circulates bound to transport plasma proteins, *transcobalamins*.

The pathogenetic lesion in pernicious anemia is severe gastric atrophy of unknown etiology with failure to secrete intrinsic factor, which is necessary for vitamin B$_{12}$ absorption in the terminal ileum. Autoantibodies to both parietal cells of the stomach and intrinsic factor are usually formed, suggesting an autoimmune basis for the disease. There may also be a genetic basis for pernicious anemia, because the family history is often positive.

The clinical features of vitamin B$_{12}$ deficiency are similar to those of folic acid deficiency, except for the occurrence in the former of neurologic abnormalities resulting from spinal-cord demyelination. The metabolic basis for the neurologic lesion is not established.

### OTHER CAUSES OF VITAMIN B$_{12}$ DEFICIENCY

Total gastrectomy results in loss of the source of intrinsic factor. Consequently, no further vitamin B$_{12}$ is absorbed. Stored vitamin B$_{12}$ is depleted in 5 years to 6 years. Loss of the specific site of vitamin B$_{12}$ absorption in the terminal ileum also leads to vitamin B$_{12}$ deficiency. This may follow surgical resection or intestinal disease such as regional ileitis, tropical sprue, lymphoma, or tuberculosis. In these disorders there is no associated lack of intrinsic factor or gastric acid. Decreased availability of vitamin B$_{12}$ occurs with anatomic abnormalities of the GI tract that lead to stasis and pooling of the intestinal contents. Such blind loop syndromes—strictures, surgically created bypasses, fistulas, and large diverticula—have in common intestinal bacterial overgrowth and steatorrhea. In these disorders, ingested vitamin B$_{12}$ is depleted by increased numbers of intestinal bacteria. A similar mechanism of vitamin B$_{12}$ consumption occurs with infestation by the fish tapeworm, *Diphyllobothrium latum.*

## LABORATORY FINDINGS

### All Megaloblastic Anemias

*Peripheral Blood*
Normochromic macrocytic (mean corpuscular volume [MCV] 100 $\mu$m$^3$–150 $\mu$m$^3$) anemia (7 g/dl–8 g/dl) with many oval macrocytes (macroovalocytes)

Moderate to marked poikilocytosis and anisocytosis

Basophilic stippling, Howell-Jolly bodies, Cabot's rings

Nucleated RBC when hematocrit is low (<20%); these show typical megaloblastic features

Reticulocytes are usually decreased, indicating ineffective erythropoiesis.

Hypersegmented enlarged neutrophils are often seen before RBC changes. These cells reflect abnormal nuclear division.

Thrombocytopenia; variably sized platelets

Leukopenia

*Bone Marrow*
Increased cellularity, which is predominantly erythrocytic; this changes the myelocytic–erythrocytic (M–E) ratio from 3:1 to 1:1

Predominance of promegaloblasts; there are also many other megaloblastic RBC precursors, which reflect impaired DNA metabolism

Enlarged granulocytic bands and metamyelocytes reflect impaired DNA metabolism.

Enlarged megakaryocytes reflect impaired DNA metabolism.

Increased stainable iron

*Other Laboratory Findings*
Increased serum iron reflects ineffective erythropoiesis and decreased RBC formation.

Normal or slightly decreased total iron binding capacity

Markedly increased lactate dehydrogenase (LDH) (predominance of $LDH_1$) reflects ineffective erythropoiesis, marrow destruction of blood-cell precursors, and release of LDH from RBC; the magnitude of the increase is related to the degree of anemia.

Slight increase in unconjugated bilirubin reflects ineffective erythropoiesis and RBC destruction in the marrow.

**Pernicious Anemia**

Decreased serum vitamin $B_{12}$—this is the single most important diagnostic test

Increased vitamin $B_{12}$ binding capacity

Lack of gastric acid, even following stimulation with betazole (Histalog) or pentagastrin; $pH$ of gastric juice >3.5; this does not decrease by more than 1 $pH$ unit after stimulation

Abnormal Schilling test—decreased absorption of radioisotope-labeled vitamin $B_{12}$ with normalization of absorption when oral intrinsic factor is given. The various intestinal disorders that may lead to vitamin $B_{12}$ deficiency show *no* correction of impaired vitamin-$B_{12}$ absorption following intrinsic-factor administration.

Antibodies to intrinsic factor (56%–60% of patients) and to parietal cells (84%–90% of patients).

## FOLIC ACID DEFICIENCY

Folate deficiency occurs primarily as a result of dietary lack. Other causes include increased folate requirements, impaired folate absorption, and drug blockage of folate activation.

Folates are especially present in green leafy vegetables. They are also present in fruits, meats, and eggs. The amount of folic acid in the average diet is not much in excess of the nutritional requirements. Because body folate reserves are relatively meager, folic acid deficiency develops frequently in persons with inadequate diets. It takes only 3 months to 4 months for a person to become folate deficient after intake is interrupted (Fig. 8-1). Megaloblastic anemia occurring in chronic liver disease is usually caused by folic acid deficiency resulting from a poor diet and from impaired hepatic storage of folates.

Folic acid deficiency anemia occurs with pregnancy, neoplastic diseases, and hemolytic anemia associated with chronic overactivity of the bone marrow. The anemia in these conditions is the consequence of increased folate requirements.

Intestinal disorders affecting extensive areas of jejunal absorptive surface frequently lead to folate deficiency. Such disorders include gluten enteropathy (nontropical sprue), tropical sprue, lymphoma, scleroderma, amyloidosis, Whipple's disease, and extensive surgical resection of the small intestine.

The drug that most commonly produces folate deficiency is alcohol. Alcohol

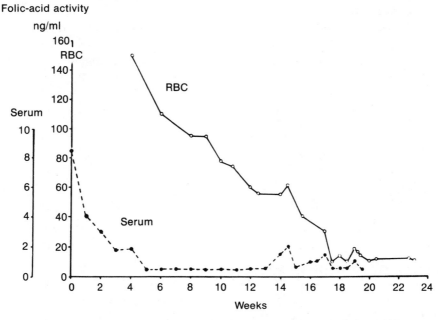

**Fig. 8-1.** Fall in serum folate and red cell folate in a subject on a folate-deficient diet. (Redrawn from Herbert V: Experimental nutritional folate deficiency in man. Trans Assoc Am Phys, 75:307, 1962)

interferes with folate absorption, metabolism, and hepatic storage and is also associated with deficient dietary intake of folate. Intestinal malabsorption of folate may be induced by various anticonvulsants such as phenytoin (Dilantin), phenobarbital, and primidone. Certain drugs such as methotrexate are used in cancer chemotherapy because they block folate metabolism and impede tumor cell growth. By interfering with DNA synthesis, the drugs also produce megaloblastic anemia.

The clinical and hematologic features of folic acid deficiency and vitamin $B_{12}$ deficiency are identical except for the neurologic abnormalities that occur with only vitamin $B_{12}$ deficiency.

## LABORATORY FINDINGS

### Peripheral Blood

Findings identical to those in vitamin $B_{12}$ deficiency

### Bone Marrow

Findings identical to those in vitamin $B_{12}$ deficiency

### Other Laboratory Findings

Decreased serum folate—this is the most sensitive indicator of folate deficiency, falling within a month of deficient intake (Fig. 8-1). This falls many weeks before megaloblastic anemia appears. Serum folate levels may change abruptly with changes in diet.

Decreased RBC folate—this appears after 3 months–4 months of folate deficiency (Fig. 8-1). RBC folate is an index of tissue folate stores.

When folate stores are depleted, megaloblastic anemia occurs.

Findings of ineffective erythropoiesis—increased serum iron, unconjugated bilirubin, and $LDH_1$

Normal gastric acid; normal Schilling test; normal serum vitamin $B_{12}$

*Laboratory Findings of Impaired Intestinal Absorption or Its Causes*
Gluten enteropathy (see Chap. 3)

Lymphoma (see Chap. 8)

Amyloidosis (see Chap. 10)

Scleroderma (see Chap. 9)

Whipple's disease (see Chap. 3)

## ANEMIA OF CHRONIC DISEASE

The chronic diseases that are frequently accompanied by anemia include chronic infections of any type and various chronic inflammatory disorders. The former group, which includes tuberculosis, osteomyelitis, and subacute bacterial endocarditis, is not commonly seen today. The latter group is chiefly represented by rheumatoid arthritis, but also includes other collagen diseases, inflammatory bowel diseases, and malignant diseases.

Anemia usually develops within two months of sustained infection. The degree of anemia tends to correlate with the activity and severity of the underlying disorder.

The mechanisms resulting in anemia include the following:

1. A slight decrease in RBC survival due to extracellular factors.
   Normal RBC transfused to these patients have decreased survival, presumably caused by inflammatory factors.
2. Impaired release of iron from iron storage sites. (Fig. 8-2).
   Iron from broken down RBC tends to be retained in reticuloendothelial (RE) cells rather than released to circulating transferrin. Furthermore there is decreased formation or availability of transferrin for iron transport. As a consequence there is a decrease in serum iron transported to the marrow for reutilization in hemoglobin synthesis (Fig. 8-3).
3. Impaired marrow response to the anemia.
   The low serum iron level is considered to be the main factor accounting for impaired marrow response to erythropoietin. Impairment of marrow response results in subnormal compensation for the slight hemolysis. Marrow iron is not utilized by developing normoblasts but accumulates in marrow macrophages.

## LABORATORY FINDINGS

### Peripheral Blood

Normochromic, normocytic anemia (8 g/dl–12 g/dl; occasionally <7 g/dl); many patients have microcytosis (MCV <80 $\mu$m³) and hypochromia (mean corpuscular hemoglobin concentration (MCHC) <31 g/dl)

Usually normal reticulocyte count; may occasionally be reduced or slightly increased

### Bone Marrow

Normal cellularity and maturation

Increased bone marrow RE iron—reflects impaired marrow utilization of stored iron. The increase in storage iron in the presence of decreased serum iron and marrow sideroblasts is characteristic of this disorder.

Decreased sideroblasts

**Fig. 8-2.** Impaired release of iron from iron storage sites in anemia of chronic disease (Hillman RS, Finch CA: Red Cell Manual, 4th ed, p 17. Philadelphia, FA Davis, 1974)

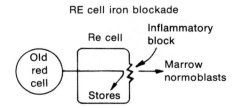

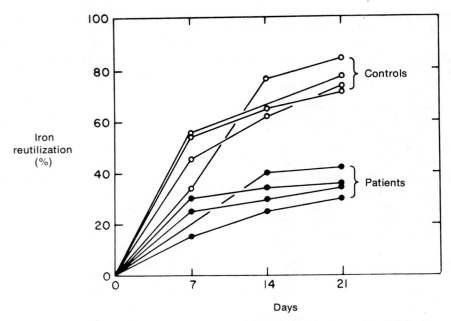

**Fig. 8-3.** Reutilization of [59]Fe-tagged hemoglobin solution in normal individuals and in patients with anemia of chronic disease. (Redrawn from Haurani Fl, Burke W, Martinez EJ: Defective reutilization of iron in the anemia of inflammation. J Lab Clin Med 65:560–570, 1965)

**Other Laboratory Findings**

Decreased serum iron—characteristic finding; precedes anemia

Decreased transferrin, which is usually measured as total iron binding capacity—occurs after the decrease in serum iron. This contrasts with increased total iron binding capacity in iron deficiency.

Decreased transferrin saturation (mean 15%, range 10%–25%); not as low as in iron deficiency

Normal or increased serum ferritin—because ferritin increases in inflammatory disorders, the level is disproportionately elevated for the amount of marrow iron.[11] This contrasts with decreased ferritin in iron deficiency.

**Laboratory Findings of Underlying Disease**

See diseases discussed above.

## ANEMIA OF CHRONIC RENAL INSUFFICIENCY

Chronic renal failure is consistently associated with anemia, but the degree of azotemia and the severity of the anemia are only roughly correlated.

The chief mechanism for the anemia is deficient production of erythropoietin by the kidney. There are also ineffective RBC production, diminished marrow responsiveness to erythropoietin, and decreased RBC survival. The shortened survival of the RBC in chronic renal disease is probably due to mechanical disruption of metabolically impaired RBC. A plasma factor affects RBC metabolism, causing formation of burr cells and irregularly contracted and fragmented RBC. The toxic plasma substances in azotemia have not been identified.

## LABORATORY FINDINGS

### Peripheral Blood

Normochromic, normocytic anemia (hemoglobin 5 g/dl–10 g/dl)—characteristic finding

Microcytic anemia occurs when there is iron deficiency due to bleeding secondary to various platelet dysfunctions. It may also be due to iron loss in hemodialysis fluid.

Macrocytic anemia—due to loss of folate in hemodialysis fluid

Occasional burr or helmet cells

Acanthocytes and schistocytes, especially in hemolytic-uremic syndrome

Usually normal reticulocyte count; might be slightly decreased; a moderate increase in reticulocytes may occur with higher blood urea nitrogen (BUN) levels.

### Bone Marrow

Normal bone marrow appearance; might appear somewhat hypoplastic

### Other Laboratory Findings

Usually normal serum iron, total iron binding capacity, transferrin saturation; these may all be decreased if iron deficiency occurs.

Laboratory findings of chronic renal insufficiency (see Chap. 5)

## *ANEMIA OF HYPOMETABOLISM*

Anemia commonly accompanies hypofunction of the pituitary gland, thyroid gland, adrenal cortex, and gonads.

Hypothyroidism is the most frequent endocrine disturbance accompanied by anemia. The anemia of hypothyroidism is an appropriate response to decreased cellular demand for oxygen. Hypothyroid patients may also have increased uterine bleeding or malabsorption of vitamin $B_{12}$ or folic acid. These factors also contribute to anemia.

Androgens increase the production of erythropoietin and account for the higher hemoglobin level in men than in women. Androgen deficiency occurring in male hypogonadism results in a hemoglobin level lowered to that of the normal woman.

In Addison's disease, mild anemia is partially obscured by dehydration. Treatment and correction of dehydration renders the anemia more evident.

Hypopituitarism results in anemia as a consequence of impaired stimulation of the thyroid, adrenal glands, and gonads and of deficiencies of their hormones.

### LABORATORY FINDINGS

Normocytic, normochromic anemia (>10 g/dl)—characteristic of hypothyroidism

Microcytic, hypochromic anemia is a consequence of uterine bleeding in hypothyroidism

Laboratory findings of anterior pituitary insufficiency, hypothyroidism, Addison's disease, or secondary testicular failure (see Chap. 6)

## *HEREDITARY SPHEROCYTOSIS*

Hereditary spherocytosis is probably the most common type of hereditary hemolytic anemia among persons of Northern European origin. Since it is inherited as an autosomal dominant disorder, it would be expected to affect one of the patient's parents; each of the patient's children has a 50% chance of inheriting the disorder.

This disorder is characterized by abnormally shaped RBC, which result from inherited defects of the RBC membrane. The intrinsic defect in the RBC of hereditary spherocytosis appears to reside in the protein portion of the membrane. These defective RBC are also characterized by the loss of lipids from the cell membrane and by an accompanying loss of membrane surface area. The reduction in surface area without commensurate volume loss converts the biconcave erythrocytes into microspherocytes, which are small, densely stained, round, and lacking in central pallor. The spherocytic RBC has a limited capacity for volume expansion. The RBC membrane is leaky and allows sodium to enter the cells at a faster than normal rate. RBC osmotic balance requires increased cellular energy to pump out the excess sodium. This can be accomplished as long as the RBC have an adequate supply of glucose available for anaerobic glycolysis. If the osmotic balance cannot be maintained, water enters the cells and causes them to swell and, eventually, rupture.

The decreased survival of spherocytic RBC is largely a result of splenic entrapment. This is a consequence of slowed circulation through the spleen and increased numbers of RBC therein. The splenic pulp has a lower glucose concentration and a more acid $p$H than has the circulating blood. These factors limit glucose metabolism and cause lipid loss from the RBC membrane. Splenic damage may not be fatal to the erythrocytes during their first passage through the spleen, but with repeated passages the RBC lose so much membrane surface area that they become microspherocytes. These cells now lack the extreme pliability of normal erythrocytes and are finally trapped in the tiny splenic vessels. The retained spherocytes are destroyed and phagocytosed by splenic macrophages. Following splenectomy, spherocytes persist but have almost normal survival. One may conclude that the inherited intrinsic RBC defect causes significant erythrocyte destruction only in the presence of the spleen.

The major clinical manifestations of spherocytosis are anemia, jaundice, and splenomegaly. The chronic hemolytic state may range from an asymptomatic compensated hemolysis to a moderately severe chronic anemia. The latter usually occurs only when another medical condition, such as infection, causes temporary bone marrow failure, or *aplastic crisis*. Less commonly, there may be acute hemolytic crises. Because of an increased turnover of bilirubin, patients have a high incidence of gallstones.

## LABORATORY FINDINGS

### Peripheral Blood

Increased spherocytes with decreased cell diameter (microspherocytes)

Normocytic, or slightly microcytic, hyperchromic (MCHC 36 g/dl–40 g/dl) anemia (hemoglobin [Hb] 9 g/dl–12 g/dl)—the increased MCHC reflects cell membrane loss

Increased reticulocytes (5%–20%)—reflects marrow response to RBC destruction

Macrocytes and polychromatophilia reflect reticulocytosis.

Increased RBC distribution width and anisocytosis reflect two RBC populations.

### Bone Marrow

Normoblastic hyperplasia

Hypoplasia may occur in the presence of an aplastic crisis.

Megaloblasts may occur with complicating folate deficiency, which may supervene in any severe chronic hemolytic anemia. This is the result of accelerated folic acid utilization and DNA synthesis in response to normoblastic hyperplasia.

Moderate hemosiderin deposits

### Other Laboratory Findings

Indicators of extravascular hemolysis—increased LDH (especially $LDH_1$ and $LDH_2$), unconjugated (indirect) bilirubin, urine hemosiderin; decreased or absent serum haptoglobin

Negative Coombs' test

*Increased Osmotic Fragility Test*
The osmotic fragility test is always abnormal in hereditary spherocytosis because spherocytic cells cannot increase their volume as water enters the cells during exposure to hypotonic solutions. At times it may be necessary to enhance the RBC abnormality by incubating the blood in graded saline concentrations for 24 hours at 37°C.

*Abnormal Autohemolysis Test*
Spherocytic erythrocytes consume glucose at an increased rate and show increased autohemolysis when sterile whole blood is incubated at 37°C for 48 hours. The addition of supplemental glucose prior to incubation will reduce the degree of autohemolysis, even to normal levels.

## GLUCOSE-6-PHOSPHATE
## DEHYDROGENASE DEFICIENCY

Glucose-6-phosphate dehydrogenase (G6PD) deficiency is by far the most common RBC enzyme abnormality. This inherited sex-linked condition affects 11% of black men in the United States.

About 10% of glycolysis for RBC energy occurs through the oxidative hexose monophosphate shunt (pentose phosphate pathway), which bypasses the early steps of the main anaerobic glycolytic (Embden-Meyerhof) pathway. G6PD catalyzes the first step in the pentose phosphate pathway of glycolysis. When the pathway is functionally deficient, the amount of reduced glutathione becomes insufficient to neutralize the effects of oxidizing drugs.

Some oxidizing drugs interact with Hb and generate intracellular hydrogen peroxide. G6PD-deficient RBC are unable to break down the hydrogen peroxide. The peroxide oxidatively damages both the RBC membrane and the Hb molecule. Hb is oxidized to methemoglobin, and globin is denatured. Denatured globin precipitates as Heinz bodies, which are attached to the inner surface of the RBC membrane. Heinz bodies damage the cell membrane and reduce cellular pliability. As affected RBC pass through the spleen, Heinz bodies, along with that portion of the RBC membrane to which they are attached, are removed by RE cells. If the process inflicts sufficient membrane damage, the entire cell is destroyed as it traverses the spleen. Hemolysis preferentially affects only older RBC because these RBCs' level of enzyme is lower than that in young RBC. This process only partially explains the multiple mechanisms of RBC destruction. The complete reasons for premature destruction of G6PD-deficient cells is not known.

Most patients with this disorder are asymptomatic. In a person with mild enzyme deficiency, oxidative destruction of RBC occurs only when there is an increased oxidant load on the RBC. Thus, hemolysis characteristically occurs in an apparently healthy person. A person with severe enzyme deficiency has lifelong chronic hemolytic anemia.

The life span of G6PD-deficient RBC is shortened under many circumstances such as drug administration, the neonatal period, and infection. The most common manifestation of G6PD deficiency is that of a self-limited episode of drug-induced hemolysis beginning 1 day to 3 days after administration of an oxidant drug (Fig. 8-4). Examples of such oxidant drugs include antimalarials, sulfonamides, nitrofurans, analgesics, and sulfones. Hemolytic episodes may also occur within a few days of onset of a febrile illness. Because infection impairs reticulocytosis, recovery from this anemia does not occur until the infection has subsided.

### LABORATORY FINDINGS

#### Diagnostic Laboratory Tests

Positive fluorescent screening test—this is a specific and sensitive screening test for the detection of both severe and mild types of G6PD deficiency in homozygous males not undergoing hemolysis. This does not identify people who are heterozygous. False-negative results occur following a recent transfusion or hemolytic episode with reticulocytosis. In these situations, many

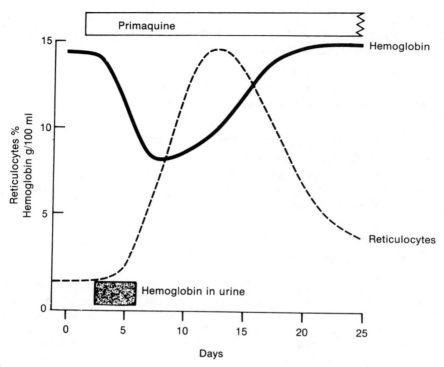

**Fig. 8-4.** Primaquine given to treat malaria in a G6PD-deficient subject caused acute hemolysis with a fall in hemoglobin and the appearance of free hemoglobin in urine. There is reticulocytosis. Despite continuation of the drug, hemolysis stops because the new red cells are more resistant to the drug. (Chanarin I, Brozovic M, Tidmarsh E, Waters DAW: Blood and its Diseases, p 122. Edinburgh, Churchill Livingstone, 1976)

circulating RBC will have normal enzyme levels and will not be detected by this test.

Positive ascorbate cyanide test—this is probably the most sensitive screening procedure for the heterozygous state

**No Hematologic Findings in the Absence of Hemolysis**

**Hematologic Findings in the Presence of Hemolysis**

*Phase 1*

Acute hemolysis (1 day–3 days after oxidative drug exposure)

Normocytic, normochromic anemia—rapid occurrence, severe

Indicators of hemolysis—increased LDH, unconjugated bilirubin, reticulocytes; decreased haptoglobin

Increased Heinz bodies (characteristic feature), basophilic stippling, polychromatophilia

Fragmented RBC and spherocytes, if hemolysis is severe

Marrow shows normoblastic hyperplasia.

*Phase 2*

Recovery (5 days–15 days after oxidative drug exposure)

Reticulocytosis (8%–12%)

Macrocytes reflect reticulocytosis.

Increase in Hb and hematocrit over earlier values

Absent haptoglobin reflects chronic hemolysis.

*Phase 3*

Resistance (more than 7 days–10 days after oxidative drug exposure)

Hemolysis stops and anemia disappears.

Young cells produced in response to hemolysis have nearly normal levels of enzyme and are relatively resistant to hemolysis. This phase continues as long as the same dose of the drug is administered.

## PYRUVATE KINASE DEFICIENCY

Pyruvate kinase deficiency is inherited as an autosomal recessive disorder. This is relatively rare in comparison to G6PD deficiency. It is the most common of the RBC enzyme deficiencies involving the main anaerobic glycolytic energy pathway and is the most common cause of nonspherocytic hemolytic anemia.

The severity of anemia varies widely from case to case. Hemolysis occurs only in the homozygous state and is the consequence of impaired RBC glycolysis. Splenectomy is not as effective in eliminating hemolysis as it is in spherocytosis.

### LABORATORY FINDINGS

#### Peripheral Blood

Normochromic, normocytic anemia (hematocrit 18%–36%)

Slight macrocytosis reflects reticulocytosis.

Increased reticulocytes, up to 2.5%–15% with hemolysis and up to 56% following splenectomy

Polychromatophilia, poikilocytosis, anisocytosis, irregularly contracted or crenated RBC, occasional nucleated RBC

No spherocytes

No Heinz bodies

#### Bone Marrow

Normoblastic hyperplasia

#### Other Laboratory Findings

Positive fluorescence screening test

Decreased RBC pyruvate kinase (5%–25% of normal). This is the only specifically diagnostic test.

Variably positive autohemolysis test—the abnormality is not corrected by the addition of glucose, because these cells cannot metabolize glucose.

Findings of hemolysis—increased LDH, unconjugated bilirubin; decreased or absent serum haptoglobin

Normal osmotic fragility test

## THE THALASSEMIAS

In the thalassemias, globin chains are structurally normal, in contrast to HbS and HbC, but are produced in inadequate amounts. The $\alpha$-thalassemias have decreased or absent synthesis of $\alpha$-globin chains and the $\beta$-thalassemias have decreased or absent $\beta$-globin chain synthesis. Because normal adult hemoglobin (HbA) is comprised of two $\alpha$ chains and two $\beta$ chains, there are varying degrees of impairment of HbA formation in both types of thalassemia. Thalassemia may be inherited in combination with an Hb variant such as sickle Hb (see Sickle-Cell Disease).

Each healthy adult has two pairs of $\alpha$-chain genes. $\alpha$-thalassemia results from a lack or defect of one to four of these genes. The defect in $\alpha$-chain synthesis results in accumulation of $\gamma$ chains in the fetal–neonatal period and of $\beta$ chains thereafter. Tetramers of $\gamma$ chains (Bart's Hb) and tetramers of $\beta$-chains (HbH) are unstable, thermolabile Hb that bind to oxygen more than 10 times as strongly as does HbA. This degree of impairment of oxygen release results in tissue hypoxia. Absence of all four $\alpha$-chain genes results in fetal or neonatal death with hepatosplenomegaly and severe anemia. This is termed *hydrops fetalis* with Bart's Hb. Absence of three $\alpha$-chain genes results in HbH disease, which is a moderately severe, chronic hemolytic anemia. If two of the four $\alpha$-chain genes are abnormal, the consequence is a mild hypochromic anemia designated as $\alpha$-thalassemia minor. The presence of only one abnormal $\alpha$ chain does not result in a clinically detectable abnormality, but rather produces a silent carrier of the $\alpha$-thalassemia trait. Persons with any of the $\alpha$-thalassemias show no increase in levels of $HbA_2$ ($\alpha_2\delta_2$) or HbF ($\alpha_2\delta_2$), because formation of these Hb, in common with HbA ($\alpha_2\beta_2$), are affected by the decreased formation of $\alpha$ chains. This contrasts with the frequent occurrence of increased levels of $HbA_2$ and HbF in the $\beta$-thalassemias.

$\beta$-thalassemia is a common disorder, particularly among Mediterranean populations. When only one $\beta$-thalassemia gene has been inherited (*thalassemia minor*) there is usually no clinical disability except in circumstances of stress such as pregnancy or severe infection. At these times a moderate degree of anemia can occur. This condition invariably shows an increase in $HbA_2$ to compensate for impaired formation of normal adult Hb.

When two $\beta$-thalassemia genes have been inherited, *thalassemia major* results. In this serious disorder there may be total absence of $\beta$-chain production or reduction in $\beta$-globin chain synthesis of 5% to 30% of normal. Consequently, HbA formation is markedly impaired. HbF becomes the major Hb type produced, usually exceeding 50% and often approaching 95% of the total. $HbA_2$ levels are variably increased, but are always elevated when expressed as a proportion of HbA. Many RBC have considerably shortened survival in the circulation. Severe hemolysis is explained by excessive production of $\alpha$ chains. The surplus of unpaired $\alpha$ chains is exceedingly unstable and precipitates as globin inclusion bodies within nucleated RBC precursors, damaging the RBC membrane and rendering erythrocytes less pliable. This causes marked erythrocyte destruction within the bone marrow and in the spleen. No more than 15% to 30% of marrow normoblasts escape destruction. RBC that have a greater proportion of HbF produce abundant γ chains, which combine with α chains preventing the precipitation of unpaired α chains. These RBC with HbF thus have less membrane damage and longer survival. Defective globin chain synthesis results in impaired heme production, in an accumulation of increased iron within RBC, precursors and in ineffective RBC formation. Excess α-chain production in thalassemia major is thus responsible for both hemolysis and for ineffective erythropoiesis. These processes combine to produce a severe degree of anemia. The presence of increased HbF, which has a higher oxygen affinity than has HbA, results in tissue hypoxia, stimulation of erythropoietin production, and consequent marked increase in marrow erythropoiesis.

Physical disfigurement occurs because of bony deformities brought on by the extreme erythroid hyperplasia of the marrow. Massive marrow hyperplasia also causes thinning of bones, which readily fracture. Ineffective marrow erythropoiesis stimulates extramedullary hematopoiesis, resulting in enlargement of the liver and spleen. Iron overload from RBC destruction, increased iron absorption, and repeated transfusions results in increased iron deposits in the

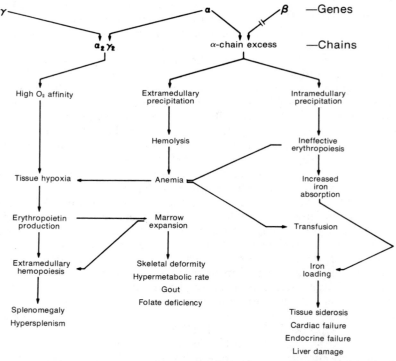

**Fig. 8-5.** Interrelationship of clinical features in homozygous β-thalassemia. Impaired β-chain formation is the basic defect. (From Hematology, 2nd ed, p 398 by Williams WJ, Beutler E, Erslev AJ, Rundles RW. Copyright © 1977 McGraw-Hill Book Company. Used with the permission of McGraw-Hill Book Company)

liver, ultimately causing cirrhosis. Excess iron deposits in the heart result in heart failure. Infection is a common cause of death. The pathophysiology of all the clinical findings in homozygous $\beta$-thalassemia is related to the basic defect in $\beta$-chain production (Fig. 8-5).

## LABORATORY FINDINGS

### $\beta$-thalassemia Minor

*Peripheral Blood*
Target cells, polychromatophilia, basophilic stippling, occasional nucleated RBC, anisocytosis, poikilocytosis

Slight hypochromic (MCH 20 pg–22 pg), microcytic (MCV 50 $\mu$m$^3$–70 $\mu$m$^3$) anemia (hemoglobin 9 g/dl–11 g/dl), with normal to increased RBC (>5.7 million/$\mu$l)

Increased reticulocytes (2%–10%)

*Bone Marrow*
Slight normoblastic hyperplasia; abundant iron deposits

*Other Laboratory Findings*
Electrophoresis shows increased HbA$_2$ (3.5%–8%); increased HbF (1%–5%) in 50% of patients; increased HbA$_2$ is diagnostic

Decreased osmotic fragility; this has been used as a rapid screening test

Normal to increased serum iron; normal serum ferritin

### $\beta$-thalassemia Major

*Peripheral Blood*
Marked anisocytosis, poikilocytosis, target cells (10%–35%), spherocytes, fragmented RBC; occasional nucleated RBC, basophilic stippling, siderocytes; inclusion bodies representing aggregated $\alpha$ chains

Marked hypochromic, microcytic anemia (Hb 2.5 g/dl–6.5 g/dl)

Increased reticulocytes (4%–10%)—this increase is lower than that which normally occurs with severe anemia and indicates inadequate marrow response

Increased white blood cell (WBC) count (10,000/$\mu$l–25,000/$\mu$l) with occasional immature granulocytes

Occasional thrombocytopenia—reflects effect of secondary hypersplenism

*Bone Marrow*
Marked normoblastic hyperplasia with poor hemoglobinization; basophilic stippling; abundant iron deposits; RBC cytoplasmic inclusions, which are free $\alpha$ chains; clinical severity correlates with amount of $\alpha$-chain precipitation

*Other Laboratory Findings*
Electrophoresis shows HbF 10%–100%; decreased or absent HbA; HbA$_2$ 1%–8%

Decreased osmotic fragility

Findings of hemolysis—increased unconjugated bilirubin, increased LDH, decreased haptoglobin

Increased serum iron and transferrin saturation

Decreased serum folate—reflects increased marrow utilization of folate

### α-thalassemia Minor

Mild hypochromic microcytic anemia

Peripheral blood—rare HbH inclusions in RBC after brilliant cresyl blue incubation.

Electrophoresis—newborn, Bart's Hb (2%–10%); adult, normal Hb electrophoresis

### HbH Disease

Severe hemolytic anemia (Hb 7 g/dl–10 g/dl)

Peripheral blood—hypochromic microcytes, target cells, irregularly crenated RBC; many HbH inclusions in RBC, especially following splenectomy

Increased reticulocytes (5%–10%)

Electrophoresis—newborn, increased Bart's Hb (20%–40%), which is gradually replaced during the first months of life by HbH; adult, HbA 70%–95%; HbH 5%–30%; trace of Bart's Hb

## SICKLE-CELL DISEASE

Hb is composed of globin and four heme groups; globin is composed of two polypeptide chain pairs. In HbA, the major normal adult Hb, one polypeptide pair is designated $\alpha$ and the other pair is designated $\beta$. The most common Hb variants, HbS and HbC, are $\beta$-chain mutations, which are the result of substitutions of a single amino acid. In the sickle-cell disorders, the amino acid *valine* is substituted for the amino acid *glutamic acid,* in position 6 at the N-terminal end of the $\beta$ chain. Sickle-cell variants are inherited and carried primarily in the black population. When the sickle hemoglobin gene is inherited from both parents (homozygous state), sickle cell anemia results. When the sickle gene is inherited from only one parent (heterozygous state), the other $\beta$ chain may carry normal adult HbA or an abnormal Hb. The latter might be HbC or the thalassemia gene.

Alterations in the amino-acid composition of the polypeptide chain may cause a change in the net charge of the molecule. A change in the electrical charge results in an alteration in the mobility and speed of migration of Hb in an electrical field. Consequently, some of the Hb variants may be differentiated by means of electrophoresis.

Substitution of an uncharged valine molecule for a charged glutamic-acid molecule in HbS results in an alteration of the Hb structure so that at low oxygen concentrations (as in capillaries) Hb molecules become more closely and firmly linked together. This molecular aggregation, or polymerization, distorts RBC, resulting in rigid sickle-shaped erythrocytes. The tendency toward sickling is enhanced because HbS releases its oxygen more readily than does HbA. Cells having large amounts of HbS require a small degree of deoxygenation to show sickling. The process is usually reversible and, as the oxygen tension is raised, the semisolid gelled Hb liquefies once again, and the cells reassume their normal biconcave shape. However, if the sickle shape is maintained for more than a few minutes, the RBC membrane becomes damaged, and the cells remain irreversibly sickled and are rapidly destroyed. Macrophages remove approximately two thirds of these cells. Those remaining undergo intravascular hemolysis. The severity of the hemolytic process is directly related to the number of HbS cells in the patient's circulation.

The increased rigidity of sickled RBC causes an alteration in blood flow, probably starting in postcapillary venules. The resultant decrease in blood flow eventually leads to infarction of the region supplied by the vessel. RBC in areas of vascular stasis, such as the spleen and bone marrow, are more vulnerable to sickling. Acidosis also enhances sickling. In pneumonia there is hypoxia, fever, and acidosis, which increase the occurrence of sickling. Other infections may also precipitate a sickling crisis.

The MCHC is a critical parameter related to sickling. When the MCHC of HbS in an RBC is reduced, so is the tendency to sickle.

*Sickle cell trait* refers to the heterozygous inheritance of HbA from one parent and HbS from the other parent. Patients with this trait show neither clinical disease nor abnormality of RBC morphology, life span, or function, except when they experience arterial oxygen saturation below 40%. This degree of hypoxia might occur with a severe respiratory infection, under administration of anesthesia, or during an airplane flight in a nonpressurized cabin. Persons with sickle cell trait have hematuria as a consequence of renal microinfarcts. The microinfarcts occur at the tips of the renal medullary papillae, owing to sickling secondary to hypoxia and acidosis.

*Sickle cell anemia* refers to the homozygous inheritance of sickle genes from both parents. The RBC contain 90% to 100% HbS, with the remainder comprising HbF. The higher the HbF content, the milder the disease. The presence of fetal Hb protects RBC from sickling by retarding gelation. Thus, newborn infants with sickle cell anemia do not have symptoms of the disease because they have increased levels of HbF. Symptoms only appear after 6 months of age as the level of fetal Hb diminishes and is gradually replaced by HbS. Sickle cell anemia is characterized by chronic hemolytic anemia and vascular occlusions, which may affect any organ of the body. RBC in these patients sickle at the oxygen tension normally found in venous blood. Consequently, there are periodic bouts of capillary occlusions resulting in painful infarctive crises due to tissue necrosis. Patients with sickle cell anemia have an increased susceptibility to infection. This is a consequence of splenic infarction and atrophy and the accompanying loss of splenic immunologic functions. Multiple organ damage is cumulative over the years. Death may result from infection, from a sudden major vascular occlusion affecting a vital organ, or from gradual failure of the liver, kidneys, or heart.

When HbS is associated with HbC (HbSC disease) or with $\beta$-thalassemia, this interaction increases the propensity of RBC to sickle and occlude vessels. The cardiac changes that are commonly observed in sickle cell anemia, representing largely a response to chronic anemia, are not a prominent finding in HbSC disease. Sickle cell $\beta$-thalassemia resembles sickle cell anemia when there is complete suppression of $\beta$-chain formation. When there is incomplete $\beta$-chain suppression, the disease resembles sickle cell trait.

The occurrence of $\alpha$-thalassemia and sickle cell anemia diminishes the severity of sickle-cell disease.[12] Compared with the levels in homozygous sickle cell anemia, there are higher Hb and hematocrit levels and lower reticulocyte counts, reflecting reduced hemolysis. There is a lower proportion of irreversibly sickled cells and greater deformability of RBC. The most likely explanation for the beneficial effect of $\alpha$-thalassemia is the reduction of MCHC, which reflects a reduced intracellular concentration of HbS.

## LABORATORY FINDINGS

### Sickle Cell Trait (HbAS Disease)

Normal peripheral smear and bone marrow

No anemia

Positive sickle cell test—when more than 25% HbS is present, sickling of RBC may be demonstrated in a blood suspension by deoxygenation of the blood

Positive solubility test for HbS—sickle cell Hb is insoluble in a phosphate buffer solution

Hb electrophoresis—HbA 70%–80%; HbS 30%–40%; HbF <2%. Preponderance of HbA over HbS is a prerequisite for this diagnosis. (The reverse occurs in sickle cell $\beta$-thalassemia)

Low fixed urine specific gravity and hematuria occur as a result of renal medullary microinfarcts.

### Sickle Cell Anemia (HbSS Disease)

*Peripheral Blood*
Sickle cells, ovalocytes, marked poikilocytosis, anisocytosis, nucleated RBC, Howell-Jolly bodies, target cells, spherocytes, polychromatophilia, stippled RBC, siderocytes. These abnormal cells appear in the circulation because the infarcted spleen is no longer able to remove them from the circulation.

Normocytic, normochromic anemia (Hb 5 g/dl–11 g/dl)

Increased reticulocytes (5%–30%)—decreased during aplastic crisis

Increased WBC with left shift (10,000/$\mu$l–30,000/$\mu$l)—does not necessarily signify an infection

Increased platelets (300,000/$\mu$l–500,000/$\mu$l)—may fall during an infarctive crisis

*Bone Marrow*
Hyperplasia of all elements but especially of RBC precursors

Increased iron deposits

*Other Laboratory Findings*
Positive sickle cell test—RBC transform to sickled form in an oxygen-poor environment

Positive solubility test for HbS—sickle cell Hb is insoluble in a phosphate buffer solution

Hb electrophoresis—HbS 80%–100%, HbF 0%–20%; because there is no normal $\beta$ polypeptide chain, there is no HbA.

Findings of hemolysis—increased unconjugated (indirect) bilirubin, LDH (especially $LDH_1$ and $LDH_2$), urine hemosiderin; decreased serum haptoglobin

Decreased sedimentation rate—reflects failure of sickle cells to undergo rouleaux formation

Decreased osmotic fragility—the sickled RBC resist hemolysis by hypotonic salt solutions

Increased serum alkaline phosphatase—result of bone and liver infarcts

Hematuria and fixed urine specific gravity (1.010–1.020)—due to repeated microinfarcts in the renal medulla

Laboratory findings of complications: infarction of lungs, spleen, kidneys; osteomyelitis, usually due to *Salmonella;* iron deficiency anemia (decreased ferritin and MCV)

### HbSC Disease

Peripheral blood—sickle cells, many target cells (20%–85%); HbC crystals in 1%–2% of RBC, especially following splenectomy

Mild anemia

Slight reticulocytosis (about 3%)

Hemoglobin electrophoresis—HbS 40%–50%, HbC 40%–50%, HbF 2%–15%, HbA absent

### Sickle Cell $\beta$-Thalassemia Disease

Many target cells (20%–40%)

Hypochromic, microcytic anemia

Hb electrophoresis—complete $\beta$-chain suppression: HbS 50%–80%, HbF 2%–30%, $HbA_2$ >3.6%; incomplete $\beta$-chain suppression: HbS 50%–80%, HbF 2%–20%, HbA 15%–35%, $HbA_2$ >3.6%

Other laboratory findings are those of HbSS disease.

## HEMOGLOBIN C DISEASE

HbC differs from adult Hb (HbA) in that the $\beta$-globin chains contain the amino acid *lysine* in place of glutamic acid in position 6.

Inheritance of HbC variant from both parents results in homozygous HbC (HbCC) disease. If the HbC variant is inherited from one parent, it results in heterozygous HbC (HbAC) trait (or in HbSC disease if the other parent transmits HbS).

Persons with homozygous HbC disease have mild chronic hemolytic anemia associated with splenomegaly. The abnormal Hb spontaneously crystallizes, particularly in aged RBC. The RBC then become rigid, fragment in the circulation, and possibly form microspherocytes. These cells are subject to entrapment and destruction by the spleen. The abnormal Hb aggregates in the central portion of RBC, resulting in marked target-cell formation.

Persons with HbAC trait have fewer target cells than do those with HbCC disease, and they do not show signs of hemolysis or anemia.

For a discussion of HbSC disease, see Sickle Cell Disease.

## LABORATORY FINDINGS

### HbAC Trait

Peripheral blood—moderately increased number of target cells (5%–30%)

Hb electrophoresis—HbA 55%–70%, HbC 30%–45%, HbA$_2$ slightly increased

### HbCC Disease

*Peripheral Blood*
Many target cells (about 90%), variable microspherocytes, polychromatophilia, a few RBC contain tetragonal HbC crystals. The crystals increase up to 10% following splenectomy and after incubation in 3% NaCl.

Mild normocytic anemia (Hb 8 g/dl–12 g/dl)

*Bone Marrow*
Normoblastic hyperplasia

*Other Laboratory Findings*
Hemoglobin electrophoresis—HbC 95%–100%, HbF 0%–5%, HbA absent

Findings of slight hemolysis—increased reticulocytes (2%–10%), LDH, unconjugated bilirubin

Osmotic fragility test shows two cell populations; target cells have decreased fragility and microspherocytes have increased fragility.

### HbSC Disease

See Sickle Cell Disease.

## *AUTOIMMUNE HEMOLYTIC ANEMIAS*

Autoimmune hemolytic anemia (AIHA) is caused by antibody to one's own RBC antigens. The mechanism of the antibody formation is unknown, although some abnormality of the normal immune pathways is suspected. RBC destruction is mediated by coating of the RBC with IgG or IgM antibodies and, in certain conditions, by complement. In the case of IgG antibodies, circulating monocytes and tissue phagocytes bind the Fc portion of the IgG molecule. This initiates a process of accelerated fragmentation and RBC membrane loss, which results in cell destruction. Phagocytosis occurs throughout the RE system, but especially in the spleen. The coated RBC are sequestered in the spleen and withdrawn from the circulation over several days. The process is greatly augmented when complement is present on the RBC surface. RBC destruction is predominantly extravascular. RBC coated with IgM antibodies, in contrast, characteristically fix complement and are hemolyzed intravascularly or are destroyed in the liver.

The autoimmune hemolytic anemias are classified as warm AIHA or cold AIHA on the basis of the temperature required for maximal activity of the autoantibody. Usually, warm autoantibodies are IgG and cold autoantibodies are IgM. Warm AIHA is far more common than is cold AIHA. The former is frequently associated with lupus erythematosus or with other autoimmune diseases, infectious diseases, chronic lymphocytic leukemia, or lymphocytic lymphoma.

Cold AIHA may manifest as cold agglutinin disease or paroxysmal cold hemoglobinuria. Cold agglutinin disease is most commonly associated with *Mycoplasma pneumoniae* infections but may also occur with malignant lymphomas or in the absence of any known underlying cause. As a rule, only patients with cold agglutinins at titers over 1:1000 and with a wide thermal range of activity develop active hemolysis. Paroxysmal cold hemoglobinuria is a rare disorder characterized by the sudden passage of Hb in the urine following local or general exposure to cold. This is characteristically found in association with syphilis and with various viral infections. Paroxysmal cold hemoglobinuria differs from cold agglutinin disease by showing a positive result to the Donath-Landsteiner test.

## LABORATORY FINDINGS

### Findings of Hemolysis

Increased unconjugated (indirect) bilirubin (2.5 mg/dl–5.0 mg/dl), decreased haptoglobin, slight increase in plasma hemoglobin.

Occasionally massive hemoglobinemia, hemoglobinuria, and hemosiderinuria in fulminant disease and in paroxysmal cold hemoglobinuria.

### Peripheral Blood

Moderately severe anemia, increased reticulocytosis unless there is impaired marrow function, anisocytosis, nucleated RBC; marked polychromatophilia and increased MCV reflect increased numbers of reticulocytes

*Warm type*—microspherocytes due to piecemeal ingestion of antibody-coated RBC membrane by macrophages in the RE system. Minimal autoagglutination, which is not enhanced by cooling.

*Cold type*—clumping of RBC on cooling and even at room temperature; clumps dissolve upon warming to 37°C.

Leukocytosis—may be slight but might reach leukemoid proportions (>50,000/$\mu$l) as a result of stress response to acute hemolysis

### Bone Marrow

Marked hypercellularity—result of normoblastic hyperplasia in response to hemolysis

Increased iron deposits—result of accelerated RBC turnover

Megaloblasts may occur; these are secondary to folic acid deficiency following prolonged severe hemolysis

Underlying lymphoma or lymphocytic leukemia may be present.

### Direct Antiglobulin (Coombs') Test

A positive direct Coombs' test indicates that an antibody is attached to the surface of the patient's RBC. This will be indicated by broad-spectrum antiglobulin reagents. Using monospecific Coombs' reagents, warm AIHA will react maximally at 37°C with anti-human IgG serum alone (30%–40% of patients) or with both anti-IgG and anticomplement sera (40%–50% of patients). When only IgG is detected, it is usually an antibody reacting with Rh antigenic sites. These sites are separated so that two IgG molecules will not be close enough to activate the complement system. When IgG and complement are both detected, the antibody is usually directed against non-Rh antigens that are spaced so that two IgG molecules can fix complement.

Cold AIHA reacts maximally at 4°C and reacts only with anti-complement serum. The IgM antibody is rarely detected because it quickly separates from RBC, especially on warming. The bound complement may be detected at 37°C.

### Indirect Antiglobulin (Coombs') Test

The indirect Coombs' test indicates the presence of free autoantibody in the patient's serum, which occurs when there are large amounts of autoantibody and low RBC binding affinity. Warm autoantibodies are usually IgG, they agglutinate test cells at 37°C, and they show no increase in reactivity at 4°C. Cold autoantibodies are IgM, they strongly agglutinate test cells at 4°C, but they may sometimes react at up to 33°C. This indicates a wide thermal range of reactivity.

### Eluates of RBC

In warm AIHA, antibody eluted from the RBC surface is usually the same as that identified in the patient's serum in the indirect Coombs' test. In cold AIHA, no antibody can be eluted from RBC surface because the antibody usually has already eluted spontaneously.

### Cold Agglutinin Titer

See Table 8-1 for examples of conditions showing increased cold agglutinin titers.

### Other Laboratory Findings

Positive Donath-Landsteiner test in paroxysmal cold hemoglobinuria. An IgG antibody initially adsorbs to the surface of RBC along with complement at a low temperature. The antibody then causes intravascular hemolysis and hemoglobinuria as the temperature is increased to 37°C. This antibody is termed a *biphasic hemolysin.*

Decreased serum complement—this is usually associated with cold AIHA because IgM, which occurs in this disorder, binds complement. Decreased complement also occurs in paroxysmal cold hemoglobinuria during an attack because the Donath-Landsteiner antibody binds complement. Complement is occasionally decreased in warm AIHA.

**Table 8-1.** Conditions Showing Increased Cold Agglutinin Titers*

| DISORDER | USUAL TITER |
| --- | --- |
| Idiopathic cold AIHA | >1 : 256 |
| Mycoplasmal pneumonia | 1 : 1000–1 : 8000 |
| Cold agglutinin disease | >1 : 10,000 |

* The hemolytic activity of the serum correlates more closely with the thermal amplitude of the antibody than with the titer. Thermal amplitude refers to the extent of temperature range of activity, even up to 33°C.

Positive antinuclear antibody suggests lupus erythematosus as the basis of warm AIHA.

Increased osmotic fragility test—this reflects the presence of spherocytes, which usually occur in warm AIHA; the osmotic fragility is not enhanced by incubation at 37°C.

Increased autohemolysis test—this occurs during periods of active hemolysis; it is not corrected by the addition of glucose.

## DRUG-INDUCED IMMUNE HEMOLYSIS

Drugs may damage RBC by interacting with intrinsic enzyme systems, such as in G6PD deficiency, and by inducing formation of extrinsic antibodies. The latter may be caused by several mechanisms and is classified as follows:[10]

### IMMUNE-COMPLEX TYPE

Certain drugs, such as quinidine and phenacetin, act as antigens and stimulate formation of an IgM antibody. This antibody then reacts with the circulating drug antigen to form an immune complex. The antibody–drug complex nonspecifically adsorbs to the RBC membrane and fixes complement (Fig. 8-6). The RBC is considered to be an innocent bystander. The RBC-bound complement accounts for the occurrence of intravascular hemolysis. Characteristically, the patient needs to take only a small quantity of the drug if he has been sensitized by prior exposure. Hemolysis is often acute in onset and fulminant in severity. This is an infrequent cause of hemolytic anemia in general and of drug-associated immune hemolysis in particular.

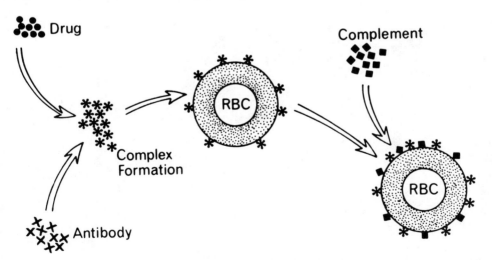

**Fig. 8-6.** The immune-complex mechanism. (Petz LD, Garraty G: Acquired Immune Hemolytic Anemias, p 474. Edinburgh, Churchill Livingstone, 1980)

### DRUG-ADSORPTION (HAPTEN-FORMATION) TYPE

Penicillin and penicillin derivatives account for most cases of this type of immune hemolysis. Penicillin, when given in very high doses, nonspecifically adsorbs to the RBC membrane (Fig. 8-7). If a patient develops a potent antibody against the adsorbed drug, this antibody will be fixed to the RBC surface. These RBC will yield a positive direct Coombs' test. Complement is usually not activated by these antibodies. Extravascular agglutination may occur; this results in sequestration and increased destruction of RBC in the spleen.

### WARM AUTOIMMUNE HEMOLYTIC ANEMIA TYPE

Methyldopa (Aldomet) is the drug most frequently responsible for this type of immune hemolysis. The drug appears to inhibit suppressor T-cell function; this leads to unregulated autoantibody production by B cells in some patients.[7] An IgG autoantibody forms and binds to an Rh site on the RBC membrane. RBC survival is shortened as a result of extravascular agglutination and splenic sequestration. One percent of patients have intravascular hemolysis. Approximately 10% to 36% of patients receiving Aldomet have positive direct Coombs' tests after receiving the drug for 3 months to 6 months. The autoimmune state persists for months after discontinuation of the drug.

### NONIMMUNOLOGIC PROTEIN-ADSORPTION TYPE

Cephalothin and its derivatives are most frequently responsible for this type of disorder. The drug alters the RBC membrane and causes nonspecific and

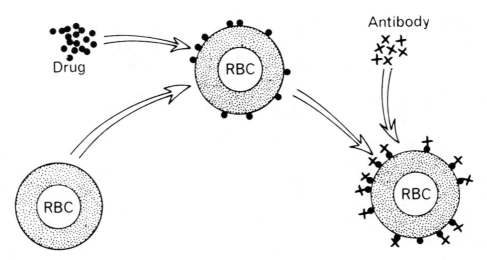

**Fig. 8-7.** The drug-adsorption mechanism. (Petz LD, Garraty G: Acquired Immune Hemolytic Anemias, p 470. Edinburgh, Churchill Livingstone, 1980)

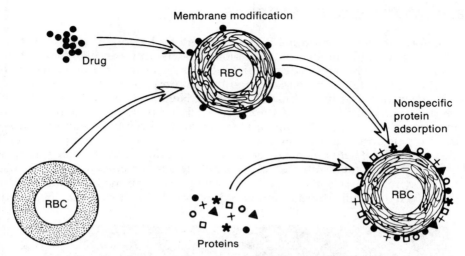

**Fig. 8-8.** Nonimmunologic protein adsorption. (Petz LD, Garraty G: Acquired Immune Hemolytic Anemias, p 473 Edinburgh, Churchill Livingstone, 1980)

nonimmunologic adsorption of serum proteins to the RBC (Fig. 8-8). The adsorbed proteins give a positive direct Coombs' test. Hemolysis is rare.

## LABORATORY FINDINGS

Normochromic anemia—severity is variable

Macrocytosis (MCV 105 $\mu m^3$–110 $\mu m^3$)—reflects reticulocytosis

Findings of hemolysis (increased unconjugated bilirubin, reticulocytosis, increased LDH; decreased haptoglobin)—usually brief, stopping when the drug is withdrawn

Positive direct Coombs' test—this finding is essential to establish an immune basis of the hemolysis. The adsorbed globulin may be IgG or complement, depending on the mechanism:[10]
    Immune complex—usually complement only
    Drug adsorption—IgG or IgG and complement
    Warm autoimmune hemolytic anemia—IgG only; strongly positive
    Nonimmunologic protein adsorption—IgG and complement (and other serum proteins)

Antibody identification:[10]
    Immune complex—serum usually reacts with RBC in presence of drug; eluate nonreactive
    Drug adsorption—serum reacts with drug-treated RBC to high titer; eluate reacts with drug-treated RBC
    Warm autoimmune hemolytic anemia—antibody in serum and eluate is similar to that found in warm antibody AIHA
    Nonimmunologic protein adsorption—no serum antibody; eluate nonreactive

## HEMOLYTIC-UREMIC SYNDROME

The hemolytic-uremic syndrome is characterized by hemolytic anemia, thrombocytopenia with thrombosis of small blood vessels, intravascular coagulation, and renal failure. The hemolytic anemia is due to intravascular fragmentation of RBC. The fragmentation is characterized by the presence of schistocytes on the blood smear and by intravascular hemolysis. Hemolysis is the result of traumatic disruption of RBC forced through vessels partially obstructed by fibrin strands (Fig. 8-9). Glomerular capillaries show fibrin thrombi and multiple areas of ischemic necrosis throughout the kidneys. The renal lesions appear to be a consequence of the hematologic disorder. Although the cause of the syndrome is unknown, disseminated intravascular coagulation is considered to play a role.

This syndrome is a major cause of acute renal failure in children. It is characterized clinically by sudden bleeding, oliguria, hematuria, hemolytic

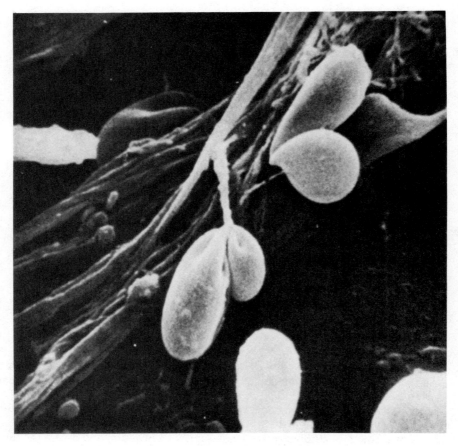

**Fig. 8-9.** Red-cell fragmentation by fibrin strands (scanning electron micrograph). (Bull BS, Kuhn IN: The Production of schistocytes by fibrin strands. Blood 35:104–111, 1970. Reproduced by permission of publisher and author.)

anemia, and often by neurologic signs. Hypertension is present in about 50% of patients. Typically, the disease begins a few days to 2 weeks after an episode of gastroenteritis or an upper respiratory tract infection.

Adult hemolytic-uremic syndrome occurs in pregnant women with septic abortion or other complications of pregnancy; following delivery after an uneventful pregnancy; in association with the use of oral contraceptives; or in association with various infections.

## LABORATORY FINDINGS

### Peripheral Blood

This characteristically shows burr and fragmented RBC and occasional nucleated RBC

Decreased Hb—often <6 g/dl

Increased reticulocytes—reflects bone-marrow response to hemolysis

### Other Laboratory Findings

Absent serum haptoglobin—reflects chronic hemolysis

Findings of disseminated intravascular coagulation—increased fibrin split products and decreased platelet count

Urine—moderate to massive protein, RBC, WBC; granular, hyaline, and RBC casts

Azotemia—BUN frequently >100 mg/dl

Oliguria

## *PAROXYSMAL NOCTURNAL HEMOGLOBINURIA*

Paroxysmal nocturnal hemoglobinuria is a relatively rare, acquired chronic hemolytic disorder classically characterized by episodes of intravascular hemolysis with passage of red or brownish black urine on arising in the morning. The mechanism of the nocturnal exacerbation is poorly understood. The usual presentation is that of chronic hemolysis with little or no hemoglobinuria.

The disorder seems to be caused by an acquired abnormality of the RBC membrane; the exact nature of the abnormality is unknown. The abnormal RBC have a markedly increased sensitivity to lysis by complement. Affected persons have differing proportions of erythrocyte populations, one sensitive and the other insensitive to complement hemolysis. The sensitive RBC population perhaps comprises the offspring of stem cells with a somatic mutation. The degree of hemolysis reflects the proportion of complement-sensitive RBC. There is evidence that platelets and granulocytes also have complement-sensitive membrane abnormalities and show increased lysis.

The membrane defects involving several types of blood cells probably reflect a type of bone-marrow dysplasia. This suggests that injured marrow, or marrow that has lost the ability to proliferate normally, could provide the setting for the development of a clone of defective cells. This condition often occurs in association with aplastic or hypoplastic anemia.

The disorder is activated following infections, exercise, surgery, or other physical or emotional stresses. The most serious consequences are intravascular thromboses, especially of the mesenteric and portal veins. Thrombophlebitis may occur in the arms or legs and may lead to thromboembolism. Venous thromboses probably reflect platelet activation by complement.

## LABORATORY FINDINGS

### Peripheral Blood

Normocytic, normochromic anemia, moderate to severe—Hb often <6 g/dl

Increased macrocytes and polychromatophilia—reflect reticulocytosis

Microcytic, hypochromic anemia—iron deficiency results from recurrent hemoglobinuria

Decrease in platelets (approximately 67% of patients)—reflects marrow hypoplasia

Decreased WBC (approximately 60% of patients)—reflects marrow hypoplasia

### Bone Marrow

Normoblastic hyperplasia

Lack of iron late in course of the disease

Possible aplasia or leukemia

### Other Laboratory Findings

Findings of hemolysis—reticulocytosis (10%–35%); decreased haptoglobin; increased unconjugated (indirect) bilirubin and LDH; increased urine hemosiderin and Hb; hemoglobinemia, especially during sleep

Decreased leukocyte alkaline phosphatase reflects dysplastic WBC.

Decreased serum iron—result of continuous urinary loss of iron

Abnormal autohemolysis test, which probably reflects lysis due to complement

Negative direct Coombs' test indicates the nonimmunologic basis of the hematologic disorder.

### Diagnostic Tests

These demonstrate lysis of complement-sensitive RBC.

Positive sucrose hemolysis test—in this screening test a sucrose solution of low ionic strength maintains osmotic equilibrium while complement fixes to and hemolyzes paroxysmal nocturnal hemoglobinuria erythrocytes. This test is sensitive but not specific.

Positive acid hemolysis test (Ham test) (definitive test)—paroxysmal nocturnal hemoglobinuria erythrocytes hemolyze when suspended in fresh, normal, compatible complement-containing serum acidified to pH 6.8. Verified pH is critical for optimal complement activation. Spherocytes will also hemolyze and will give a false-positive test.

# HEMOLYTIC DISEASE OF THE NEWBORN

In hemolytic disease of the newborn (HDN), the RBC of the fetus and newborn are coated with maternal IgG antibody and undergo immune destruction in the infant's RE system. Cases vary in severity, ranging from intrauterine death to a clinically inapparent condition that can be detected only by serologic tests in a healthy baby. The most severe form of HDN is that due to anti-D; next in severity is that due to other Rh antibodies. Least severe is HDN due to ABO antibodies (ABO HDN).

Except for ABO antibodies, maternal antibodies result from previous immunization by transfusion or pregnancy. When immunization follows pregnancy, the antigenic stimulus is fetal RBC possessing antigens foreign to the mother; these cells escape through the placenta and gain access to the mother's circulation. Small numbers of cells characteristically enter the mother's circulation during the last half of pregnancy, but these are usually insufficient to induce immunization. Intrapartum sensitization may occur. Most immunizations result from larger amounts of fetomaternal hemorrhage that occurs during placental separation at the time of delivery. Approximately half of all women have fetal cells in their circulation in the postpartum period, but the absolute volume of fetomaternal hemorrhage at delivery usually is small.

Rh-negative women probably experience primary immunization during the delivery of an Rh-positive child but do not produce detectable levels of antibody. For immunization to take place, fetal RBC must remain in the maternal circulation long enough to stimulate the mother's antibody-producing mechanisms. The small numbers of fetal cells that enter the circulation during a subsequent Rh-positive pregnancy constitute a secondary stimulus sufficient to produce antibody while the pregnancy is in progress.

The incidence of Rh immunization is much lower following delivery of an ABO-incompatible child than when the fetal cells are ABO compatible with the mother. ABO incompatibility between mother and fetus results in the destruction of many fetal cells in the maternal circulation before they can stimulate Rh-antibody production.

Only about 12% of Rh-negative mothers become immunized. Type ABO incompatibility, poor antibody formation by the mother, or an insufficient antigenic stimulus (small volume of fetal-maternal bleeding) protects most Rh-negative mothers from sensitization.

In ABO HDN there is, in the mother's circulation, anti-A, anti-B, or anti-A, B of the IgG class without requisite prior immunization by foreign RBC. IgG is the only maternal immunoglobulin to cross the placenta. ABO HDN may occur in any pregnancy, including the first. Type ABO incompatibility is the most common cause of HDN, but the hemolysis is minimal and does not require treatment. Group O women are far more likely to produce the IgG class of anti-A and anti-B than are group A or B women. Consequently, ABO HDN usually is limited to group A or B babies born of group O mothers. Most of the maternal A and B antibodies are absorbed or neutralized by fetal tissues diminishing their impact on fetal RBC. Owing to the small number of antibody molecules sensitizing the fetal cells, the antibody attachment is weak and only minimal fetal RBC destruction occurs. The first indication of ABO HDN may be the appearance of jaundice at 24 to 48 hours of life, later than its appearance in Rh HDN. No tests are available for the accurate prenatal prediction of ABO HDN.

When fetal RBC are coated with maternal antibody, they are removed from the circulation by the fetal liver and spleen, resulting in varying degrees of anemia. Fetal hematopoietic tissue responds to the RBC destruction with increased production of new RBC, many of which prematurely enter the circulation as reticulocytes and nucleated RBC. The liver and spleen enlarge primarily because of their role in forming blood cells to supplement bone-marrow activity. If the immune destruction is severe, increased RBC production cannot completely compensate for the loss of RBC, and the fetus becomes increasingly anemic. Severe anemia may lead to heart failure with generalized edema, sometimes resulting in intrauterine or neonatal death. If the severely affected baby is liveborn, the major risk during the first few hours of life is heart failure from severe anemia.

*In utero*, the bilirubin resulting from the RBC destruction crosses the placenta to the maternal circulation, where the maternal liver excretes it. After birth, the infant continues to experience increased RBC destruction. However, the liver of the premature and newborn infant is unable to conjugate and excrete bilirubin effectively because glucuronyl transferase, the enzyme necessary to conjugate bilirubin, is poorly developed. If the serum level of unconjugated bilirubin exceeds the binding capacity of plasma albumin, the unbound, unconjugated bilirubin leaves the circulation and tends to deposit in certain brain cells. This condition is called *kernicterus*, which can cause permanent brain damage or even death.

At birth there is an inverse relationship between the concentrations of cord Hb and bilirubin. Infants who are severely anemic tend to have high bilirubin levels. The clinical severity of HDN correlates better with cord blood Hb levels than with the cord bilirubin level. The former is the most important laboratory test to be done at birth. Fifty percent of infants with HDN will have normal cord Hb values. Following delivery, the placental transfer of blood tends to falsely elevate newborn Hb values. When blood is obtained by heel prick, the Hb values may average up to 4 g/dl higher than in cord blood. The cord blood bilirubin value is important because it serves as a baseline for evaluation of the rate of increase of jaundice.

## LABORATORY FINDINGS

### Rh Incompatibility

Fetal blood group Rh$_o$(D)-positive

Maternal blood group Rh$_o$(D)-negative

Positive direct antiglobulin test on cord RBC indicates maternal antibody which is attached to fetal RBC. Antibody should be eluted and identified.

Maternal antibody screening positive—the antibody must match that eluted from fetal RBC. The antibody titer does not correlate with the severity of HDN.

Normal cord Hb is 14 g/dl–20 g/dl. Capillary blood may be up to 4 g/dl higher.

Cord blood Hb indicates the degree of anemia and reflects the severity of the disease.

Macrocytic anemia (8 g/dl–16 g/dl)—not usually present at birth, maximal at 3–4 days

Peripheral blood: Increased nucleated RBC (>10/100 WBC)—this reflects the rapid formation and release from the marrow, liver, and spleen of immature RBC in response to the RBC destruction. Macrocytes and polychromatophilia reflect reticulocytosis.

Reticulocytosis (10% to 60%) reflects marrow response to hemolysis.

Leukocytosis (15,000/$\mu$l–30,000/$\mu$l) reflects marrow response to stress.

Increased serum unconjugated (indirect) bilirubin—present at birth or very shortly thereafter; rises rapidly

**ABO Incompatibility**

Fetal blood group A or B

Maternal blood group O

Weak direct antiglobulin test on cord RBC, which becomes negative within 12 hours after birth. The weak reaction is due to the small number of antibody molecules attached to the RBC.

Eluted IgG, anti-A, or anti-B from infant's RBC are tested against adult A and B RBC.

Anti-A may be found in Group A infant's serum; anti-B may be found in Group B infant's serum.

Marked microspherocytosis—not seen in Rh hemolytic disease

Increased osmotic fragility reflects presence of spherocytes

Increased unconjugated (indirect) bilirubin—this is less elevated and of shorter duration than in Rh incompatibility

Minimal anemia

# APLASTIC ANEMIA

*Aplastic anemia* refers to pancytopenia associated with a decrease in all hematopoietic precursors of the bone marrow. Committed stem cells are decreased or absent. Evidence suggests that the stem cells are deficient, defective, or suppressed. Other possible mechanisms include abnormalities of the bone-marrow microenvironment, ineffective cell-to-cell interactions, and immune disorders. In addition to anemia, granulocytopenia and thrombocytopenia always occur. Because of the insidious onset of the disease, it is difficult to assess the sequence of appearance of the various cytopenias. However, the platelet level is usually the last marrow function to recover when the disease process remits.

There is a decrease in the volume of active blood-cell-producing bone marrow; there is also extensive marrow replacement by fat. The remaining marrow becomes confined to small, often intensely active islands. These hyperplastic foci contain functionally abnormal blood-cell precursors.

The reduced and impaired bone marrow clears iron from the plasma slowly. This allows extramedullary tissues, such as the liver and spleen, more time to compete with the marrow for circulating iron. The decreased utilization of iron by marrow RBC results in an increased concentration of serum iron and increased transferrin saturation. RBC have increased oxygen affinity, resulting in tissue hypoxia. This stimulates the kidneys to form increased erythropoietin.

No cause can be found for approximately 50% of cases of aplastic anemia. Most cases of known origin are due to drugs used for cancer chemotherapy, an industrial hydrocarbon such as benzene, or a medical drug such as chloramphenicol. Generally, the mode of action of drugs leading to aplastic anemia may be divided into three categories: dose-dependent reversible toxicity, individual increased sensitivity, and drug-induced immune reactions.[5] Other causes of aplastic anemia include radiation therapy, viral hepatitis, miliary tuberculosis, and Fanconi's anemia, which is associated with multiple congenital anomalies. Aplastic anemia develops in approximately 25% of patients with paroxysmal nocturnal hemoglobinuria.

Pure RBC aplasia frequently appears to be part of an autoimmune disorder, and 50% of these cases are associated with thymoma, a tumor of the thymus gland.

## LABORATORY FINDINGS

### Peripheral Blood

Normocytic, normochromic anemia (Hb <9 g/dl); occasional macrocytosis

Leukopenia (<2,000/$\mu$l)—granulocytes especially decreased; 70%–90% lymphocytes

Thrombocytopenia (<70,000/$\mu$l)—decrease persists long after WBC and RBC return to normal levels

Decreased reticulocytes

### Bone Marrow

Aspiration and biopsy—several biopsies may be required because there may be foci of normal cellularity

Decreased cellularity, especially granulocytes and megakaryocytes

Increased fat is a characteristic finding.

Focal hypercellularity showing relative lymphocytosis (60%–100%).

Usually increased iron in RE cells

### Other Laboratory Findings

Increased serum iron due to impaired marrow utilization of iron

Decreased serum iron-binding capacity

Increased transferrin saturation, marked (may be almost 100%)—this is often the first sign of reduced marrow utilization of iron

Increased serum and urine erythropoietin—levels are higher than in most other types of anemia

Prolonged bleeding time and poor clot retraction reflect thrombocytopenia.

Increased infections reflect impaired defenses associated with severe granulocytopenia.

## SIDEROBLASTIC ANEMIA

*Sideroblastic anemia* refers to a rare anemia characterized by ineffective erythropoiesis, two RBC populations in the peripheral blood, normoblastic hyperplasia of the bone marrow, increased marrow iron, and a large number of ringed sideroblasts in the bone marrow. A sideroblast is a normoblast with cytoplasmic iron granules. When the granules are arranged in a ring around the nucleus, the resulting cell is called a ringed sideroblast.

The ringed sideroblast is caused by iron accumulation in the mitochondria of RBC precursors. Iron-loaded mitochondria are morphologically and functionally abnormal. It is thought that this form of iron accumulation is secondary to disturbances in heme metabolism. Studies reveal increase in plasma iron turnover, with decreased RBC iron utilization and normal to slightly decreased RBC survival. There is premature destruction of marrow RBC precursors. These features all indicate ineffective erythropoiesis. Many RBC formed from the maturation of the ringed sideroblasts are nonviable.

Sideroblastic anemia may be hereditary or acquired. When acquired, it may be drug-induced or associated with leukemia, myeloma, thyroid dysfunction, carcinoma, uremia, or rheumatoid arthritis. The hereditary form of the disease may be due to one or more inborn errors of metabolism. Sideroblastic anemia has also been found in malnourished, chronic alcoholic patients, some of whom respond to pyridoxine (vitamin $B_6$) therapy. Pyridoxine-responsive sideroblastic anemia occurs as both a primary and a secondary disorder.

### LABORATORY FINDINGS

#### Peripheral Blood

Normocytic to slightly macrocytic anemia (Hb 7 g/dl–10 g/dl)

Increased RBC distribution width indicates two RBC populations; most RBC are normochromic, and some are hypochromic.

Marked anisocytosis with many bizarre forms

Occasional basophilic stippling, siderocytes, target cells, normoblasts

Usually normal reticulocytes—this is inappropriately low for the degree of anemia

Normal WBC and platelet counts; occasionally decreased WBC, especially neutrophils

Decreased WBC alkaline phosphatase (50% of patients)

#### Bone Marrow

Increase in ringed sideroblasts (>25% of nucleated RBC)—characteristic finding

Normoblastic hyperplasia, marked, with a shift to younger forms; occasional megaloblastoid maturation

Increased stainable iron (hemosiderin)

**Other Laboratory Findings**

Increased serum iron and normal or decreased total iron-binding capacity

Increased transferrin saturation

Increased serum ferritin

## ANEMIA OF MARROW INFILTRATION

Marrow infiltration anemia is also known as myelophthisic anemia. Whenever the bone marrow is infiltrated by cells that are either foreign to the marrow or present in abnormally excessive numbers, replacement of normal hematopoietic cells occurs. This most frequently results in anemia, with or without thrombocytopenia. Less commonly there is leukoerythroblastosis, which is the occurrence of immature granulocytes and nucleated RBC in the peripheral circulation. The explanation for release of immature marrow cells may be a mechanical disruption of the marrow architecture. Immature circulating cells may also arise from sites of blood cell formation in the liver and spleen. Pancytopenia may occur owing to slowly progressive hypersplenism secondary to depression of marrow function.

The most common infiltrative marrow processes are leukemia, lymphoma, myeloma, and metastatic cancer. Cancer usually originates in the breast, prostate, lung, or GI tract. Less common causes of marrow infiltration include myelofibrosis, granulomatous disorders, lipid storage diseases, tuberculosis, and fungus infections.

### LABORATORY FINDINGS

**Peripheral Blood**

Normochromic, normocytic anemia (Hb >9 g/dl)

Nucleated RBC, even in absence of anemia; this suggests marrow invasion

Marked anisocytosis and poikilocytosis; "teardrop" erythrocytes occur with myelofibrosis; polychromatophilia, basophilic stippling

WBC are normal to decreased; occasional immature cells suggest marrow invasion

Platelets are normal to decreased; giant platelets or fragments of megakaryocytes suggest marrow invasion.

**Bone Marrow**

Bone marrow shows the infiltrates of leukemia, metastatic cancer, fibrosis or plasma cells. Marrow biopsy is usually more diagnostic than is a marrow aspirate.

**Laboratory Findings of Underlying Disease**

See diseases discussed above.

## HEMOPHILIA A

Hemophilia A (classical hemophilia or Factor VIII deficiency), although a rare disease, is the most commonly inherited coagulation disorder. It is transmitted as a sex-linked recessive trait, being carried on the X chromosome. The disease is transmitted to males by their mothers who, despite having the defective gene on one X chromosome, show no bleeding tendency.

Hemophilia A is due to a deficiency or functional abnormality of the small-molecular-weight subunit of the factor-VIII (antihemophilic factor [AHF]) molecule. This is the portion of AHF having coagulant activity.

The severity of the disease closely parallels the level of AHF. The disease may be so mild that a patient is able to live a completely normal life or so severe that a patient must be frequently hospitalized. Patients with severe classic hemophilia have virtually no AHF as measured in clotting assays. Patients with moderate hemophilia have less than 3% AHF, and mild hemophiliacs have 5% to 15% AHF. Spontaneous bleeding does not occur unless the level of AHF falls below 10%.

Except when mild, hemophilia appears in infancy. The joints are the most frequent site of hemorrhage, followed by the muscles. Bleeding occurs less frequently from the skin, GI tract, genitourinary tract, nose, and mouth. Hemophiliacs who bleed from these sites do so after injury or surgery, including dental extraction. The injury that initiates bleeding may be so slight as to go unnoticed and the bleeding may appear to be spontaneous. Bleeding does not occur immediately after the injury but only after a variable time interval. Without treatment, bleeding continues for prolonged periods.

Antibodies against AHF develop in about 7% of patients with hemophilia A. The titer of the antibody increases after transfusions of plasma, cryoprecipitate, or AHF concentrates. Antibody detection is important because the patient may become unresponsive to treatment.

### LABORATORY FINDINGS

Prolonged activated partial thromboplastin time (APTT) when factor VIII is below 25%–30%; corrected by normal plasma

Normal prothrombin time, bleeding time, thrombin time, fibrinogen

Decreased AHF—definitive test

Normal von Willebrand antigen and ristocetin-induced platelet agglutination

Possible presence of antibody against AHF—reflects reaction to repeated administration of AHF

## VON WILLEBRAND'S DISEASE

In von Willebrand's disease there is an abnormality or deficiency in the production or release of factor VIII related antigen/Willebrand factor.[2] Some patients also have decreased levels of coagulant activity of AHF. As a consequence, platelets do not adhere normally to collagen or to damaged blood vessel lining cells. Platelets are present in normal numbers.

The disease is inherited as an autosomal dominant trait affecting both sexes. Many of the cases are so mild that bleeding symptoms are only manifested following some precipitating factor, such as ingestion of aspirin or slight thrombocytopenia following an infection.

### LABORATORY FINDINGS

Decreased AHF (6%–60% of normal levels)—occurs in less than 50% of patients

Marked increase in AHF following transfusion of normal plasma.

Decreased von Willebrand's factor (factor VIII related antigen)—characteristic finding

Prolonged bleeding time reflects level of von Willebrand's factor.

Decreased platelet retention by glass bead columns

Decreased or absent ristocetin-induced platelet agglutination—characteristic finding. In the presence of normal plasma, the patient's platelets aggregate with ristocetin; the patient's plasma impairs agglutination of normal platelets in the presence of ristocetin.

Normal platelet agglutination with adenosine diphosphate (ADP), epinephrine, and collagen

Abnormal activated partial thromboplastin time if AHF is less than 25%–30% of normal level

Normal prothrombin time, fibrinogen, thrombin time, platelet count, and clot retraction

## HEMOPHILIA B

Hemophilia B, or Factor IX deficiency, is commonly known as Christmas disease, which is named for the family in whom it was originally described.

Christmas disease is clinically indistinguishable from classical hemophilia; however, bleeding is less severe than in classical hemophilia. Inheritance and transmission are similar to those in classical hemophilia. Hemophilia A is four to eight times more common than hemophilia B.

### LABORATORY FINDINGS

Decreased factor IX level—titer <5% in severe cases; titer >30% in mild cases

Prolonged APTT—corrected by aged plasma, normal plasma, and normal serum

Normal prothrombin time, bleeding time, thrombin time, fibrinogen

## DISSEMINATED INTRAVASCULAR COAGULATION

Disseminated intravascular coagulation (DIC) occurs when there is a disturbance of the normal balance between the procoagulant factors and the natural inhibitors that maintain blood in the fluid state. When this balance is upset, there is widespread formation of thrombi in small blood vessels and capillaries. The consequent depletion of platelets, fibrinogen, prothrombin, and factors V and VIII causes bleeding. This process resembles that of *in vitro* conversion of plasma to serum. Thrombi are removed by fibrinolysis, which aggravates the bleeding tendency. Fibrinolysis results in formation of several fibrin or fibrinogen degradation or split products.

The following mechanisms may initiate DIC: endothelial injury, which activates Hageman factor and the intrinsic clotting system; tissue injury, which activates the extrinsic clotting system; and RBC or platelet injury with release of coagulant phospholipids. Plasminogen activators, which result in secondary fibrinolysis, are apparently released as a result of fibrin deposition on endothelial surfaces, endothelial injury, or hypoxia.

DIC may be caused by a great variety of clinical disorders, including systemic infections, sepsis, various obstetric conditions, shock, metastatic carcinoma, tissue injury, extensive burns, hemolysis, liver diseases, antigen–antibody reactions, and snake bites.

If not fatal, the process may be acute and self-limited or chronic and compensated, depending on the underlying cause. The coagulation profile differs between the acute and chronic forms.

Rapid fibrinolysis removes fibrin deposits from small blood vessels. Consequently, there is minimal tissue damage from blocked capillaries. Renal failure is a serious consequence of diminished circulation. Fragmented RBC, or schistocytes, occur as RBC are forced through an obstructing fibrin meshwork within small blood vessels (Fig. 8-9, p 246). The occurrence of fragmented RBC with vascular hemolysis is termed *microangiopathic hemolytic anemia*.

### LABORATORY FINDINGS

Increased fibrin or fibrinogen degradation products—these reflect lysis and breakdown of fibrin or fibrinogen; this finding is necessary for definitive diagnosis

Decreased platelets

Decreased fibrinogen—may be normal if the prior level was elevated

Prolonged thrombin time—only if fibrinogen <75 mg/dl

Additional findings in severe, acute DIC:
  Prolonged prothrombin time and APTT
  Schistocytes on peripheral blood smear
  Findings of intravascular hemolysis—hemoglobinemia, increased LDH, decreased haptoglobin

## *IDIOPATHIC THROMBOCYTOPENIC PURPURA*

Idiopathic thrombocytopenic purpura (ITP) refers to thrombocytopenia of unknown cause, with associated sites of purpura, or cutaneous bleeding. ITP is now considered to be an autoimmune disease.

In childhood, ITP is usually acute and often follows a viral infection. Such infections include rubella, measles, chickenpox, and mild respiratory or GI upset. Thrombocytopenia occurs about 1 week to 3 weeks after the infection has subsided; this suggests that platelet injury is caused by platelet antibodies or by immune complexes rather than by the virus itself. Immune complexes produce platelet damage in a manner similar to immune-mediated leukopenia and hemolytic anemia (see Drug-Induced Immune Hemolysis). Antibody production and action depend on the presence of circulating viral antigen and are thus of limited duration. The disease usually undergoes spontaneous remission within 2 weeks to 6 weeks.

In adults, the disorder is chronic and has an insidious onset in an otherwise healthy person. The agent responsible for the production of platelet autoantibodies is unknown. The pathogenesis is comparable to that of AIHA, but ITP is more common. ITP follows a fluctuating course that lasts months or years.

## LABORATORY FINDINGS

### Peripheral Blood

Decreased platelets (<20,000/$\mu$l in the acute form; 10,000/$\mu$l–80,000/$\mu$l in the chronic form)—thrombocytopenia is due to shortened platelet survival (1–2 days versus 10 days). Platelets are coated by an IgG antibody and removed from the circulation, primarily by the spleen but also by the liver and other reticuloendothelial organs.

Large platelets are seen on smear—the early release of large immature platelets and megakaryocytic fragments from the bone marrow reflect an increased rate of platelet production.

### Bone Marrow

Increased numbers of megakaryocytes that are less granular, smoother in contour, and more basophilic than normal megakaryocytes; immature large megakaryocytes with increased numbers of nuclei; absence of attached platelets indicate rapid release from the marrow

### Other Laboratory Findings

Increased bleeding time and impaired clot retraction—reflect effect of thrombocytopenia

Findings due to bleeding: anemia, reticulocytosis, leukocytosis

## CHRONIC GRANULOMATOUS DISEASE

Chronic granulomatous disease of childhood is a sex-linked disorder of granulocyte function in boys. Infants with this disorder have repeated bacterial or fungal infections of the skin or lungs with low-virulence organisms. Infections begin early in life and usual life expectancy is 5 years to 7 years.

The defective granulocytes are capable of phagocytosing microorganisms but are incapable of forming hydrogen peroxide, which is necessary for the destruction and disposal of the ingested organisms. Bacterial metabolism generates some hydrogen peroxide, which kills ingested non–catalase-producing bacteria, such as pneumococci or streptococci. Organisms that form catalase, such as *Staphylococcus aureus,* most gram-negative enteric bacteria, *Candida albicans,* and *Aspergillus* species, inactivate bacterially produced hydrogen peroxide. Thus, catalase-producing organisms multiply within granulocytes because granulocytic hydrogen peroxide is unavailable for their destruction. The intracellular organisms are protected from most circulating antibiotics and may be transported to distant sites and released to establish new foci of infection. *S. aureus* is the most common pathogen.

## LABORATORY FINDINGS

Leukocytosis; increased sedimentation rate and C-reactive protein—reflect presence of infection

Increased granulocytes in the bone marrow

Negative nitroblue tetrazolium test reflects the inability of chronic granulomatous disease leukocytes to reduce the dye to blue crystals.

Normal serum complement and immunoglobulins

Laboratory evidence of recurrent infections

## *SECONDARY ERYTHROCYTOSIS*

Erythrocytosis is an absolute increase in the total number of circulating RBC. Erythrocytosis may be secondary to increased production of erythropoietin, which regulates the differentiation of committed erythroid stem cells in the bone marrow. The rate of erythropoietin production determines the rate of RBC production by the bone marrow.

Erythropoietin production may be physiologically appropriate or inappropriate. Appropriate erythropoietin formation is that formed chiefly in the kidneys in response to tissue hypoxia. The hypoxia results from anemia, arterial hypoxemia, increased affinity of Hb for oxygen, or reduced tissue blood flow. Specific causes of such conditions include chronic obstructive pulmonary disease, congenital heart disease with a right-to-left shunt, high altitude, increased carboxyhemoglobin (in smokers), and high oxygen affinity in persons with abnormal Hb.

Physiologically inappropriate secondary erythrocytosis is uncommon and occurs without tissue hypoxia. Causes include increased erythropoietin production by renal carcinoma, by renal cysts, or by hydronephrosis. Erythropoietin may also be produced by such nonrenal lesions as hepatoma, cerebellar hemangioma, or uterine fibroids. When such lesions are removed, the increased RBC returns to normal.

## LABORATORY FINDINGS

### Peripheral Blood

Increased Hb, hematocrit, and RBC; these parameters are markedly increased in congenital heart disease with right-to-left shunt

Increased reticulocyte count

*Normal WBC and platelet counts

**Bone Marrow**

Normoblastic hyperplasia

*No increase in granulocyte precursors or megakaryocytes

*Normal stainable iron

**Other Laboratory Findings**

*Decreased arterial oxygen saturation (<92%)—appropriate type

Normal arterial oxygen saturation (>92%)—inappropriate type

*Normal leukocyte alkaline phosphatase

*Increased serum erythropoietin

*Normal serum unbound vitamin $B_{12}$ binding capacity

Normal serum iron

Increased serum uric acid

Increased RBC mass (total number of circulating RBC)

Laboratory Findings of Underlying Disorders

## MYELOFIBROSIS WITH MYELOID METAPLASIA

Myelofibrosis with myeloid metaplasia is also known as agnogenic (meaning *unknown origin*) myeloid metaplasia or idiopathic myelofibrosis. Myelofibrosis is one of the myeloproliferative disorders, which include polycythemia vera, chronic myelocytic leukemia, acute myelocytic leukemia, essential thrombocythemia, and erythroleukemia. The basic defect in the myeloproliferative disorders is believed to be an abnormal proliferation of the bone marrow stem cells. In myelofibrosis, there is formation of fibrous tissue in the bone marrow. The fibrosis is thought to be a response or reaction to the abnormally proliferating cells. The fibrous tissue gradually obliterates the marrow cavity and interferes with the formation of all blood cells. Accompanying this process in the bone marrow, there is evidence of hematopoiesis in the liver and spleen. Conversion of these organs to perform a marrow function is called *myeloid metaplasia*. The metaplasia might be a compensatory mechanism for the profound pancytopenia seen in this disease. More likely, it is indicative of a neoplastic or abnormal growth process involving the liver and spleen. The process of hematopoiesis results in massive enlargement of the spleen and causes hepatomegaly in 75% of patients.

Myelofibrosis with myeloid metaplasia is an uncommon disorder that usually has an insidious onset with symptoms of anemia or splenomegaly. It generally affects persons over the age of 40 years. This condition may be the terminal event in chronic myelocytic leukemia or polycythemia vera or may itself termi-

---

* These findings help in differentiating secondary erythrocytosis from polycythemia vera.

nate in acute myelocytic leukemia. The causes of death include infection, hemorrhage, cardiac failure, and conversion to leukemia.

## LABORATORY FINDINGS

### Peripheral Blood*

Normocytic anemia, which becomes more severe as the disease progresses; microcytic anemia occurs if the patient has had considerable bleeding. The anemia reflects the combined effects of increased plasma volume, reduced RBC survival and ineffective erythropoiesis.

Marked poikilocytosis, anisocytosis, polychromatophilia, "teardrop" cells, and nucleated RBC are common findings—these all reflect impaired erythropoiesis

Slightly increased reticulocytes (<10%)

Mild or moderate leukocytosis (<30,000/$\mu$l); immature granulocytic elements. This reflects ineffective granulocytopoiesis.

Platelet count is increased early, but decreased later; giant and bizarrely shaped platelets and megakaryocyte fragments reflect impaired platelet formation.

### Bone Marrow

Aspirate frequently results in a "dry tap"; biopsy is necessary.

Early, the marrow is hypercellular with hyperplasia of all cell types; later, the marrow becomes progressively less cellular and more fibrotic.

A special stain of the marrow biopsy for reticulin shows an increase in reticulin fibers; this is diagnostic of myelofibrosis. These fibers are later replaced by collagen fibers.

Megakaryocytes are numerous, often occur in clusters, frequently are abnormal in size and shape, and are the last hematopoietic element to disappear.

Increased stainable iron reflects hemolysis due to hypersplenism or is the consequence of multiple transfusions for unresponsive anemia.

### Other Laboratory Findings

Elevated leukocyte alkaline phosphatase (about 67% of patients); the level tends to fall as the disease progresses

Increased serum uric acid reflects leukocytosis and WBC breakdown.

Increased unconjugated (indirect) bilirubin reflects increased RBC destruction.

Increased LDH reflects ineffective hematopoiesis and increased hematopoietic cellular destruction within the bone marrow.

Moderate increase in serum vitamin $B_{12}$ and in unsaturated $B_{12}$ binding capacity

Needle biopsy of spleen or liver shows evidence of hematopoiesis.

---

* The combination in the peripheral blood of immature RBC, WBC, and platelets is known as *leukoerythroblastosis* and is characteristic of myelofibrosis with myeloid metaplasia. These morphologic abnormalities may be a consequence of damage to the normal cellular release system of the marrow, of extramedullary blood-cell formation, or of both.

## POLYCYTHEMIA VERA

Polycythemia vera is a chronic myeloproliferative disorder characterized by an uncontrolled proliferation of erythrocytic, myelocytic, and megakaryocytic bone-marrow elements. RBC production is independent of the action of erythropoietin, in contrast to RBC production in secondary erythrocytosis. The low levels of serum erythropoietin in polycythemia vera have been attributed to feedback inhibition by the increased RBC mass. The ability of the kidneys to produce erythropoietin remains intact. Marrow proliferation is predominantly erythroid, and the circulating RBC mass and blood volume are usually increased early in the disease. The plasma volume shows little or no change. Because of the increased RBC concentration, the viscosity of the blood becomes increased. Increased platelets, together with increased blood viscosity, account for the frequent formation of thrombi in this disorder.

Most of the early symptoms are caused by circulatory disturbances secondary to the increased RBC mass and consequent increased blood volume and hyperviscosity. As the disease progresses, patients develop complications that are not seen in the secondary erythrocytoses. The paradoxical combination of thromboses and hemorrhages occurs quite frequently. Cerebral, coronary, mesenteric, and portal thromboses may be seen along with nasal, gastric, and cutaneous hemorrhages.

Splenomegaly, which is seen in 75% of patients, is caused in part by vascular engorgement, but is probably more closely related to splenic formation of marrow cellular elements, especially granulocytes.

In a considerable number of patients, the disease changes slowly, over 5 years to 25 years, into myelofibrosis with myeloid metaplasia. Reduction in available bone-marrow space due to increased fibrous tissue and an increase in splenic size and blood cell destruction result in anemia. Eventually there is pancytopenia and marrow failure. A picture resembling that of acute myelogenous leukemia ultimately develops in about one third of patients with polycythemia vera. Prior radiation therapy for polycythemia may contribute to this conversion.

### LABORATORY FINDINGS

#### Peripheral Blood

Increased hematocrit (60%); RBC (7 million/$\mu$l–12 million/$\mu$l); and Hb (18 g/dl–24 g/dl)

Normal RBC indices

Increased WBC (12,000/$\mu$l–25,000/$\mu$l)

Increased platelets (450,000/$\mu$l–1 million/$\mu$l)

Early in the disease, the blood cell morphology is usually normal. Later, the blood smear shows nucleated RBC, anisocytosis, poikilocytosis, "teardrop" RBC, polychromatophilia, immature WBC, bizarre and clumped platelets. As the disease progresses, these findings become more striking, reflecting increasing extramedullary hematopoiesis.

**Bone Marrow**

Increased cellularity of all elements; the megakaryocytic increase is prominent; no stainable iron; normal M–E ratio—the absence of marrow iron is characteristic, reflecting increased iron uptake, utilization, and release

**Other Laboratory Findings**

Increased RBC mass, marked—this is the most characteristic finding and is essential for diagnosis.

Increased serum uric acid—result of increased formation of uric acid from metabolized hematopoietic nucleoprotein

Increased leukocyte alkaline phosphatase—occurs in 80% of patients

Increased serum vitamin $B_{12}$ or unsaturated $B_{12}$ binding capacity—the latter increase is greater and more characteristic than the former

Normal arterial oxygen saturation (>92%)—this is essential for diagnosis

Poor clot retraction

Decreased sedimentation rate reflects increased hematocrit and blood viscosity.

Absent or reduced serum erythropoietin; may not be decreased when the hemoglobin is only moderately increased.

**Diagnostic Criteria of the Polycythemia Vera Study Group***

*Category A*
1. Increased RBC mass
2. Normal arterial $O_2$ saturation
3. Splenomegaly

*Category B*
1. Thrombocytosis
2. Leukocytosis
3. Elevated leukocyte alkaline phosphatase score
4. Elevated serum vitamin $B_{12}$ or unsaturated $B_{12}$ binding capacity

## ESSENTIAL THROMBOCYTHEMIA

Several synonyms have been used for this myeloproliferative disorder characterized by persistently increased platelets: idiopathic thrombocythemia, hemorrhagic thrombocythemia and primary thrombocythemia.

This uncommon disorder of abnormally increased platelet production affects persons over the age of 50 years. It is characterized by bleeding, throm-

---

* Diagnosis of polycythemia vera is acceptable if the following criteria are present:

$$A_1 + A_2 + A_3$$

*or*

$$A_1 + A_2 + \text{any 2 criteria in Category B}$$

boembolic phenomena, and splenomegaly. The most common site of bleeding is the GI tract. Bleeding is due to impaired platelet function. Bleeding usually ceases when the platelet count falls below 1 million. Thromboemboli occur less frequently than hemorrhage.

## LABORATORY FINDINGS

### Peripheral Blood*

Increased platelet count ($>$1 million/$\mu$l)—many platelet clumps; large and abnormal platelets; megakaryocyte fragments may be seen.

Increased WBC ($<$40,000/$\mu$l)—mature granulocytes occur

Microcytic, hypochromic anemia—reflects bleeding

### Bone Marrow

Increase in all cellular elements, but especially in megakaryocytes, which are large and bizarre in shape

Decreased stainable iron

Mild to moderate increase in reticulin fibers are seen in a bone-marrow biopsy

### Other Laboratory Findings

Abnormal platelet aggregation or adhesiveness reflects impaired platelet function.

Increased leukocyte alkaline phosphatase

Increased serum uric acid and vitamin B$_{12}$—reflect leukocytosis and increased WBC metabolism

Increased serum potassium reflects increased platelet breakdown.

# LEUKEMIAS

## ACUTE LEUKEMIAS

Leukemia is a neoplastic disorder of leukocytes, which proliferate in and eventually replace the bone marrow. Leukemic cells also proliferate in lymph nodes, spleen, and liver. These cells may also be found in the meninges, ovaries, testes, skin, GI tract, and kidneys.

*Acute leukemia* is defined as a leukemia that, if left untreated, runs a rapidly fatal course with an expected life span for the patient of fewer than 6 months. Leukemic cells consist predominantly of blasts and closely related immature cells such as promyelocytes or prolymphocytes. In most patients, the peripheral blood and bone marrow have more than 30% blasts. These blast cells generally retain the capacity to proliferate but lose the ability to differentiate.

The cause of leukemia is unknown, but many factors play a role. Some of these factors are viruses, radiation, chemical agents, chromosomal and genetic factors, and abnormal immunologic function. Certain acquired hematologic disorders are associated with an increased frequency of acute leukemia. These

---

* This combination of laboratory findings is characteristic of essential thrombocythemia.

include the myeloproliferative disorders, such as chronic granulocytic leukemia, polycythemia vera, myelofibrosis with myeloid metaplasia, and sideroblastic anemia.

Acute leukemia is the most common malignant disease of childhood. In children, acute leukemia is usually of the lymphoblastic type; in adults, it is usually of the myeloblastic type.

All forms of acute leukemia are associated with decreased production of normal granulocytes, erythrocytes, and platelets. Ineffective hematopoiesis occurs even before the bone marrow is significantly replaced by blast cells. Disruption of normal marrow function is not a consequence of the overgrowth of leukemic cells. Impaired hematopoiesis results in the serious complications of anemia, hemorrhage, and infections. Leukemic infiltrates into various tissues produce bone or joint pain, neurologic symptoms, enlarged lymph nodes, and enlargement of the liver and spleen.

Infections, which are the most frequent cause of death, increase with the degree and duration of granulocytopenia. Infections are enhanced by impairment of cellular and humoral immunity due to both the leukemia and antileukemic therapy. Treatment suppresses granulocytes and also the immune defense mechanisms. Infections are due to a great variety of bacteria, fungi, protozoa, and viruses.

Acute leukemias have been classified by a French–American–British (FAB) committee of hematologists.[1] In this classification, myeloid acute leukemias are separated from the nonmyeloid, or lymphoblastic, leukemias. These two groups are further subdivided into six myeloblastic and three lymphoblastic categories. The myeloblastic subcategories are based on the direction of differentiation along one or more cell lines and the degree of maturation of the cells. The lymphoblastic characteristics used for subclassification include cell size, nuclear chromatin, nucleoli, and amount and basophilia of cytoplasm.

## LABORATORY FINDINGS

### Peripheral Blood

Normocytic anemia, occasionally macrocytic—progressive, severe

Thrombocytopenia—progressive, severe

Leukocyte count—normal or decreased (aleukemic leukemia) or increased (50,000/$\mu$l–100,000/$\mu$l). Therapy usually produces granulocytopenia.

Differential count—occasional blast to 100% blasts; lymphoblasts or myeloblasts; immature leukocytes

Auer bodies may be seen in the cytoplasm of myeloblasts; they do not occur in lymphoblasts.

In acute myelocytic leukemia, granulocytes may have failure of normal nuclear lobe development, resembling Pelger–Huët anomaly.

Nucleated RBC, polychromatophilia

Decreased leukocyte alkaline phosphatase

Cytochemical staining may help differentiate the various blast cells: nonlymphoblasts stain for myeloperoxidase, chloroacetate esterase, nonspecific esterase, Sudan Black B. Lymphoblasts do not show these staining reactions.

### Bone Marrow

Hypercellular marrow with increased blasts, even when none are found in the peripheral blood; increased immature leukocytes; increased M–E ratio.

Rarely, the marrow is hypocellular with only clusters of blasts.

Occasionally, megaloblastic changes are seen in RBC precursors.

Decreased RBC and megakaryocytic elements

### Other Laboratory Findings

Positive cultures of blood, urine, sputum—various indigenous and opportunistic organisms occur as infectious complications of leukemia

Cerebrospinal fluid (CSF) may contain leukemic cells (25%–50% of children).

Increased serum uric acid—this is the end product of nucleic acid catabolism and is seen with high WBC and during chemotherapy.

*Terminal deoxynucleotidyl transferase (TdT)*
This is a biochemical marker of some leukemic cells. It is found in 95% of patients with acute lymphocytic leukemia and 5–10% of patients with acute myelocytic leukemia.

*Immunologic Characteristics*
The identification of cell surface markers helps to categorize normal and leukemic lymphocytes as thymus-derived (T cells) or bursal type (B cells). Lymphocytes without surface markers have been termed *null cells.*

*Cytogenetic Studies*
No consistent findings occur in the acute leukemias. The presence of the Philadelphia chromosome (Ph$^1$ chromosome) in adult acute leukemia indicates that the acute leukemia arose as an acute transformation or blast crisis from chronic myelocytic leukemia.

### CHRONIC MYELOCYTIC LEUKEMIA

Chronic myelocytic leukemia is a malignant disorder of granulocytes, which proliferate in the blood, bone marrow, and spleen. The onset is insidious and is characterized by fatigue, loss of appetite, weight loss, fever, and enlargement of the spleen. This usually occurs in patients between 30 years and 50 years of age.

An abnormality found in approximately 90% of cases is the loss of much of the longer arm of chromosome 22 and its translocation, usually to chromosome 9. The abnormal chromosome 22 is referred to as the *Philadelphia* (Ph$^1$) *chromosome* because it was first observed in that city. The granulocytic, erythrocytic, and megakaryocytic cells are all Ph$^1$-positive. This indicates that chronic myelocytic leukemia is a neoplastic disorder of the hematopoietic stem cell. Growth and function of RBC and platelet precursors do not appear to be affected by the defective chromosome. The clinical effects appear to be a function of the total amount of proliferating leukemic tissue and the early release of marrow granulocytes. Two years to three years after the initial diagnosis, about 80% of patients develop an accelerated phase called a *blast crisis,* with features indistinguishable from acute myelocytic leukemia. This is the cause of death in 60% to 90% of patients with chronic myelocytic leukemia.

## LABORATORY FINDINGS

### Peripheral Blood

Leukocytosis (50,000/$\mu$l–500,000/$\mu$l). All granulocytic precursors are present, with mature granulocytes and metamyelocytes predominating. <10% blasts are present. Increased eosinophils, basophils, and monocytes.

Normocytic anemia (Hb 9 g/dl–12 g/dl) due to marrow displacement and impaired erythropoiesis. Severity of the anemia is proportional to the degree of leukocyte proliferation.

Normal or slightly increased reticulocyte count

Few nucleated RBC, slight polychromatophilia

Normal platelet count (50%) or increased platelet count (40%) in early stages; this is not related to the WBC count; thrombocytopenia occurs in later stages

### Bone Marrow

Hypercellular bone marrow with predominance of all granulocytic elements showing orderly maturation; M–E ratio is 10:1–30:1; increased basophils and eosinophils

Increased megakaryocytes, some of which are atypical

Increased reticulin fibers and fibrosis may appear in a biopsy taken late in the course of the disease (30%–40% of patients).

Decreased stainable iron

### Other Laboratory Findings

Decreased or absent leukocyte alkaline phosphatase in approximately 90% of patients

Presence of Ph[1] chromosome in 70%–90% of patients

Increased serum and urine uric acid, especially when chemotherapy is given, reflects WBC breakdown.

Increased serum vitamin $B_{12}$ and unsaturated $B_{12}$ binding capacity reflect elevated vitamin $B_{12}$ binding protein derived from breakdown of leukemic granulocytes.

Increased serum LDH reflects RBC and WBC breakdown.

Presence of terminal deoxynucleotidyl transferase (TdT) in 20%–30% of patients with chronic myelocytic leukemia in blast crisis. This enzyme is usually found in lymphoblasts.

## CHRONIC LYMPHOCYTIC LEUKEMIA

Chronic lymphocytic leukemia is a neoplastic disorder characterized by an uncontrolled proliferation, usually of B-lymphocytes, probably originating in the bone marrow. Abnormal lymphocytes accumulate also in lymph nodes and spleen. The majority of patients with chronic lymphocytic leukemia is over 60 years of age. The onset is usually insidious and the disease may be discovered by chance during a routine physical examination or blood test. Fatigue, loss of appetite, weight loss, fever, or enlargement of lymph nodes or spleen may cause the patient to seek medical attention. Massive splenic enlargement adds to the severity of the cytopenia by trapping and destroying many of the circulating blood cells. About 5% to 10% of patients have associated autoimmune hemolytic anemia.

In this disease, there are marked decreases in the normal defense mechanisms. Complications reflect disorders of immunologic functions. Patients with chronic lymphocytic leukemia have an increased susceptibility to a variety of bacterial and viral infections as a result of severe neutropenia and impaired production of circulating antibodies. Most patients die of uncontrolled infection.

## LABORATORY FINDINGS

### Peripheral Blood

Leukocytosis (20,000/$\mu$l–250,000/$\mu$l)—over 90% of cells are small lymphocytes; many smudge cells, which are fragile leukemic cells. The total lymphocyte count does not correlate with the degree of organ involvement.

Mild normocytic anemia, early; severe anemia in later stages due to decreased RBC production and shortened RBC survival

Normal or decreased reticulocytes

Normal platelets in the early stage; thrombocytopenia in the later stage

### Bone Marrow

Early, slight lymphocytosis

Later, lymphocytes gradually replace the entire marrow and all other cellular elements are decreased.

### Other Laboratory Findings

Immunologically, the lymphocytes in 98% of patients are B-lymphocytes.

Decrease in serum proteins, especially immunoglobulins, contributes to increased susceptibility to bacterial, fungal, and viral infections

Monoclonal $\gamma$-globulin (5% of cases), usually IgM

AIHA, IgG type (5%–10% of cases)—increased LDH, spherocytes, and reticulocytes reflect the hemolytic process.

## LEUKEMIC RETICULOENDOTHELIOSIS

Leukemic reticuloendotheliosis (hairy-cell leukemia) is a rare form of leukemia characterized by splenomegaly, minimal lymph-node enlargement, pancytopenia, and the presence of atypical mononuclear cells in the peripheral blood and bone marrow. The tumor cells have features of both lymphocytes and monocytes and have characteristic hair-like cytoplasmic projections. These cells are thought to be of stem-cell origin. Infection is common and is a frequent cause of death.

## LABORATORY FINDINGS

### Peripheral Blood

Decreased WBC, RBC, and platelets

Small to medium-sized mononuclear cells with moderate to abundant cytoplasm showing hairlike projections

Tumor cells contain acid phosphatase, which is not removed by incubation with tartrate—this is a common but not consistent finding.

### Bone Marrow

Aspirate often yields no cells.

Biopsy shows focal or diffuse infiltrate of the characteristic leukemic cells. Bone-marrow biopsy usually is diagnostic.

## MALIGNANT LYMPHOMAS

Malignant lymphomas are tumors of the solid lymphoid tissues. The disease usually starts in lymph nodes but frequently also involves the liver, spleen, and bone marrow. Far less common are extranodal lymphomas, in which the disease originates in the GI tract, thyroid, breast, gonads, or bone.

Malignant lymphoma differs from leukemia mainly in the distribution and dissemination of tumor cells. *Lymphoma* denotes initial tumor involvement of the solid lymphoid tissues, whereas *leukemia* implies origin in the bone marrow and dissemination through peripheral blood. As a lymphoma spreads, the bone marrow may become involved and occasionally tumor cells appear in the peripheral blood. Hence, in some stages of lymphoma there may be leukemoid features.

### NON–HODGKIN'S LYMPHOMAS

The lymphomas are usually divided into two major groups: Hogdkin's disease and the non–Hodgkin's lymphomas. The non–Hodgkin's lymphomas have been separated morphologically by cell type into four categories, each of which shows a nodular or diffuse pattern on tissue biopsy: (Rappaport classification)*

1. Well-differentiated lymphocytic lymphoma
2. Poorly differentiated lymphocytic lymphoma
3. Histiocytic lymphoma
4. Mixed histiocytic–lymphocytic lymphoma

In recent years, advances in immunology, cytochemistry, and electron microscopy have given us much new information about the biologic activity and morphology of the lymphoreticular cells. It has been shown that all nodular lymphomas arise from follicular, or germinal center, B-lymphocytes and that the histiocytic lymphomas do not comprise true histiocytes; in most instances,

* Rappaport H: Tumors of the Hematopoietic System. Washington, Armed Forces Institute of Pathology. Fasc 8, 1966

they are tumors of transformed B-lymphocytes. A more recent classification of the non-Hodgkin's lymphomas uses various categories of B cell types and T cell types.* There recently appeared a working formulation of non-Hodgkin's lymphomas for clinical usage. This classified the malignant lymphomas into low, intermediate, and high grades of clinical severity.†

The clinical manifestations of malignant lymphoma are varied, but the most common presenting complaint is enlarged, usually painless lymph nodes or an abdominal mass. Non–Hodgkin's lymphomas are frequently disseminated at the time of initial diagnosis. Clinical staging, or the determination of the extent of involvement includes physical examination; bone marrow aspiration and biopsy; radiologic studies to detect disease in the mediastinum, retroperitoneum, and bones; laboratory tests; and, in selected cases, exploratory abdominal surgery. Infection is the most frequent cause of death.

## LABORATORY FINDINGS

Biopsy of lymph node or other tissue that shows morphologic cell type in a nodular or diffuse pattern—required for definitive diagnosis

Anemia, normocytic (50% of patients)—due to one or more of the following: lymphoma involvement of bone marrow, bone marrow suppression resulting from therapy, hypersplenism, autoimmune hemolytic anemia, bleeding from GI lymphoma, or secondary to a low platelet count

Peripheral blood rarely shows circulating lymphoma cells; 5%–10% of cases may evolve into leukemia.

Bone-marrow biopsy may show involvement by lymphoma.

Serum protein electrophoresis shows decreased albumin as the disease progresses; there may be a monoclonal gammopathy, usually IgM type, or occasionally hypogammaglobulinemia.

Cytologic examination of pleural or peritoneal fluid may show lymphoma tumor cells.

Classification of tumors into B cell, T cell, or null cell types uses immunofluorescent, immunoperoxidase, or cell suspension techniques.

Cytochemical studies of tumor cells helps differentiate lymphocytes from histiocytes.

### *HODGKIN'S DISEASE*

Hodgkin's disease is a malignant lymphoma that differs from non–Hodgkin's lymphomas in patterns of organ involvement. This usually originates from one focus rather than from multiple foci. Hodgkin's disease generally begins in the lymph nodes of the neck. Patients up to the age of 40 years to 50 years tend to present with well-defined local tumors and, except for some intermittent fever or symptoms of mild anemia, appear to be in excellent health. Disease may be

* Lukes RJ, Collins RD: Lukes-Collins classification and its significance. Cancer Treat Rep 61:971, 1977
† National Cancer Institute Sponsored Study of Classifications of Non-Hodgkins Lymphomas. Cancer 49:2112–2135, 1982

restricted to a few foci and spread locally to involve the next nearest group of nodes. Older patients usually have no evidence of disease localization but have severe systemic symptoms. Symptoms include weakness, loss of appetite, fever, night sweats, itching, and weight loss.

In contrast to the non–Hodgkin's lymphomas, one histopathologic classification is generally accepted. Reed-Sternberg cells are the characteristic tumor cells. These multinucleated cells may be transformed lymphocytes or histiocytes. Reed-Sternberg cells are found in one of the following cellular backgrounds, which determines the category of Hodgkin's disease: lymphocyte predominance, lymphocyte depletion, mixed cellularity, or nodular sclerosis. The type, extent, and severity of the disease give an indication of prognosis and appropriate therapy.

## LABORATORY FINDINGS

### Lymph Node Biopsy

Required for definitive diagnosis.

### Peripheral Blood

Normocytic or microcytic anemia, moderate; worsens as disease progresses

Hemolytic anemia occasionally occurs in advanced disease; the Coombs' test is usually negative.

Leukocytosis, which is characterized by increased granulocytes and decreased lymphocytes

Pancytopenia reflects extensive bone marrow involvement, the effect of therapy, or hypersplenism.

### Bone Marrow

Requires biopsy to demonstrate involvement, which occurs in approximately 11% of cases

### Other Laboratory Findings

Increased sedimentation rate reflects disease activity.

Increased leukocyte alkaline phosphatase during the active phase of disease; not increased during remission

Protein electrophoresis—decreased albumin, increased globulins; reflects active disease

Decreased serum iron and increased ferritin reflect chronic disease anemia.

## IMMUNOPROLIFERATIVE DISORDERS

### MULTIPLE MYELOMA

Multiple myeloma is a malignant immunoproliferative disease characterized by aggregations of both immature and mature plasma cells that are of the same family or clone.[6,8,9] The plasma-cell aggregates usually occur in the bone marrow but occasionally may be found in other sites. The bone-marrow tumors commonly cause extensive bone destruction. Malignant plasma cells are derived from B-lymphocytes and form abnormal amounts of monoclonal immunoglobulins. These proteins are responsible for the hyperviscosity syndrome, cryoglobulinemia, amyloidosis, and hemostatic abnormalities.

The disease affects patients over 40 years of age and usually becomes evident with one or more of the following findings: anemia, an abnormal serum protein electrophoresis, bone pain and x-ray evidence of unsuspected bone fractures, increased infections, nephrotic syndrome, acute spinal-cord compression from vertebral collapse, and hypercalcemia. Other symptoms may include weakness, fever, weight loss, abnormal bleeding, nausea, vomiting, and diarrhea. Infection, which is usually due to gram-negative organisms, is the most frequent cause of death. Increased vulnerability to infection seems to be due to deficient antibody responses. Even though monoclonal B-lymphocytes are increased, their immunoglobulin-synthetic functions are impaired, especially during periods of disease activity. Some degree of renal insufficiency occurs in approximately one half of patients with multiple myeloma, and renal failure is the second most common cause of death, (see Myeloma Nephropathy, Chap. 5). Bence Jones proteins, which are monoclonal light chains, are directly toxic to proximal tubular cells and are the major factor in the pathogenesis of renal failure. Other factors that contribute to renal failure include hypercalcemia, hyperuricemia, amyloid deposits, hyperviscosity, dehydration, and pyelonephritis.

## LABORATORY FINDINGS

### Peripheral Blood

Normochromic, normocytic anemia, mild to moderate (Hb 7 g/dl–10 g/dl), reflects the number of plasma cells in the marrow; anemia is also due to shortened RBC survival, increased blood loss, increased plasma volume, renal insufficiency, and the effects of radiation therapy or chemotherapy.

Rouleaux formation due to increase in serum protein

Blue-gray background of blood smear when observed macroscopically is due to increase in serum protein.

Mild degree of leukopenia and thrombocytopenia

Relative lymphocytosis; rare plasma cells

Nucleated RBC and immature granulocytes—this leukoerythroblastic reaction, or pancytopenia, might occur late in the disease as a result of myeloma replacement of the bone marrow.

### Bone Marrow

Increased plasma cells, >20% (average 36%); immature atypical plasma cells are termed *myeloma cells.* The percentage of plasma cells is not a reliable indicator of the extent of disease. Marrow biopsy may be necessary to show plasma-cell aggregates.

Increased lymphocytes (>20%)

### Protein Abnormalities

Increased serum total protein due to increased globulins (8 g/dl–15 g/dl); decreased albumin

*Serum protein electrophoresis*—Monclonal protein in the $\beta$ or $\gamma$ zone, usually IgG or IgA. There might be decreased $\gamma$-globulin, which suggests IgD myeloma or light-chain myeloma. In light-chain myeloma, no heavy chains are formed.

Serum protein immunoelectrophoresis—Identifies the heavy and light chains of the monoclonal protein. Approximately 11% of plasma-cell tumors form only light-chain proteins. Presence of free light chains in the serum reflects impaired renal excretion.

Marked increase in the monoclonal protein (5–10 times > normal)—produced by a single clone of malignant plasma cells. The most frequently produced monoclonal protein is IgG.

Moderate to marked decrease in the nonmonoclonal immunoglobulins. Impaired synthesis of normal immunoglobulins is a characteristic finding.

Proteinuria

Urine protein electrophoresis—May show one or more of the following: a monoclonal protein similar to that in the serum; multiple proteins similar to normal serum proteins, indicating nephrosis; and albumin, reflecting a glomerular filtration defect.

Urine protein immunoelectrophoresis—Identifies the specific monoclonal protein present, which is usually similar to that in the serum. Monoclonal light chains of either the $\lambda$ or $\kappa$ type are termed *Bence Jones proteins.* These proteins occur in 60% of IgG myelomas, 70% of IgA myelomas, 100% of IgD myelomas, and 100% of light-chain myelomas.

### Other Laboratory Findings

Increased serum viscosity, evidenced as cryoglobulins or cryofibrinogens; most frequently seen in IgA myeloma, which tends to polymerize readily.

Increased sedimentation rate—result of increased immunoglobulin or fibrinogen

Increased BUN and serum creatinine; decreased creatinine clearance—indicate impaired renal function, chiefly due to Bence Jones protein damage to renal tubules

Urine casts and renal epithelial cells reflect progressive renal failure.

Increased serum calcium reflects bone resorption by myeloma infiltrates and tumor-cell secretion of an "osteoclast-stimulating factor." Hypercalcemia is usually associated with extensive bone disease, azotemia, and hyperuricemia.

Positive cultures of sputum, blood, and urine usually yield gram-negative bacteria—reflect increased susceptibility to infection

## MACROGLOBULINEMIA

Waldenström's macroglobulinemia is a malignant immunoproliferative disorder characterized by increased lymphocytes that produce IgM monoclonal protein.

Lymphocytes diffusely involve the bone marrow and lymph nodes. Enlargement of the liver and spleen may be present. This disorder typically affects people in their sixth and seventh decades with a clinical picture resembling that of malignant lymphoma of the lymphocytic type. Initial symptoms are usually weakness and fatigue or bleeding.

Because of the large size of IgM proteins (they are six times the molecular weight of IgG), they cause a marked increase in serum viscosity. The clinical consequences of hyperviscosity include visual disturbances, retinal venous congestion, renal impairment, mental confusion, stupor, and even coma. Vascular thrombosis and gangrene may also occur. Bleeding is a consequence of IgM impairment of platelet and clotting-factor functions. Another complication of macroglobulinemia is cold agglutinin hemolytic anemia.

## LABORATORY FINDINGS

### Peripheral Blood

Normochromic, normocytic anemia, marked (Hb 6 g/dl–9 g/dl)—this is primarily due to decreased RBC formation; other factors contributing to the anemia include increased plasma volume, RBC destruction, and blood loss

Rouleaux formation, marked—this is due to adhesion of RBC to each other in the viscous serum

Immature lymphocytes, late in disease

### Bone Marrow

Hypercellular; marrow is diffusely replaced by lymphocytes with features resembling plasma cells

### Other Laboratory Findings

Increased sedimentation rate, marked—due to RBC aggregation

Increased total serum protein and globulins

Serum protein electrophoresis—monoclonal protein present in $\beta$ or $\gamma$ region

Serum protein immunoelectrophoresis—the abnormal protein is IgM $\kappa$ or IgM $\lambda$.

Immunoglobulins, quantitative—increased IgM, decreased IgG and IgA

Proteinuria

Urine protein electrophoresis and immunoelectrophoresis—25%–40% of cases show free $\kappa$ or $\lambda$ light chains (Bence Jones proteins) in the urine

Presence of serum cryoglobulins, cryofibrinogens, or pyroglobulins

Increased serum viscosity—this may cause false-positive results in tests using latex particles, such as tests for rheumatoid arthritis, pregnancy, fibrin split products

Increased cold agglutinins

Impaired platelet adhesion, aggregation, platelet-factor-3 release; prolonged bleeding time—these are the result of IgM coating of platelets

Impaired function of coagulation factors II, V, VII, or VIII prolonging prothrombin time or partial thromboplastin time—this may be the result of immune-complex formation with IgM

Prolonged thrombin time—this frequent finding is thought to be due to immunoglobulin binding to fibrin during clot formation and polymerization

### HEAVY-CHAIN DISEASE

Heavy-chain disease comprises a rare group of malignant immunoproliferative disorders characterized by lymphocytes or plasma cells that produce heavy-chain fragments ($\gamma, \alpha, \mu$) without associated light chains. This may be caused by deletion of the area in the heavy chain that is responsible for attaching to light chains.

Gamma heavy-chain disease resembles non–Hodgkin's lymphomas. Patients show increased susceptibility to infection and have enlarged lymph nodes, spleen, and liver. Edema of the palate occurs as a consequence of involvement of lymph nodes of the throat and neck.

Alpha heavy-chain disease is characterized by infiltration of the small intestine and abdominal lymph nodes with lymphocytes and plasma cells, resulting in severe intestinal malabsorption. This results in marked weight loss, steatorrhea, and excessive fecal losses of water and electrolytes.

Mu heavy-chain disease is rare and occurs in association with chronic lymphocytic leukemia.

## LABORATORY FINDINGS

### All Heavy-Chain Diseases

Serum protein electrophoresis—decreased albumin and $\gamma$-globulin; abnormal broad heterogeneous protein in $\alpha$, $\beta$, or $\gamma$ region

Urine protein electrophoresis—identical pattern to that of serum.

### Gamma Heavy-Chain Disease

Normocytic anemia, leukopenia, thrombocytopenia—due to hypersplenism

Eosinophilia and atypical lymphocytes or plasma cells in peripheral blood

Increased sedimentation rate

Proteinuria—up to 1 g/day

Increased lymphocytes and plasma cells in the bone marrow

Immunoelectrophoresis of serum and urine shows increased $\gamma$ chains but no light chains—this is the diagnostic finding.

Decreased serum IgA and IgM

### Alpha Heavy-Chain Disease

Normal peripheral blood and bone marrow

Immunoelectrophoresis of serum and urine shows increased $\alpha$ chains but no light chains—this is the diagnostic finding.

Laboratory findings of intestinal malabsorption (see Chap. 3)

### Mu Heavy-Chain Disease

Peripheral blood resembles that of chronic lymphocytic leukemia.

Bone marrow shows 70%–80% lymphocytes and vacuolated plasma cells.

Immunoelectrophoresis shows $\mu$ chains but no light chains in serum—this is the diagnostic finding.

$\kappa$ light chains present in the urine

**Table 8-2.** Immunodeficiency Disorders

| SYNDROME | CLINICAL FEATURES | LABORATORY FINDINGS |
|---|---|---|
| *Predominant Humoral Abnormality* | | |
| X-linked agammaglobulinemia | Increased bacterial sinus and pulmonary infections; rheumatoid arthritis; affects males | All Ig decreased or absent; absence of plasma cells in all sites |
| IgA deficiency | Steatorrhea and nontropical sprue | Absence of serum and secretory IgA, may have IgA antibodies |
| Ig deficiencies with hyper-IgM | Increased bacterial respiratory infections; increased autoimmune diseases | Increased IgM and decreased IgA and IgG |
| *Predominant Cell-Mediated Abnormality* | | |
| Thymic dysplasia (Nezelof's syndrome) | Increased fungal and viral infections | Decreased granulocytes; 50% of patients have decreased IgA or IgG |
| Congenital thymic aplasia (DiGeorge's syndrome) | Increased fungal and viral infections; absent parathyroids, thymus; cardiovascular, tracheal, and esophageal malformations | Normal serum Ig levels; decreased calcium; diminished cell-mediated immunity |
| *Combined Immunologic Abnormalities* | | |
| Wiskott-Aldrich syndrome | Thrombocytopenia and eczema; increased bacterial and viral infections; bleeding | Decreased IgM, increased IgA; decreased lymphocytes and cellular immunity |
| Ataxia–telangiectasia | Cerebellar ataxia; telangiectasia in skin and eyes; ovarian dysgenesis; sinus and pulmonary infections | Decreased serum and secretory IgA and IgE; impaired cellular immunity |
| Severe combined immunodeficiency | Overwhelming widespread bacterial and viral infections; failure to thrive; malabsorption | Marked decrease in all Ig; decreased to absent lymphocytes and plasma cells; impaired cellular immunity |
| Common variable hypo-gammaglobulinemia | Recurrent bacterial respiratory infections and GI disorders including malabsorption; frequent occurrence of autoimmune diseases | Absence of plasma cells; variable decrease in immunoglobulins, especially IgG |

(Adapted from Thaler MS, Klausner RD, Cohen HJ: Medical Immunology. Philadelphia, JB Lippincott, 1977)

## IMMUNODEFICIENCY DISORDERS

The congenital immunodeficiency disorders are rare.[4] The major clinical and laboratory features are listed in Table 8-2.

## REFERENCES

1. Bell A, Hippel T, Goodman H: Use of cytochemistry and FAB classification in leukemia and other pathological states. Am J Med Tech 47:437–471, 1981
2. Bloom AL: The von Willebrand syndrome. Semin Hematol 17:215–227, 1980
3. Camitta BM, Storb R, Thomas ED: Aplastic anemia. N Engl J Med 306:645–652, 712–718, 1982
4. Denman AM: Immunodeficiency and general medicine. Br Med J 281:1376–1378, 1980
5. Heimpel H, Heit W: Drug-induced aplastic anemia. Clin Haematol 9:641–662, 1980
6. Kapadia SB: Multiple myeloma: A clinicopathologic study of 62 consecutively autopsied cases. Medicine 59:380–392, 1980
7. Kirtland HH, Mohler DN, Horwitz DA: Methyldopa inhibition of suppressor-lymphocyte function. N Engl J Med 302:825–832, 1980
8. Kyle RA: Multiple myeloma: Review of 869 cases. Mayo Clin Proc 50:29–40, 1975
9. Paredes JM, Mitchell BS: Multiple myeloma: Current concepts in diagnosis and management. Med Clin North Am 64:729–742, 1980
10. Petz LD: Drug-induced immune haemolytic anemia. Clin Haematol 9:455–482, 1980
11. Reeves WB, Haurani FI: Clinical applicability and usefulness of ferritin measurement. Ann Clin Lab Sci 10:529–535, 1980
12. Schechter AN, Bunn HF: What determines severity in sickle cell disease? N Engl J Med 306:295–296, 1982

## BIBLIOGRAPHY

**Erslev AJ, Gabuzda TG:** Pathophysiology of Blood. Philadelphia, WB Saunders, 1975
**Hillman RS, Finch CA:** Red Cell Manual, 4th ed. Philadelphia, FA Davis, 1974
**Maslow WC, Beutler E, Bell CA et al:** Practical Diagnosis: Hematologic Disease. Boston, Houghton Mifflin, 1980
**Williams WJ, Beutler E, Erslev AJ et al:** Hematology, 2nd ed. New York, McGraw-Hill, 1977
**Wintrobe MM, Lee GR, Boggs DR et al:** Clinical Hematology, 8th ed. Philadelphia, Lea & Febiger, 1981

# 9

# MUSCULOSKELETAL AND CONNECTIVE-TISSUE DISEASES

Systemic Lupus Erythematosus
Scleroderma
Sjögren's Syndrome
Polymyositis
Mixed Connective Tissue Disease
Infectious Arthritis
Reiter's Syndrome
Rheumatoid Arthritis

Juvenile Arthritis
Ankylosing Spondylitis
Polymyalgia Rheumatica
Osteomyelitis
Paget's Disease
Osteogenic Sarcoma
Metastatic Carcinoma of Bone

## SYSTEMIC LUPUS ERYTHEMATOSUS

Systemic lupus erythematosus (SLE) is a chronic multisystem disease of unknown etiology. It usually involves the skin and is often associated with arthritis or arthralgia, fever, glomerulonephritis, pericarditis, pleuritis, central nervous system (CNS) disease, and enlargement of the spleen and lymph nodes (see Lupus Nephritis, Chap. 5). The most common cause of death is active nephritis. Anemia, leukopenia, and dysproteinemia are common laboratory findings.

The major pathologic changes appear to be due to circulating autoimmune complexes of antinuclear antibodies and their antigens. The major immune complexes are anti-DNA bound to DNA. Deposits of immune complexes have been identified in the glomerular capillary basement membranes and at the dermal–epidermal junction of the skin. Immune-complex deposition is followed by fixation of complement at that site; this leads to activation of the complement system, an inflammatory reaction, and tissue injury. All of the clinical and pathologic abnormalities in SLE are considered to be related to these autoimmune phenomena.

The etiologic events leading up to the formation of autoantibodies and circulating immune complexes are unknown. Some contributing factors might be chronic viral infection, heredity, environmental factors, and hormonal influences. No specific or primary immune defect has been identified.

Various drugs can induce a lupuslike syndrome.[2] The mechanisms are still under study. Procainamide hydrochloride (Pronestyl) and hydralazine (Apresoline) are the drugs that are most frequently implicated. Antinuclear antibodies and lupus erythematosus (LE) cells develop in approximately 90% of patients, but antibodies to native DNA do not occur. Patients with drug-related lupus rarely show immune complexes, decreased serum complement, or antilymphocyte antibodies. Clinical features of lupus occur infrequently (10% of cases) and are mild. The syndrome regresses on withdrawal of the drug. Renal involvement rarely, if ever, occurs.

## LABORATORY FINDINGS

### Immunologic Abnormalities

*Presence of antinuclear antibodies (98%)

*Presence of anti-DNA antibodies (double stranded or native)—highly specific for SLE; found in most patients with active renal disease (90%) and in patients with active disease but without renal involvement (50%); titers reflect disease activity; these do not occur in drug-induced LE.

*Antibodies against extractable nuclear antigens. These antigens include nuclear ribonuclear protein (nRNP) and nuclear nonnucleic acid glycoprotein (Smith [Sm] antigen). The latter appears to be highly specific for patients with SLE; present in 25%–30% of patients with SLE

*Positive test for LE cells (70%–85%)—specific for SLE but not as sensitive as the presence of antinuclear antibodies; LE cells may be seen in synovial, pleural, and pericardial fluid

*Presence of circulating immune complexes—indicates active disease.

Decreased serum complement (75%)—reflects consumption by immune complexes and implies active disease

Increased serum γ-globulins (80%)—reflects increased immunologic activity

Presence of rheumatoid factor (20%–35%)—reflects increased immunoglobulins

False-positive nontreponemal test for syphilis (15%–20%)—reflects increased immunoglobulins

### Hematologic Findings

Mild normocytic anemia (50%–80%)—usually chronic disease type; occasionally there is an autoimmune hemolytic anemia with a positive direct Coombs' test

Moderate leukopenia—autoimmune mechanism

Lymphocytopenia—due to lymphocytotoxic antibodies; this is the most frequent initial laboratory finding

Thrombocytopenia—autoimmune mechanism; often reflects disease activity

Increased fibrin split products—seen in lupus nephritis

### Plasma Proteins

Decreased serum albumin (50%–60%)—reflects chronic disease or loss of albumin in urine in the nephrotic form of lupus nephritis

* This finding is of diagnostic significance.

Increased sedimentation rate and C-reactive protein—usually reflects disease activity

**Urinalysis**

Hematuria, cellular casts, and proteinuria reflect active lupus nephritis.

**Synovial Fluid**

Low white blood cell (WBC) count (<3000/$\mu$l); predominant lymphocytes

LE cells and antinuclear antibodies

Decreased complement

**Spinal Fluid**

Findings of aseptic meningitis

***Biopsy of Kidney and Skin**

Immunofluorescent studies show deposits of immunoglobulins and complement.

## SCLERODERMA

Scleroderma (*i.e.*, hard skin) is an uncommon multisystem disorder involving primarily connective tissue and small blood vessels. The disease may be limited to the skin or it may involve many organs. When there is multiple organ involvement, the disorder is known as *systemic sclerosis*. Although skin involvement is the most prominent feature, the most severe manifestations result from scarring, vascular involvement, and inflammation of various internal organs. The diverse clinical features of the disease include Raynaud's phenomenon (pallor, cyanosis, reddening, and then swelling of the fingers and toes); skin thickening of the hands, forearms, and legs; impaired swallowing and gastrointestinal (GI) motility; and disorders of the lungs, heart, kidneys, and musculoskeletal and neurologic systems. About 40% of all deaths in patients with scleroderma are due to malignant hypertension and renal failure (see Scleroderma Renal Disease, Chap. 5).

Although the etiology of scleroderma is unknown, various studies have suggested that vascular, metabolic, and immunologic events may play pathogenetic roles.[3,4] One hypothetical model states that immunologically mediated injury to small blood vessels and capillaries leads to vascular occlusion and decreased blood flow. Diminished circulation results in injury to the surrounding connective tissues, stimulating fibroblast proliferation and increased collagen deposition. The tissue changes are similar to scar formation. Perivascular accumulation of scarlike tissue alters blood-vessel distensibility and contractility, further impairing blood flow. The injured connective tissue might possibly stimulate an immunologic reaction, which continues the disease process.

### LABORATORY FINDINGS

*Presence of antinuclear antibodies (60%)—nucleolar and speckled patterns are characteristic

* This finding is of diagnostic significance.

Increased sedimentation rate (30%) reflects disease activity.

Normochromic, normocytic anemia (25%–30%)—chronic disease type

Increased serum γ-globulin, especially IgG—indicates immunoglobulin stimulation

Presence of small amounts of cryoglobulins (50% of patients)

Absence of antibodies to native DNA and Sm antigen.

Biopsy of skin—usually of help only late in the disease

### Laboratory Findings that Reflect Specific Organ Involvement

Kidney—scleroderma renal disease (see Chap. 5)

Small intestine—malabsorption (see Chap. 3)

Heart—pericarditis (see Chap. 1)

Lung—diminished gas diffusion due to interstitial fibrosis; pneumonia (see Chap. 2)

Muscle—polymyositis (see p. 282)

## SJÖGREN'S SYNDROME

Sjögren's syndrome is an autoimmune disease characterized by oral and ocular dryness, which result from partial to complete destruction of the salivary and lacrimal glands by lymphocytic and plasma-cell infiltrates.[6] Approximately 50% of patients also have rheumatoid arthritis. Sjögren's syndrome also occurs in association with SLE, scleroderma, polymyositis, and other autoimmune disorders.

One theory suggests that certain histocompatibility antigens might be genetically linked to immune-response genes. These genes could predispose a person to the development of Sjögren's syndrome. Antigenic alteration of salivary-gland tissue might lead to autoimmune sensitization, lymphocytic infiltration, production of autoantibodies against the salivary and lacrimal glands, and ultimately damage to these glands.

### LABORATORY FINDINGS

#### Immunologic Abnormalities

Positive rheumatoid factor (75%–90%)—this is not associated with clinical rheumatoid arthritis

*Presence of antinuclear antibodies (50%–80%)—characteristically nucleolar or speckled pattern

*Presence of antibody to nonhistone antigen, SS-B (60% of patients)

Presence of antibody to nonhistone antigen, SS-A (70% of patients)

Presence of salivary-duct antibody, occasionally

*Lip biopsy showing lymphocytic infiltration of the salivary glands

---

* This finding is of diagnostic significance.

### Other Laboratory Findings

Mild normocytic anemia

Leukopenia

Increased sedimentation rate (>90%)

Markedly increased serum γ-globulins (50%), especially IgA—usually polyclonal pattern

## *POLYMYOSITIS*

Polymyositis is a disease of unknown etiology in which there are diffuse inflammation and weakness of the skeletal muscles. It may occur alone, in association with malignant tumors, or as a manifestation of another connective tissue disorder such as SLE, scleroderma, or Sjögren's syndrome. When polymyositis is associated with skin involvement (40% of cases), the condition is termed *dermatomyositis*. This form of the disease is usually seen in children and in adults with occult neoplasms. Approximately 17% of patients with polymyositis who are older than 40 years have an associated carcinoma.

Polymyositis is generally considered to be an autoimmune disorder. This concept is supported by the occurrence of antinuclear antibodies, the clinical association of SLE and Sjögren's syndrome, and the response to immunosuppressive therapy. Muscle inflammation has been experimentally produced from T-lymphocytes specifically sensitized to striated muscle antigens.

### LABORATORY FINDINGS

Slightly to moderately increased sedimentation rate—correlates with disease activity; may be normal in the chronic form of disease

*Increased creatine phosphokinase (CPK) (MM and MB isoenzymes†) and aldolase reflect muscle injury, enzyme release, and disease activity.

Increased lactate dehydrogenase (LDH), serum glutamic-oxaloacetic transminase (SGOT) (AST [aspartate aminotransferase])—usually elevated

*Increased LDH isoenzymes $LDH_2$–$LDH_5$, especially $LDH_5$—indicates active skeletal-muscle necrosis in acute polymyositis

Slightly increased serum γ-globulin, polyclonal pattern

Occasionally, positive rheumatoid factor

Presence of antibody against PM-1 antigen—this is a nonhistone acid nuclear antigen often associated with polymyositis

Occasionally, presence of antinuclear antibody

Mild normocytic anemia

*Muscle biopsy shows characteristic inflammation and muscle degeneration and regeneration.

Increased urinary creatine–creatinine ratio reflects increased release and excretion of creatine from necrotic muscle.

* This finding is of diagnostic significance.
† See definition on page 12 in Chapter 1.

# MIXED CONNECTIVE TISSUE DISEASE

Mixed connective tissue disease shows varying features of SLE, scleroderma, and polymyositis.[5] The clinical pattern consists of polyarthalgia or polyarthritis, diffuse swelling of the hands, Raynaud's phenomenon, impaired esophageal motility, muscle inflammation, and a reduction in pulmonary diffusing capacity. In some patients, these findings appear simultaneously; in others, the clinical manifestations of the syndrome develop over a period of many months to years. Many cases evolve into a clear-cut picture of scleroderma or SLE.

Although the etiology and pathogenesis of mixed connective tissue disease are unknown, an immunologic basis of the disorder is suggested by the characteristic laboratory findings.

Patients who die with this disorder frequently have thickening of blood-vessel walls, resulting in narrowing of the lumina of many arteries and arterioles.

## LABORATORY FINDINGS

*High titer of antinuclear antibody, which usually has a speckled pattern

*Very high titer of antibody to extractable nuclear antigen

*High titers of antibody to nRNP, frequently >1:100,000. This is the characteristic serologic finding, occurring in 95%–100% of patients with this disorder.

Absent antibody to nuclear Sm antigen

Absent antibody to DNA

Normal serum complement

Increased serum γ-globulin (2 g/dl–5 g/dl) in 75% of patients

Positive rheumatoid factor in 50% of patients

Increased sedimentation rate reflects active inflammation.

Moderate anemia, occasional

Moderate leukopenia, occasional

Increased SGOT (AST), aldolase, and CPK reflect muscle involvement.

# INFECTIOUS ARTHRITIS

Infectious arthritis is an infection of joints. Infection may be caused by bacteria, mycobacteria, fungi, or possibly some viruses. Bacterial infections are more virulent than are infections produced by other microorganisms. In classic suppurative arthritis, the organisms usually enter the joint through the bloodstream or, less commonly, by direct penetration from the outside. The organisms first involve the subsynovial connective tissues; they then multiply and penetrate into the synovial fluid. Within an hour after bacteria enter the joint space, they are phagocytized by the synovial lining cells and polymorphonuclear leukocytes that have migrated to the site of infection. Subsequently, bacteriolysis occurs within these cells, releasing lysosomal enzymes that result

---

* This finding is of diagnostic significance.

in synovial-membrane necrosis, accumulation of increased synovial fluid, and damage to joint cartilage. Later, the resulting inflammatory exudate fills the entire joint cavity, obliterating the joint space. In chronic joint inflammation, there are regeneration and increased growth of cells lining the synovial cavity. These proliferating reparative tissues invade cartilage and bone. This results in marked joint destruction and, ultimately, in ankylosis or fusion and immobility of the joint.

Nongonococcal or classic septic arthritis is most frequently due to *Hemophilus influenzae* in children 6 months to 2 years old, to *Staphylococcus aureus, Streptococcus pyogenes,* and *Streptococcus pneumoniae* in children from 2 years old to adolescence, and to *Staphylococcus aureus* in adults over 40 years of age. Factors that seem to predispose adults to joint infection include diabetes mellitus, rheumatoid arthritis, malignancy, cirrhosis, chronic debilitating disease, and immunosuppressive therapy.

*Neisseria gonorrhoeae* is the most common cause of bacterial arthritis in patients between the ages of 16 and 40, accounting for 75% of cases in this age group. Gonococcal arthritis is classified separately from classic septic arthritis because of its different clinical presentation. Approximately 1% of patients with gonorrhea have disseminated gonococcal infection with involvement of the joints and skin (see Chap. 11). If treated appropriately, gonococci rarely cause permanent joint destruction.

About 1% of patients with tuberculosis develop joint involvement. Tuberculous arthritis is secondary to reactivation of a primary pulmonary infection, which then disseminates through the bloodstream. Fungi rarely cause arthritis.

The most frequent cause of viral arthritis occurs in the early stages of viral hepatitis. Arthritis and the accompanying skin rash are considered to be due to viral immune complexes or to direct viral invasion of joints and blood vessels. Serum and synovial fluid have been shown to contain hepatitis B surface antigen ($HB_sAg$) and decreased levels of complement. Antigen–antibody complexes have been identified in serum and synovial fluid by immunologic techniques and by electron microscopy.

## LABORATORY FINDINGS

### Synovial Fluid

Turbid, yellow; decreased viscosity; fibrin clot present; poor mucin clot; increased protein

*Gonococcal Arthritis*
WBC 1,500/$\mu$l–108,000/$\mu$l (avg 14,000); predominantly neutrophils

Decreased glucose

Positive Gram's stain >25%

*Positive culture 35%

*Septic Arthritis*
WBC usually >50,000/$\mu$l; neutrophils usually >90%

Low or undetectable glucose

---

* Positive blood culture, when there is systemic dissemination, may be the only source of microbial identification.

Positive Gram's stain up to 60%

*Positive culture >90%

Increased lactic acid

*Tuberculous Arthritis*
WBC 15,000/$\mu$l–25,000/$\mu$l; lymphocytes and neutrophils

Low glucose

Rarely positive smear and culture of synovial fluid

Frequently positive culture of synovial-tissue biopsy

*Viral Arthritis*
WBC 5,000/$\mu$l–25,000/$\mu$l; predominantly lymphocytes

Normal glucose

Presence of $HB_sAg$ in serum and synovial fluid (50%–80%)

**Blood**

Leukocytosis—often 15,000/$\mu$l; usually normal in nonbacterial infections

Increased sedimentation rate and C-reactive protein indicate active inflammation.

## REITER'S SYNDROME

Reiter's syndrome is a nonsuppurative peripheral polyarthritis of more than 1 month's duration. It is associated with urethritis or cervicitis. Conjunctivitis occurs in one third to two thirds of cases. Skin lesions occur in over one half of patients. The arthritis occurs several weeks following GI or genital infections. This disorder predominantly affects young men and usually involves joints below the waist. The cause is unknown and the course ranges from mild and transient to severe and incapacitating. Relapses and chronic illness are common.

Ankylosing spondylitis and arthritis with psoriasis are frequently found in the families of persons with Reiter's syndrome. There is a strong association between this disease and the histocompatibility antigen HLA-B27. The antigen is present in 75% of patients with the syndrome, but is present in only 8% of normal persons. Patients with this antigen have an increased familial occurrence of the disorder, indicating that genetic factors might play a role in this syndrome.

### LABORATORY FINDINGS

**Synovial Fluid**
WBC 100/$\mu$l–43,000/$\mu$l (avg 18,500); 60% neutrophils

Poor mucin clot

Increased protein

Glucose usually normal but may be low when the leukocyte count is high

* Positive blood culture, when there is systemic dissemination, may be the only source of microbial identification.

Normal or increased complement

Presence of "Reiter's cells" (macrophages with partially digested neutrophils)

**Blood**

Leukocytosis ($10,000/\mu l$–$20,000/\mu l$)

Increased sedimentation rate—parallels the clinical course

Increased serum complement—reflects active inflammation

Increased serum globulins—in chronic disease

Presence of HLA-B27 antigen in 75% of patients

Negative rheumatoid factor

**Other Laboratory Findings**

Increased WBC in urine and prostatic fluid—reflects urethritis.

Negative cultures of blood, synovial fluid, and urethral discharge

# RHEUMATOID ARTHRITIS

Rheumatoid arthritis is a chronic disease of the joints. It is of unknown etiology. Beginning with inflammation in the synovial lining of the joint, it usually runs an intermittent course or progresses to a proliferative synovitis with erosion of bone and destruction of cartilage and tendons.

The most widely held hypothesis for the pathogenesis of rheumatoid arthritis is that synovial tissue in a susceptible patient produces IgG in response to an unknown antigenic stimulus. The IgG antibody reacts with the unknown antigen and becomes altered or aggregated, so that the body no longer recognizes it as "self." IgM (rheumatoid factor) is then formed as an antibody against the altered IgG. Rheumatoid factor combines with IgG to form soluble immune complexes which are found both in the synovial membrane and in the synovial fluid. The complement system is activated, liberating chemotactic factors that attract leukocytes. The leukocytes ingest immune complexes; this triggers the release of enzymes and other mediators of inflammation into the synovial fluid. Fibrin, fibrin degradation products, and fibrinogen are found in the joints of patients with rheumatoid arthritis. Leukocytes engulf these substances, perpetuating the inflammatory process. Continued inflammation stimulates the synovium to proliferate and spread over the joint surface, interfering with joint function. Synovial tissue forms and releases large quantities of the enzyme collagenase, which destroys cartilage and connective tissue, resulting in permanent joint damage. Figure 9-1 compares an involved joint with a normal joint.

Rheumatoid disease is not always confined to joints. Extra-articular manifestations that might accompany rheumatoid arthritis include subcutaneous rheumatoid nodules, Felty's syndrome (splenomegaly and neutropenia), vasculitis, lung disease, pericarditis, Sjögren's syndrome, eye involvement, enlarged lymph nodes, and neuromuscular disorders. Patients with rheumatoid involvement of extra-articular sites usually have high titers of rheumatoid factor, soluble immune complexes, and decreased levels of complement.

Amyloidosis of a mild degree may occur as a complication in up to 25% of patients. This is diagnosed by biopsy of the gums, rectal mucosa, liver, or kidneys (see Chap. 10).

## LABORATORY FINDINGS

### Synovial Fluid

Yellow to white; turbidity reflects increased WBC; fibrin clot indicates chronicity

Mucin clot may be fair or poor; a poor clot and decreased viscosity indicates that hyaluronic acid is decreased.

WBC—usually 5,000/$\mu$l–50,000/$\mu$l—reflects the degree of inflammation

Differential WBC—usually 65% neutrophils, which increase along with the total WBC

Glucose—normal or low—there is interference with normal glucose transport

*Positive rheumatoid factor—usually present in higher concentration than in serum; inversely related to the synovial-fluid complement level

Decreased complement—reflects consumption in immunologic reaction

Increased IgG and immune complexes

Ragocytes—neutrophils with ingested immune complexes

### Peripheral Blood

WBC are usually normal or slightly elevated (<12,000/$\mu$l). WBC are decreased in the presence of splenomegaly; this suggests Felty's syndrome.

Normocytic or microcytic anemia—chronic disease type

### Other Laboratory Findings

*Positive rheumatoid factor (IgM)—75% of patients; occurs in 95% of patients with subcutaneous nodules

Presence of antinuclear antibodies (10%–50% of patients)—titers are lower than in SLE

Negative anti-DNA antibodies

Increased C-reactive protein, fibrinogen, and sedimentation rate—reflect disease activity

Increased $\alpha_1$- and $\alpha_2$-globulins—acute phase reactants

Increased $\gamma$-globulin—reflects accelerated protein breakdown in chronic disease

Normal serum complement; decreased complement in the presence of severe extra-articular disease, such as vasculitis

Presence of circulating immune complexes—frequent when there are systemic manifestations

---

* This finding is of diagnostic significance.

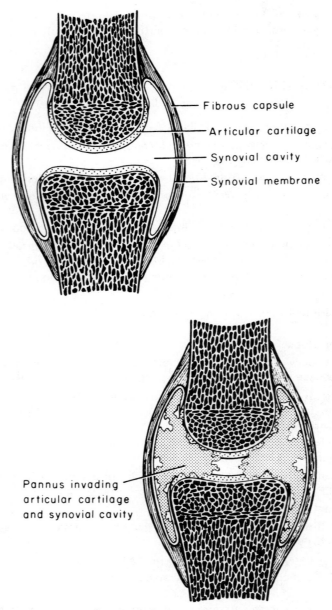

Fibrous capsule

Articular cartilage

Synovial cavity

Synovial membrane

Pannus invading
articular cartilage
and synovial cavity

**Fig. 9-1.** Normal joint (*top*) and rheumatoid arthritis (*bottom*). *Pannus* is the term for hyperplastic synovial tissue. (Gilbert EE, Huntington RW: An Introduction to Pathology, pp 268, 270. New York, Oxford University Press, 1978)

## *JUVENILE ARTHRITIS*

Chronic arthritis occurring in children under 16 years of age is defined as *juvenile arthritis.*[1] There are a number of clinical and serologic findings that are different from those in the adult disease. Features more frequently found in children include persistence of a high fever, a characteristic rash, onset involving one joint, chronic eye involvement, and a low incidence of rheumatoid factor.

There are several clinically distinct patterns:

1. Acute systemic—fever, rash, lymphadenopathy, hepatomegaly, splenomegaly
2. Pauciarticular (four or fewer joints)
   A. Older boys—childhood form of ankylosing spondylitis
   B. Younger girls—50% have chronic eye inflammation
3. Polyarticular (five or more joints)
   A. Seronegative—younger girls
   B. Seropositive—older girls; typical rheumatoid arthritis; rheumatoid nodules common

The development of inflammatory arthritis often retards growth but, on occasion, may actually accelerate the rate of growth of individual bones. In advanced disease there may be joint destruction and, occasionally, joint fusion.

### LABORATORY FINDINGS

Synovial fluid—increased leukocytes; decreased glucose; negative cultures

Normal or elevated serum complement (except in seropositive polyarticular form)

#### Acute Systemic Form

Leukocytosis

Mild normocytic anemia; hemoglobin (Hb) usually 9 g/dl–11 g/dl

Decreased serum iron and total iron binding capacity

Increased sedimentation rate and C-reactive protein

Decreased serum albumin, increased $\alpha_2$-globulin

Negative test for rheumatoid factor

Negative test for antinuclear antibodies

#### Pauciarticular Form

Normal complete blood count

Increased sedimentation rate and C-reactive protein during acute inflammation

Rheumatoid factor usually negative

Antinuclear antibodies frequently present in early childhood type, especially those with eye involvement

Presence of HLA-B27 in late childhood type

**Polyarticular Form**

Rheumatoid factor negative in younger children and positive in older children

Antinuclear antibodies present more frequently in older than in younger children

## ANKYLOSING SPONDYLITIS

Ankylosing spondylitis is inflammation of the joints of the spine, often resulting in fusion and loss of spinal mobility (Fig. 9-2). (Ankylosis is abnormal immobil-

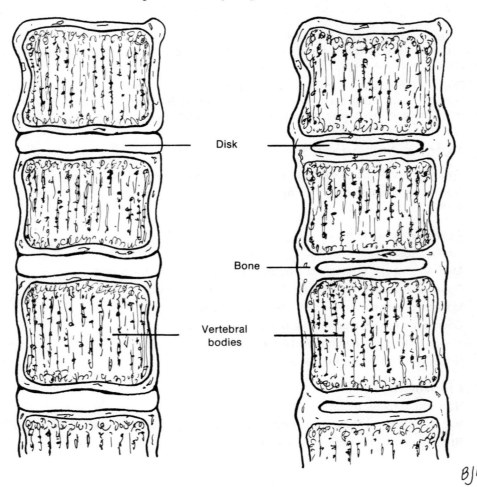

Disk

Bone

Vertebral bodies

BJH

**Fig. 9-2.** Normal spine (*left*) and spine in ankylosing spondylitis (*right*), which shows vertebral bodies united by bone at the margins of the intervertebral disks.

ity and consolidation of a joint. Spondylitis is inflammation of the vertebrae.) Although the disease is predominantly one of the spine, 30% of patients may have involvement of the hips, shoulders, and other peripheral joints. Ossification occurs in the regions of the intervertebral disks, sacroiliac joints, and other sites of attachment of ligaments and capsules to bones.

The cause of ankylosing spondylitis is unknown. There is a strong association between this disease and HLA-B27. This antigen is present in 90% of patients with ankylosing spondylitis, 50% of unaffected relatives, and 8% of normal persons. A hypothesis of the pathogenetic relationship is that the HLA-B27 gene is linked on the same chromosome to a disease-susceptibility complex.

Patients with ankylosing spondylitis may occasionally develop aortic insufficiency, iritis, pulmonary fibrosis, amyloidosis, or neurologic disorders. There is an association between ankylosing spondylitis and the occurrence of inflammatory bowel disease and psoriasis.

## LABORATORY FINDINGS

Increased sedimentation rate and C-reactive protein (90%)

Normocytic, hypochromic anemia (<30%)—chronic disease type

Presence of HLA-B27 antigen in 90% of patients

Increased alkaline phosphatase (50%)—reflects inflammation, immobilization, and resorption of bones

Synovial-fluid findings are similar to those in rheumatoid arthritis

Negative rheumatoid factor

### Laboratory Findings of Associated diseases

Ulcerative colitis*
Regional ileitis*

## POLYMYALGIA RHEUMATICA

Polymyalgia rheumatica is a common disorder affecting the elderly. The syndrome is characterized by early-morning pain and stiffness in the neck, arms, shoulders, back, and thighs. Constitutional symptoms include malaise, anorexia, fever, weight loss, and depression. The etiology and pathogenesis of this disorder are unknown. There is frequent association of this disorder with temporal arteritis (see Chap. 1).

## LABORATORY FINDINGS

Markedly increased sedimentation rate—usual finding

Increased C-reactive protein, fibrinogen, and $\alpha_2$-globulin reflect disease activity.

Increased serum $\gamma$-globulin, polyclonal pattern

Normocytic anemia (Hb 10 g/dl–12 g/dl)—chronic disease type

Normal CPK, aldolase, LDH, and SGOT (AST)

* See Chapter 3.

Negative LE test and rheumatoid factor

Temporal artery biopsy occasionally shows evidence of temporal arteritis.


# OSTEOMYELITIS

Osteomyelitis is an infection of the bone and bone marrow. This is most frequently caused by *Staphylococcus aureus*. It might also be due to other bacteria, mycobacteria, fungi, or rickettsiae.

Infection reaches the bone through the bloodstream, from a fracture or severe injury with a break in the skin, or by extension from an adjacent infection. Bacteremia is usually secondary to an acute local infection, such as pneumonia, middle-ear infection, or an abscess.

The bone marrow is the first portion of the bone to be involved. While the infection is extending through the marrow cavity, it may break through the bone cortex and spread along the bone surface. Infected periosteum, which is the covering of bone, separates from the underlying dead bone. Necrotic bone undergoes fragmentation. Bone fragments, which are deprived of their blood supply offer conditions conducive to bacterial or fungal growth. The adjacent joint may become infected or it may be the site of a sterile synovial-fluid effusion.

## LABORATORY FINDINGS

Leukocytosis, especially in acute infection; normal WBC in chronic disease

Normocytic anemia, chronic disease type

Increased sedimentation rate and C-reactive protein—indicates active disease

Decreased serum albumin and increased $\alpha_2$-globulin reflect chronic infection.

*Positive blood culture, especially in acute osteomyelitis in children

### Culture of Infected Bone

*Staphylococcus aureus* (60%–90%)—most infections of hip, skull, vertebrae, long bones

*Pseudomonas*—frequently found in drug addicts

*Candida, Aspergillus, Rhizopus*—in patients who are immunosuppressed or receiving protracted intravenous or parenteral therapy

*Salmonella*—occurs frequently in patients with sickle cell disease


# PAGET'S DISEASE

Paget's disease of bone is also known as osteitis deformans. It is a skeletal disorder of the elderly in which there is a high rate of bone destruction followed by excessive new bone formation. The cause of this condition is unknown. The

---

* This finding is of diagnostic significance.

earliest lesion appears to be haphazard absorption of bone. The response to this bone absorption is increased and inappropriate new bone formation. The new bone is irregularly formed and weak. The affected bones enlarge, soften, and bend, resulting in deformities. The most frequently involved bones are the pelvis, spine, femur, skull, and tibia. Patients with skull enlargement may experience blindness, deafness, headaches, and facial paralysis from bony compression of the cranial nerves. The disease process does not involve cartilage or joints but the bone deformity may result in degenerative arthritis. Osteogenic sarcoma may develop as a complication of Paget's disease of long duration.

### LABORATORY FINDINGS

*Increased serum alkaline phosphatase, marked—this characteristic finding is the result of excessive new bone formation, which reflects the activity of the disease; a rapid rise occurs if osteogenic sarcoma develops

Increased urinary hydroxyproline—this is the result of accelerated bone collagen resorption, breakdown, and excretion

Usually normal serum calcium and phosphorus

Increased incidence of renal calculi

## OSTEOGENIC SARCOMA

Osteogenic sarcoma is a highly malignant and rapidly fatal primary tumor of bone. It usually occurs in patients between 10 and 25 years of age. The neoplasm forms bone, which accounts for the increase in serum alkaline phosphatase.

### LABORATORY FINDINGS

Increased serum alkaline phosphatase—this reflects new bone formation by the tumor. It is usually not more than two to three times higher than normal for the age of the patient.

Increased alkaline phosphatase after surgical removal of the tumor suggests spread or recurrence of the tumor.

*Biopsy showing malignant bone tumor

## METASTATIC CARCINOMA OF BONE

Malignant tumors of various organs may spread, or metastasize, to involve bones. If the metastatic tumor destroys the involved bone, it is referred to as *osteolytic*, whereas if the tumor stimulates the involved bone to form new bone, it is referred to as *osteoblastic*.

The most common osteolytic metastases originate from cancers of the

---

* This finding is of diagnostic significance.

breast, lung, thyroid, and kidney. Osteoblastic metastases usually originate from cancer of the prostate.

## LABORATORY FINDINGS

### Osteolytic Metastases

Increased serum calcium reflects removal of calcium from destroyed bone at sites of metastatic tumor.

Increased urine calcium reflects excretion of increased serum calcium.

Increased urine hydroxyproline reflects breakdown and excretion of bone collagen.

Normal serum alkaline phosphatase

### Osteoblastic Metastases

Increased serum alkaline phosphatase reflects new bone formation stimulated by the metastatic tumor.

Increased serum acid phosphatase reflects metastases from prostatic cancer, which is the source of acid phosphatase.

## REFERENCES

1. Baum J: Juvenile arthritis. Am J Dis Child 135:557–560, 1981
2. Hess EV: Introduction to drug-related lupus. Arthritis Rheum 24, No. 8:VI–IX, 1981
3. Hochberg MC: The spectrum of systemic sclerosis: Current concepts. Hosp Pract 16:61–67, 70–72, 1982
4. Phillips RC, Wasner CK: Scleroderma, current understanding of pathogenesis and management. Postgrad Med 70:153–168, 1981
5. Sharp GC: Mixed connective tissue disease. Bull Rheum Dis 25:828–831, 1974–1975
6. Strand V, Talal N: Advances in the diagnosis and concept of Sjögren's syndrome (autoimmune exocrinopathy). Bull Rheum Dis 30:1046–1052, 1980

## BIBLIOGRAPHY

Cohen AS (ed): Rheumatology and Immunology. New York, Grune & Stratton, 1979
Currey HLF (ed): Clinical Rheumatology, 3rd ed. Philadelphia, JB Lippincott, 1980
Katz WA (ed): Rheumatic Diseases, Diagnosis and Management. Philadelphia, JB Lippincott, 1977
McCarty DJ: Arthritis and Allied Conditions, 9th ed. Philadelphia, Lea & Febiger, 1979

# 10

# *NUTRITIONAL AND METABOLIC DISEASES*

Malnutrition
Disorders of Amino-Acid Transport and
    Metabolism
  Disturbances of Amino-Acid Transport
   Cystinuria
   Hartnup Disease
  Disturbances of Amino-Acid
    Metabolism
   Phenylketonuria
   Histidinemia
   Homocystinuria
Disorders of Carbohydrate Metabolism
  Von Gierke's Disease
  Galactosemia
  Lactase Deficiency
Disorders of Lipid Metabolism
  Hypercholesterolemia
  Endogenous Hypertriglyceridemia
  Hyperchylomicronemia
  Dysbetalipoproteinemia
  Mixed Hyperlipidemia
Gout

Pseudogout
Hemochromatosis
Wilson's Disease
Osteomalacia
Cystic Fibrosis
Disorders of Porphyrin Metabolism
  Erythropoietic Porphyrias
    Congenital Erythropoietic Porphyria
    Erythropoietic Protoporphyria
  Hepatic Porphyrias
   Acute Intermittent Porphyria
   Variegate Porphyria
   Hereditary Coproporphyria
   Porphyria Cutanea Tarda
Amyloidosis
Disorders of Bilirubin Excretion
  Unconjugated Hyperbilirubinemias
   Gilbert's Syndrome
   Crigler-Najjar Syndrome
  Conjugated Hyperbilirubinemias
   Dubin-Johnson Syndrome
   Rotor's Syndrome

## *MALNUTRITION*

Generalized food deficiency is much more common than are specific nutritional deficiencies. Caloric deficiency is a more prevalent problem than is isolated protein deficiency. Malnutrition is particularly prevalent and serious among infants. In infants there is a vicious cycle of debilitation, leading to respiratory and gastrointestinal infections, which further decrease food intake. Pregnant and lactating women are also at an increased risk of developing malnutrition.

    The most important clinical feature of malnutrition is growth failure and weight loss. Edema occurs as a result of albumin loss and sodium retention.

Losses of potassium and magnesium contribute to the sodium retention. Fatty liver develops as a result of a failure of triglyceride transport to peripheral tissues and deficient lipoprotein synthesis. Anemia occurs following iron and folic acid deficiencies. There is normal immunoglobulin production; however, impaired T-lymphocyte response leads to overwhelming common infections, such as measles.

Secondary starvation may result from fasting; impaired digestion or absorption (see Impaired Intestinal Absorption, Chap. 3); impaired amino-acid metabolism due to liver disease; excessive tissue breakdown caused by thyrotoxicosis or chronic debilitating illnesses; loss of protein due to burns, draining wounds, or fistulas or to protein-losing enteropathy; or prolonged chemotherapy or radiation therapy.

When there is a deficit in energy intake, the body draws on its own stores to maintain blood glucose, which is its main fuel. Liver glycogen is depleted within a few hours, following which skeletal muscle protein is converted to glucose to maintain plasma glucose levels. Triglycerides from fat depots are converted to fatty acids as another energy source. Homeostatic mechanisms attempt to maintain the level of plasma albumin. Eventually plasma albumin concentration falls, resulting in reduced serum oncotic pressure and edema.

### LABORATORY FINDINGS[6]

Decreased plasma albumin (<3.4 g/dl) and total protein—correlates with the degree of fatty liver and edema

Decreased total iron binding capacity (<240 mcg/dl)—total iron binding capacity reflects transferrin concentration, which is a sensitive and early indicator of protein deficiency

Decreased 24-hr urine creatinine—this should be compared with the expected creatinine excretion based on the patient's height and sex

Decreased total lymphocyte count (<1500/μl)

Decreased blood urea nitrogen (BUN), magnesium, and urine urea nitrogen

Normocytic, normochromic anemia—chronic disease type

Laboratory findings of impaired intestinal absorption (see Chap. 3) and osteomalacia

## DISORDERS OF AMINO-ACID TRANSPORT AND METABOLISM

Disorders of amino-acid transport and metabolism are uncommon. This discussion includes only those disorders that occur with greatest frequency, for which testing is generally done, or that are correctable by treatment. Most of the inherited inborn errors are recessive, which implies that the affected person will have no symptoms unless he is lacking more than half of the necessary enzyme.

Disorders of amino-acid transport across cell membranes include cystinuria and Hartnup disease.[2] In these conditions there is impairment of the normal absorption of amino acids by the small intestine or impairment of the normal reabsorption of filtered amino acids by the proximal renal tubules. In the latter circumstance, aminoaciduria results. Blood levels of amino acids are normal or low. In the normal person, the kidney reabsorbs 93% to 100% of the amino acids filtered by the glomerulus. In the various transport disorders, only 50% of certain amino acids are reabsorbed, and the other 50% is lost in the urine. Until 3 months of age, the normal infant reabsorbs only 85% to 90% of filtered amino acids. This reflects immaturity of the transport mechanisms and is not pathologic.

Disorders of amino-acid metabolism include phenylketonuria, histidinemia, and homocystinuria. In these conditions, genetic impairment of specific enzyme activity results in disturbance of intracellular amino-acid metabolism. As a consequence of biochemical disequilibrium, characteristic clinical and laboratory findings occur. In this group of disorders there are increased plasma levels of various amino-acid metabolites. These increases are in contrast to the normal plasma levels of amino acids that occur in the transport disorders.

## DISTURBANCES OF AMINO-ACID TRANSPORT

### Cystinuria

Cystinuria is one of the most common genetic defects affecting amino-acid transport. It occurs in approximately 1 : 15,000 live births. Defective absorption of cystine by renal tubular epithelial cells results in greatly increased urinary excretion of cystine. Because cystine is the least soluble of the naturally occurring amino acids, the affected person forms cystine calculi in the kidneys, ureters, and bladder. The calculi contribute to obstruction and secondary infection of the urinary tract.

Aside from causing urinary cystine loss, the defect also results in increased urinary loss of lysine, ornithine, and arginine. These four amino acids have molecular similarities and share the same transport system. In addition to their impaired renal tubular reabsorption, they are incompletely absorbed by the small intestine. Consequently, there are no increases in the plasma levels of these amino acids.

### LABORATORY FINDINGS

Presence of cystine crystals in the urine

Positive cyanide–nitroprusside test on urine and on calculi indicates presence of cystine.

Amino-acid analysis of urine shows increased excretion of cystine (20–30 times normal), lysine, arginine, and ornithine.

Hematuria occurs as a result of cystine calculi.

### Hartnup Disease

Hartnup disease, which is named for the first family in which it was identified, occurs in 1 : 16,000 to 1 : 25,000 live births. Although the basic biochemical defect involves impaired intestinal and renal transport of many amino acids, the clinical abnormalities appear to be secondary to the malabsorption of only tryptophan.

Tryptophan is an essential amino acid that normally is absorbed from the small intestine and converted to nicotinamide. Impairment of this absorption and conversion is responsible for the pellagralike clinical syndrome. Pellagra also results from dietary deficiency of niacin. The clinical features are an intermittent red scaly rash appearing after exposure to sunlight, cerebellar ataxia, and occasionally psychiatric disturbances ranging from emotional instability to delirium.

The transport defect in Hartnup disease affects both the renal tubules and the small intestine. Urinary excretion of several neutral amino acids occurs because they share the same renal transport defect. Impaired intestinal absorption of these amino acids results in their retention in the intestine for abnormally long periods of time. This allows the intestinal bacteria to metabolize the amino acids. Some of the metabolites are absorbed into the bloodstream, affect the central nervous system, and may account for the neuropsychiatric disturbances.

## LABORATORY FINDINGS

Increased urine amino acids (5–10 times normal amounts)—alanine, serine, threonine, valine, leucine, isoleucine, phenylalanine, tryrosine, tryptophan, histidine

Normal to low plasma levels of the affected amino acids

### DISTURBANCES OF AMINO-ACID METABOLISM

### Phenylketonuria

Phenylketonuria (PKU) is an inherited deficiency of hepatic phenylalanine hydroxylase, resulting in interference with the normal conversion of phenylalanine to tyrosine. Phenylalanine accumulates in all body fluids. Metabolites of phenylalanine, such as phenylpyruvic acid, are excreted in large amounts in the urine. The enzyme defect occurs in 1 : 6000 to 1 : 15,000 live births.

Associated secondary biochemical abnormalities include decreased serotonin synthesis, decreased melanin synthesis, impaired cerebral protein synthesis, decreased epinephrine synthesis, decreased gluconeogenesis, and decreased glycolysis.

The major clinical characteristic of untreated patients is mental retardation. Most patients are also agitated, aggressive, and hyperactive. Muscular hypertonicity, tremors, and increased motor activity affect gait, movement, and posture. Affected persons have lighter than normal pigmentation of skin, hair, and eyes.

## LABORATORY FINDINGS

Increased urine phenylalanine and phenylpyruvic acid; the latter might not appear until 2 weeks to 3 weeks of age

Increased plasma phenylalanine and decreased plasma tyrosine occur when there is a normal phenylalanine intake. These findings might not appear until after 4 days of age, after which time any maternally transmitted enzymes will have been depleted.

Near-normal plasma phenylalanine occurs when dietary phenylalanine intake is restricted to about 250 mg/day–500 mg/day.

There is no increase in plasma tyrosine after a dietary intake of increased phenylalanine.

## Histidinemia

Histidinemia is a trait characterized by an increase in the concentration of histidine in blood and urine as a consequence of deficient histidase activity in the liver and skin. Histidine breakdown is impaired. This occurs in 1 : 12,000 to 1 : 25,000 live births. The amount of histidine in the blood is, in part, dependent on the amount of protein in the diet.

Patients with histidinemia often present with mental retardation and delayed speech development. Some patients are asymptomatic. There is no consistent association between this metabolic disorder and clinical findings.

### LABORATORY FINDINGS

Increased plasma histidine is the characteristic laboratory finding.

Increased urine histidine, especially after meals

## Homocystinuria

Classic homocystinuria is caused by a deficiency of the hepatic enzyme cystathionine synthetase. As a consquence of this deficiency, there is impaired metabolism of homocystine to cystathionine. Defective activity of this enzyme causes elevated levels of both homocystine and its precursor, methionine, in body fluids. There are decreased blood levels of cystine, which follows cystathionine in the normal metabolic pathway. This disorder occurs in 1 : 80,000 to 1 : 150,000 live births.

Patients with this disorder have the characteristics of a connective-tissue disease that is complicated by vascular thromboses. Increased homocystine in the circulation makes platelets sticky and causes damage to the endothelial lining of arteries. Both of these factors contribute to the frequent occurrence of vascular thrombi. Premature atherosclerosis also develops. An affected person may die of coronary-artery occlusion, cerebrovascular thrombosis, pulmonary embolus, or thrombosis of the renal artery or vein. Other clinical features include lens dislocation and mental retardation.

### LABORATORY FINDINGS

Increased serum, urine, and cerebrospinal fluid (CSF) methionine and homocystine

Decreased serum cystine

# DISORDERS OF CARBOHYDRATE METABOLISM

Glycogen storage diseases are disorders of carbohydrate metabolism that result from an inherited defect in glycogen metabolism. The defect causes production of an abnormal form, or excessive amounts, of glycogen. Glycogen excess occurs because it cannot be degraded in a normal fashion or because it is synthesized preferentially.

The glycogenoses have been classified into ten different types on the basis of the specific enzymes affected. Enzyme assays from biopsied tissue are required in order to categorize each type of disorder. Clinically, the diseases predominantly involve either the liver or the skeletal muscles and myocardium. In the hepatic type, the liver is greatly enlarged and there are severe hypoglycemia, marked hypertriglyceridemia and hypercholesterolemia, and increased blood lactate and uric acid. Death is common in childhood. In the muscle form of glycogenosis there are muscle cramps, weakness, and atrophy or massive muscle infiltration with glycogen. Infiltration of heart muscle results in myocardial failure and death.

## VON GIERKE'S DISEASE

The most common form of glycogenosis, and the only one that is described in this chapter, is von Gierke's disease, in which glucose-6-phosphatase activity is defective in the liver, kidneys, and intestine. Lack of this enzyme in the liver prevents conversion of glucose-6-phosphate to glucose. Consequently, patients develop severe hypoglycemia. Accumulated glucose-6-phosphate slows glycogen breakdown, but the stimulus to glycogen formation persists. The result is an excessive accumulation of glycogen in the liver and in the proximal renal tubules. Hypoglycemia inhibits insulin secretion; this affects lipid and protein metabolism. The results are hyperlipidemia and stunted growth, respectively. There is a compensatory increase in glucose metabolism in the liver; this leads to increased blood lactate and pyruvate. Patients usually present clinically with hypoglycemia, lactic acidosis, and hepatomegaly. They may also manifest bleeding due to impaired platelet function.

### LABORATORY FINDINGS

Marked decrease in blood glucose due to impaired hepatic release of glucose

Increased lactic acid, marked

Decreased bicarbonate and pH (metabolic acidosis) due to increased lactic acid

Marked increase in triglycerides and cholesterol due to impaired lipid metabolism

Increased serum uric acid due to decreased urinary excretion of uric acid

Mild anemia

Decreased serum phosphorus

Evidence of impaired platelet function—prolonged bleeding time, decreased platelet adhesion, and defective platelet aggregation

Liver biopsy shows increased glycogen and diminished glucose-6-phosphatase.

## GALACTOSEMIA

Galactosemia, which occurs in 1 : 50,000 live births, is the result of a genetic deficiency of galactokinase or galactose transferase. The classic disorder is due to transferase deficiency. Only homozygous patients have clinically evident disease.

A lack of transferase enzyme activity in the liver and red blood cells (RBC) interferes with the conversion of galactose to glucose, impairing normal glucose metabolism. This results in accumulation of galactose-1-phosphate and galactose in the liver, kidneys, and brain. The consequences of this accumulation are cirrhosis, renal tubular malabsorption, and mental retardation.

Presenting symptoms include lethargy, vomiting, diarrhea, failure to thrive, jaundice, and hepatomegaly. If diagnosis is delayed, there are continuing enlargement of the liver, cirrhosis, splenomegaly, and ascites. Cataracts develop in approximately 50% of patients as a consequence of conversion of galactose to galactitol. Galactitol is trapped in the lens, where it creates an osmotic gradient and produces degeneration of lens fibers.

### LABORATORY FINDINGS

Increased plasma galactose and galactose-1-phosphate—result of impaired conversion of galactose to glucose

Galactosuria

Aminoaciduria and proteinuria reflect renal tubular dysfunction.

Lack of galactose transferase in RBC

Hyperchloremic metabolic acidosis reflects the effect of diarrhea or renal tubular acidosis.

Increased serum glutamic-oxaloacetic transaminase (SGOT) (AST |aspartate aminotransferase|) and serum glutamic-pyruvic transaminase (SGPT) (ALT |alanine aminotransferase|)—reflects impaired liver function

## LACTASE DEFICIENCY

Lactase deficiency is the most common deficiency of intestinal disaccharide enzymes. The primary disorder is deficiency of lactase in the cellular brush border of the intestine. It commonly occurs in patients with no other intestinal disease. Secondary lactase deficiency occurs in patients with other intestinal mucosal disorders such as celiac sprue or regional enteritis. Patients with lactase deficiency are unable to hydrolyze the disaccharide lactose into its two constituent monosaccharides, glucose and galactose. Lactose is undigested and remains in the intestinal lumen. Its osmotic activity draws a large volume of fluid and electrolytes into the intestine. The osmolality of lactose is further increased in the colon, where it is converted to lactic acid by bacterial and metabolic action. There is severe diarrhea and acid stools.

### LABORATORY FINDINGS

Impaired lactose tolerance test—minimal rise in blood glucose after ingestion of lactose; diarrhea occurs

Normal tolerance test of glucose and galactose—normal rise in blood glucose when the two monosaccharides are ingested separately; no diarrhea occurs

Decreased stool *p*H due to increased lactic acid

Increased stool lactose indicated by positive Clinitest reaction of stool

## DISORDERS OF LIPID METABOLISM

The hyperlipidemias are a diverse group of disorders in which there is impaired lipid transport. This results in increased blood levels of cholesterol or triglyceride and of the lipoproteins that carry them. Rarely, the disorders are primary, occurring as a result of an inherited genetic defect. Hyperlipidemias are more commonly secondary to other medical conditions or to diet. The major medical impact of the hyperlipidemias is their role in atherosclerosis (see Chap. 1).

The most frequent exogenous conditions that may cause secondary elevation of lipids include excess calorie intake, alcoholism, diabetes mellitus, liver disease, hypothyroidism, and use of various drugs. Laboratory studies cannot differentiate the primary from the secondary forms of hyperlipidemia. Reversal of the lipid abnormality following treatment of the underlying condition indicates that the hyperlipoproteinemia had been of the secondary form.

The hyperlipoproteinemias have been classified into the following phenotypes: Type I, Type IIa, Type IIb, Type III, Type IV, and Type V. This classification is based on lipoprotein electrophoresis, measurement of plasma cholesterol and triglyceride, and the appearance of the plasma after overnight refrigeration (Fig. 10-1). The lipoproteins have also been classified on the basis of their densities following ultracentrifugation into high-density lipoproteins

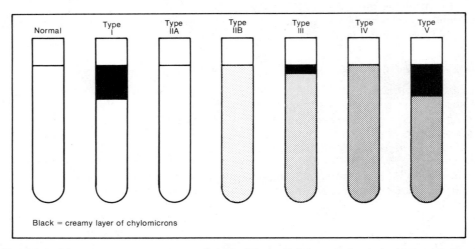

Black = creamy layer of chylomicrons

**Fig. 10-1.** The serum patterns associated with each lipoprotein phenotype are shown schematically in comparison with clear normal serum. These serum patterns are observed after serum from patients fasting 14 hours are allowed to stand overnight in a refrigerator at a temperature just above freezing. (Whayne TF Jr: The hyperlipoproteinemias. J Fam Pract 11:789–799, 1980)

(HDL), low-density lipoproteins (LDL), and very low-density lipoproteins (VLDL).

A practical classification of the hyperlipidemias is based on the findings of hypercholesterolemia alone, hypertriglyceridemia alone, or increased blood levels of both lipids. *Pure hypercholesterolemia* is exemplified by Type IIa, which is usually of dietary origin but might be hereditary. *Pure hypertriglyceridemia* occurs in Type IV, Type I, and Type V disorders. The latter two types have an impaired capacity to clear dietary triglyceride from the bloodstream and characteristically show abundant chylomicrons on electrophoresis. They also share such characteristics as grossly lipemic plasma, xanthomas, pancreatitis, and hepatosplenomegaly. Type I is usually hereditary, whereas Types IV and V are usually acquired. The *mixed hyperlipidemias* include Type III, Type IV and Type IIb. These may be differentiated by means of lipoprotein electrophoresis.

### HYPERCHOLESTEROLEMIA

Hypercholesterolemia is characterized chemically by an elevation of plasma cholesterol and clinically by deposition of cholesterol in the tendons or subcutaneum, corneas, and blood-vessel walls. The hereditary form of the disorder has an autosomal dominant inheritance and a deficiency in the LDL receptor that regulates the metabolism of LDL and the synthesis of cellular cholesterol. The LDL-receptor defect diminishes normal clearance of plasma LDL–cholesterol and results in moderate to marked increases in plasma LDL–cholesterol, depending on heterozygosity or homozygosity. Homozygotes show severe clinical disease with progressive atherosclerosis beginning in childhood and usually ending in death from myocardial infarction, often before 20 years of age. Heterozygotes have less severe disease, although their risk of coronary heart disease is five to six times that of unaffected persons.

Secondary hypercholesterolemia occurs far more frequently than does the primary hereditary form of the disorder. The most common cause of secondary increase in plasma cholesterol is an excessive dietary intake of cholesterol. Other conditions that result in a secondary elevation of plasma cholesterol include hypothyroidism, nephrotic syndrome, hepatic disease, dysgammaglobulinemias, and acute intermittent porphyria.

Persons with elevated levels of cholesterol, especially LDL–cholesterol, are at increased risk of developing coronary-artery disease.

### LABORATORY FINDINGS*

Plasma is usually clear after overnight refrigeration—the increased LDLs are too small to diffract light and produce turbidity.

Increased plasma cholesterol. 200 mg/dl–350 mg/dl—dietary, common; 400 mg/dl–600 mg/dl—heterozygous, uncommon; >600 mg/dl—homozygous, rare

Normal plasma triglyceride

Electrophoresis—increased β-lipoprotein (LDL)

---

* These findings indicate Type IIa hyperlipoproteinemia.

## *ENDOGENOUS HYPERTRIGLYCERIDEMIA*

Endogenous hypertriglyceridemia is the most commonly occurring form of hyperlipidemia. The primary disorder is inherited as an autosomal dominant trait in which heterozygotes manifest a mild form of the disease. They show moderate elevation of VLDL. This elevation is frequently associated with atherosclerotic vascular disease, diabetes, obesity, and chronic renal disease. In the severe form of the disease, the plasma triglyceride concentration and VLDL are markedly elevated and chylomicrons are present. This is termed *mixed hyperlipidemia* and commonly is associated with glucose intolerance and hyperuricemia.

Increased plasma triglyceride is more frequently a secondary than a primary hereditary disorder. The most common conditions causing secondary hypertriglyceridemia include excessive caloric intake, alcoholism, poorly controlled diabetes mellitus, hypothyroidism, nephrotic syndrome, uremia, glycogen storage disease, pancreatitis, and dysgammaglobulinemias. Among persons with markedly elevated levels of triglycerides there is an increased incidence of pancreatitis.

## LABORATORY FINDINGS

### Mild Form*

Plasma appears turbid to opaque due to increased VLDL, which diffract light but remain in stable dispersion; there is no creamy layer after overnight refrigeration.

Increased plasma triglyceride (200 mg/dl–2000 mg/dl)

Normal or slightly increased cholesterol

Electrophoresis—Increased prebetalipoprotein (VLDL), normal or slightly increased β-lipoprotein (LDL), normal chylomicrons. The latter differentiates Type IV from Type V.

### Severe Form†

Plasma is turbid to opaque due to VLDL, which diffract light but remain in stable dispersion; after overnight refrigeration the top layer is creamy owing to presence of chylomicrons.

Markedly increased plasma triglyceride (500 mg/dl–3000 mg/dl)

Increased plasma cholesterol (250 mg/dl–500 mg/dl)

Electrophoresis—Increased prebeta lipoprotein (VLDL) and chylomicrons

## *HYPERCHYLOMICRONEMIA*

Hyperchylomicronemia is a rare inherited recessive disorder in which very greatly increased concentrations of chylomicrons caused marked elevations of plasma triglyceride and lesser increases in cholesterol. The triglyceride elevation appears with ingestion of dietary fat. All abnormalities disappear after the pa-

---

* These findings indicate Type IV hyperlipoproteinemia.
† These findings indicate Type V hyperlipoproteinemia.

tient maintains a fat-free diet for 5 days. Usually detected in childhood, the disorder is associated with abdominal pain, severe pancreatitis, xanthomas (lipid deposits in the soft tissue), and enlargement of the liver and spleen. There is no evidence of premature vascular disease.

A deficiency in the enzyme lipoprotein lipase is thought to underlie the metabolic abnormalities of this disorder. As a consequence of this deficiency, chylomicrons accumulate in the bloodstream. There is also only minimal change in plasma lipids following the intravenous injection of heparin. This is in contrast to the normal precipitous drop in concentration of triglyceride and rise in free fatty acids following such an injection.

## LABORATORY FINDINGS*

Plasma shows a creamy top layer and a clear to slightly turbid lower layer after overnight refrigeration—the creamy layer consists of chylomicrons.

Massively increased plasma triglyceride (2,500 mg/dl–12,000 mg/dl)

Normal to slightly increased plasma cholesterol

Electrophoresis—Increased chylomicrons

### DYSBETALIPOPROTEINEMIA

Dysbetalipoproteinemia is a rare disorder that is usually inherited rather than acquired. It is characterized by the accumulation of an unusual class of lipoproteins with reduced electrophoretic mobility in the density range of VLDL. These lipoproteins are referred to as $\beta$-VLDL. This disorder is also known as broad-beta or floating beta lipoproteinemia. Patients have premature coronary and peripheral vascular disease and show characteristic xanthomas of the limbs, buttocks, and palms. They also demonstrate abnormal glucose tolerance tests.

## LABORATORY FINDINGS†

Plasma is clear, cloudy, or milky but rapidly becomes more turbid on chilling, and a waxy, yellowish pellicle may form after overnight refrigeration.

Markedly increased plasma cholesterol (300 mg/dl–1000 mg/dl)

Markedly increased plasma triglyceride (200 mg/dl–1000 mg/dl)

Electrophoresis—Increased $\beta$-lipoprotein (LDL); increased "floating" $\beta$-lipoprotein, which is an abnormal LDL that merges with the prebeta band—that is the characteristic finding in the disorder; increased prebetalipoprotein (VLDL)

### MIXED HYPERLIPIDEMIA

Family members affected with mixed hyperlipidemia manifest an elevation of VLDL or LDL or both. This is a commonly occurring hyperlipidemia. Dietary cholesterol excess is probably the most common cause of this disorder.

---

* These findings indicate Type I hyperlipoproteinemia.
† These findings indicate Type III hyperlipoproteinemia.

## LABORATORY FINDINGS

Plasma is slightly to moderately turbid after overnight refrigeration

Increased plasma cholesterol and plasma triglyceride

Electrophoresis is necessary to differentiate among this group of disorders:

Type IIb—increased β-lipoprotein (LDL) and prebetalipoprotein (VLDL)
Type IV—increased prebetalipoprotein (VLDL)
Type III—increased "floating" β-lipoprotein (abnormal LDL)


## *GOUT*

Gout is a metabolic disorder characterized by increased serum uric acid, recurrent attacks of acute crystal-induced arthritis, deposition of sodium urate in and around joints, and formation of uric-acid calculi.[1]

Uric acid is the chief end product of purine metabolism in man. Approximately 60% of uric acid is of endogenous origin. About two thirds of the uric acid formed each day is eliminated by the kidney. The pathways of both biosynthesis and reutilization are controlled by feedback inhibition, a mechanism whereby the concentration of the end product regulates its own rate of production. Alterations in purine intake and the extrarenal disposal of uric acid generally have relatively little influence on the serum urate level.

More than 90% of patients with gout have primary familial gout, which is thought to be due to a genetically determined metabolic defect in the regulation of purine metabolism. In these patients, the total amount of body urates may be up to 25 times normal. Eighty percent to ninety percent of patients with primary gout have impaired renal tubular secretion of urate and a consequent increase in plasma urate. In only 10% to 20% of cases is there increased synthesis of uric acid. These patients have normal renal clearance of the excessively produced uric acid and consequently have increased urinary excretion of uric acid. This group of cases more frequently includes the formation of renal calculi. Both overproduction and decreased secretion may exist in many patients.

Ten percent of patients with gout have hyperuricemia that is secondary to other disease processes. The underlying condition has accelerated nucleic-acid metabolism and increased uric-acid formation, or else there is impaired renal excretion of urates. Conditions with increased cell breakdown and uric-acid formation include myeloproliferative disorders (polycythemia, myeloid metaplasia, chronic myelocytic leukemia), lymphoproliferative disorders (chronic lymphocytic leukemia, multiple myeloma), disseminated carcinoma, sickle cell anemia, and hemolytic anemias. Impaired urate excretion may be secondary to drugs such as diuretics, chronic renal failure, ketoacidosis, lead intoxication, or thyroid or parathyroid disorders.

When serum uric-acid concentration exceeds 8 mg/dl, monosodium urate tends to precipitate in body tissues. These deposits have a striking predilection for forming on the surface and within the substance of joint cartilages as well as in the synovium, which lines joints. The marked predilection of acute gout for peripheral joints may in part be due to the lower temperature of these joints, enhancing urate precipitation. Deposits also occur adjacent to joints in bursae, tendons, and tendon sheaths. Deposits of urates in nonjoint tissues are referred to as *tophi* (Latin for *porous stone*). In general, the higher the serum urate level the earlier the appearance and more extensive the development of tophi.

Attacks of joint inflammation occur when microcrystals of monosodium urate monohydrate are discharged into the joint cavity from cartilage or synovial deposits. An intense inflammatory reaction occurs within 4 to 8 hours. Crystals become coated with immunoglobulins, which enhance their phagocytosis by granulocytes. Phagocytosis results in the formation of a chemotactic factor, which attracts additional leukocytes. Entrapment of urate crystals by leukocytes is followed by rapid degranulation and disintegration of the leukocytes, with release of both cytoplasmic and lysosomal enzymes. After repeated attacks, these enzymes dissolve articular cartilage and injure soft tissues.

Uric-acid urinary calculi occur in 15% to 20% of patients with primary gout and in 40% of those with secondary gout. In many of these patients, the stones result from urate precipitation in persistently acidic urine. Acid urine may be due to a deficiency in the production of ammonia buffer by the kidney.

Patients with gout have a higher frequency of hypertension and renal malfunction than do nongouty persons. Chronic hyperuricemia does not appear to be injurious to the kidneys, and azotemia is usually mild. Renal insufficiency, when seen in patients with gout, usually correlates with coexistence of hypertension, ischemic heart disease, or primary preexisting renal insufficiency. Hyperuricemia in hypertension appears to be related to an abnormality in uric-acid transport by the renal tubules. Diabetes mellitus, cardiac and cerebral vascular atherosclerosis, and increased serum triglycerides occur more frequently among patients with gout than in the general population.

## LABORATORY FINDINGS

Synovial fluid—white blood cells (WBC) 5,000/$\mu$l–50,000/$\mu$l (avg 13,500); neutrophils 48%–94% (avg 83%); increased complement. Monosodium urate crystals are found free and also within WBC; they are visualized when viewed microscopically under polarized light. This finding establishes the diagnosis. Urate crystals are also seen in biopsies of tophi.

Increased serum uric acid (more than 95% of patients)

Moderate leukocytosis during acute attacks

Increased sedimentation rate during acute attacks

Increased urine uric-acid crystals and amorphous urates (10%–25% of patients)

Proteinuria—this precedes other evidence of renal disease

Decreased urine $p$H throughout the day due to impaired ammonia formation

## *PSEUDOGOUT*

Pseudogout is associated with acute goutlike episodes of arthritis. This condition is also referred to as *chondrocalcinosis, pyrophosphate arthropathy,* and *calcium pyrophosphate crystal disease.* The disorder is characterized by deposition of calcium pyrophosphate dihydrate crystals in articular cartilage, fibrocartilage, ligaments, and tendons.

A proposed mechanism for the arthritis is that during an acute attack articular cartilage cells die and the surrounding pyrophosphate crystals coalesce within the thinned cartilage. Crystals subsequently are shed into the joint space, inducing an inflammatory reaction. Crystals are phagocytosed by leukocytes, following which a chemotactic factor is released from the WBC; this attracts more leukocytes. It is not known why pyrophosphate crystals are deposited in cartilage, and the relation of these deposits to degenerative arthritis is currently unresolved.

In most patients there is no evidence of any underlying biochemical or metabolic abnormality. In some patients, however, the condition occurs in association with hyperparathyroidism, hemochromatosis, hypophosphatasia, or true urate gout.

### LABORATORY FINDINGS

Synovial fluid—cloudy, yellow, low viscosity, fair to good mucin clot; WBC average 20,000/$\mu$l; increased complement; calcium pyrophosphate dihydrate crystals within WBC; these are best visualized under polarized light

Leukocytosis in an acute attack

Increased sedimentation rate and C-reactive protein reflect acute inflammation.

## HEMOCHROMATOSIS

Hemochromatosis is a genetic disorder in which there is excessive accumulation of iron in body tissues. In the normal person, when the body's need for iron is satisfied, intestinal absorption of dietary iron ceases. In hemochromatosis, however, the intestinal absorption of iron inexplicably continues, even in the presence of abundant iron stores. As dietary iron continues to be absorbed, it passes rapidly from the gut into the reticuloendothelial (RE) cells of the liver, spleen, and lymph nodes, because serum transferrin is already saturated. After many years the RE cells also become saturated and iron accumulates in the tissue cells. Excessive stored iron in the skin causes darkening of the skin. Accumulated iron in the heart causes cardiac dysfunction. Abundant iron in the liver eventually stimulates scar-tissue formation, which leads to cirrhosis. This is referred to as *pigmentary cirrhosis*, because the presence of increased iron deposits imparts a dark brown color to the liver.

The natural history of the biochemical and pathologic progression of iron overload in idiopathic hemochromatosis includes the following sequential stages: increased iron absorption, decreased serum transferrin, increased serum iron, increased hepatic iron concentration, increased total-body iron stores, progressive tissue injury, cirrhosis, and finally hepatic failure.

### LABORATORY FINDINGS

Increased serum iron and transferrin saturation, marked

Decreased total iron binding capacity

Increased serum ferritin, marked—reflects increased body iron stores; this gradually increases as the disease progresses

Increased serum glucose and decreased glucose tolerance—indicates development of diabetes as a result of pancreatic scarring from iron accumulation

Liver biopsy shows marked iron deposits in liver cells and in Kupffer's RE cells.

Laboratory findings of cirrhosis (see Chap. 4)

## WILSON'S DISEASE

Wilson's disease is a rare inherited inborn error of copper metabolism; it affects children and young adults. These patients have involvement of the basal ganglia in the brain and also of the liver. They may also have acute hemolytic anemia.

Ceruloplasmin is a plasma protein that normally binds and transports copper in the blood. This is characteristically decreased in Wilson's disease. Consequently, the unbound copper in the circulation is excreted in the urine and also is deposited in the liver, brain, kidneys, and corneas. Free copper is a potent enzyme poison that damages liver cells and brain cells. Cirrhosis occurs as a late consequence of severe liver damage caused by accumulated deposits of copper.

### LABORATORY FINDINGS

Decreased serum ceruloplasmin—characteristic finding

Decreased total serum copper—correlates with the ceruloplasmin level

Increased urinary copper—reflects increased excretion of unbound copper

Mild normochromic anemia and decreased serum haptoglobin—reflect the occurrence of hemolytic anemia

Increased urinary amino acids, glucose, and uric acid; decreased serum uric acid—reflect renal tubular damage due to copper

Liver biopsy shows increased hepatic copper

Laboratory findings of cirrhosis (see Chap. 4)

## OSTEOMALACIA

Osteomalacia, or bone softening, indicates impaired calcification of bone. This results from defective mineralization of newly forming bone, not from the loss of mineral from bone that has already been formed. Osteomalacia in childhood also produces impaired cartilage mineralization and is referred to as *rickets*. It results in characteristic dwarfing and skeletal deformities.

Osteomalacia is usually secondary to an insufficiency of vitamin D, which may be due to decreased exposure to sunlight, dietary deficiency, or impaired intestinal absorption.[5,8] Diminished vitamin D impairs calcium metabolism. This frequently stimulates secondary hyperparathyroidism (see Chap. 6). These disorders are responsive to vitamin-D therapy. Osteomalacia that is resistant to vitamin-D treatment is less common. It might be the consequence of excessive calcium or phosphorus loss in the urine due to renal tubular acidosis, familial hypophosphatemia, or uremia of any etiology. Kidney disease may also cause osteomalacia as a consequence of impaired renal formation of 1,25-dihy-

**Table 10-1.** Classification of the Main Osteomalacias

| MAIN ETIOLOGIC DEFECT | CAUSES | MAIN CLINICAL FORMS |
|---|---|---|
| Vitamin D deficiency | Dietary deficiency<br>Malabsorption<br>Sunlight deficiency | Asian<br>Elderly<br>Small-bowel disease |
| 25-hydroxyvitamin $D_3$ deficiency | 25-hydroxylase abnormality | Liver disease<br>Drugs |
| 1,25-dihydroxyvitamin $D_3$ deficiency | 1-α-hydroxylase failure<br>1-α-hydroxylase deficiency | Renal failure<br>Pseudo-vitamin D deficiency |
| Hypophosphatemia | Decreased tubular phosphate reabsorption | Familial<br>Sporadic<br>Tumoral |
|  | Phosphate depletion | Use of oral phosphate binders |

(Nordin BEC, Peacock M, Aaron J et al: Osteoporosis and osteomalacia. Clin Endocrinol Metab 9:177–205, 1980)

droxyvitamin $D_3$. This results in diminished intestinal absorption of calcium.

The most frequently encountered causes of osteomalacia are listed in Table 10-1. All of these conditions have in common impaired absorption or increased excretion of calcium and phosphorus with consequent defective calcification of bone. The usual biochemical abnormalities in various types of osteomalacia are indicated in Table 10-2.

## LABORATORY FINDINGS

Increased serum alkaline phosphatase—this is the earliest and most reliable biochemical abnormality; it parallels the severity of the disease and may remain elevated until bone healing is complete. This reflects increased new bone formation.

Decreased serum phosphorus due to impaired renal tubular reabsorption. This is the most common finding, but it is not always present.

Normal to low serum calcium due to impaired intestinal absorption

Decreased serum calcium × serum phosphorus product (<30)—this results in impaired bone calcification

Decreased serum 1,25-dihydroxyvitamin $D_3$ in osteomalacia due to renal failure

Bone biopsy showing increased osteoid, which is noncalcified bone—a definitive diagnosis requires histologic confirmation

**Table 10-2.** Usual Biochemical Abnormalities in Various Types of Osteomalacia

| FASTING PLASMA | VITAMIN-D DEFICIENT | RENAL FAILURE | HYPOPHOSPHATEMIA |
|---|---|---|---|
| Decreased calcium | ✓ | ✓ | |
| Decreased phosphorus | ✓ | | ✓ |
| Decreased calcium × phosphorus | ✓ | | ✓ |
| Increased alkaline phosphatase | ✓ | ✓ | |
| Increased parathyroid hormone | ✓ | ✓ | |
| Decreased 25-hydroxyvitamin $D_3$ | ✓ | ✓ | |

(Modified from Nordin BEC, Peacock M, Aaron J et al: Osteoporosis and osteomalacia. Clin Endocrinol Metab 9:177–205, 1980)

**Laboratory Findings of Underlying Disorders**

Renal tubular acidosis (see Chap. 4)

Impaired intestinal absorption (see Chap. 3)

Chronic renal failure (see Chap. 4)

## CYSTIC FIBROSIS

Cystic fibrosis is an inherited disease affecting the secretions of the pancreas, bronchi, and sweat glands. This condition is also termed *mucoviscidosis* and *fibrocystic disease of the pancreas*.

The disease usually begins in infancy and is characterized by chronic respiratory infections, pancreatic insufficiency, and abnormal susceptibility to heat. The latter is a consequence of high concentrations of salts lost in the sweat due to abnormal salt reabsorption by the sweat glands. Mucous obstruction of the pancreatic ducts results in pancreatic scarring and enzyme insufficiency. Fat and protein maldigestion and their loss in stool are the primary manifestations of pancreatic involvement in cystic fibrosis. These are not observed until the secretion of lipase and trypsin falls below 10% of normal, which occurs in most patients. The endocrine function of the pancreas is unaffected. Salivary glands might show obstruction of ducts, atrophy, and scarring. The earliest pulmonary change appears to be enlargement of the bronchial glands. Increased thick tenacious secretions result in bronchiolar and then bronchial obstruction, which promotes infection, tissue destruction, more infection, and ultimately bronchiectasis, abscesses, and diffuse scarring of the lungs. A later complication is heart failure secondary to the severe lung disease. Respiratory complications are the most frequent cause of death.

### LABORATORY FINDINGS

Increased sweat chloride and sodium—this is a constant and characteristic finding detectable at birth; the degree of electrolyte elevation is related neither to the severity of the disease nor to the extent of organ involvement.

Serum and urine electrolytes are normal.

Sputum culture—hemolytic *Staphylococcus aureus* and the mucoid form of *Pseudomonas aeruginosa* are commonly found.

Increased serum $\gamma$-globulins, especially IgG and IgA

Laboratory findings of emphysema, bronchiectasis, maldigestion, and chronic pancreatitis (see Chaps. 2, 3, and 4)

## DISORDERS OF PORPHYRIN METABOLISM

The porphyrias are usually hereditary disorders of porphyrin or porphyrin-precursor metabolism due to specific enzyme defects in the pathway of heme synthesis.[3] Heme formation occurs in hepatic and in nucleated RBC. Metabolic disorders of heme synthesis result in the accumulation of porphyrin compounds in the liver or bone marrow. This is the basis of classifying these disorders as either hepatic or erythropoietic. The erythropoietic porphyrias include congenital erythropoietic porphyria and erythropoietic protoporphyria. The hepatic porphyrias include acute intermittent porphyria, variegate porphyria, hereditary coproporphyria, and porphyria cutanea tarda. In the acute porphyrias, there is accumulation of porphyrin precursors; in the nonacute porphyrias, only formed porphyrins accumulate.

Clinical cutaneous photosensitivity results from the action of ultraviolet radiation on porphyrins deposited in the skin and on increased circulating porphyrins. The photosensitivity is probably related to the intense fluorescence of porphyrin compounds. Abdominal pain and neurologic symptoms result from accumulation of porphyrin precursors in nerves. Laboratory diagnosis is by detection and measurement of porphyrins and their precursors in urine, feces, or RBC. The compound that accumulates and is excreted in excess in each of the various porphyric syndromes is generally the nonmetabolized substrate of the defective enzyme.

## ERYTHROPOIETIC PORPHYRIAS

### Congenital Erythropoietic Porphyria

Congenital erythropoietic porphyria is a rare, recessively inherited disease characterized by urinary excretion of large amounts of uroporphyrin I, mutilating skin lesions, and hemolytic anemia. The cause of this disorder is a deficiency of uroporphyrinogen III cosynthetase in marrow and circulating RBC. There is an associated increased formation of uroporphyrinogen I synthetase. The enzymatic imbalance results in overproduction and accumulation of uroporphyrin I in RBC.

Exposure to light increases formation, accumulation, and excretion of porphyrins and accounts for the occurrence of cutaneous blisters. These lesions ulcerate and may become infected and then scarred. Accumulation of uroporphyrin in erythrocytes impairs their survival. Consequently, anemia is caused not only by hemolysis of circulating RBC but also by destruction of developing erythrocytes. Splenomegaly commonly occurs, reflecting extramedullary erythropoiesis.

### LABORATORY FINDINGS

Increased urine uroporphyrin I—characteristic finding

Increased urine coproporphyrin I—less elevated than uroporphyrin

Pink or red urine, which fluoresces in ultraviolet light

Increased RBC uroporphyrin I—characteristic finding

Increased plasma uroporphyrin I

Increased fecal coproporphyrin I

Bone marrow—normoblastic hyperplasia; fluorescent normoblasts indicating increased porphyrin content

Peripheral blood—anisocytosis, poikilocytosis, polychromatophilia, reticulocytosis, occasional fluorescent RBC

Normochromic, normocytic anemia, slight—hemolysis is usually well
compensated by increased RBC production

Hematologic and chemical findings of hemolysis—usually intermittent

## Erythropoietic Protoporphyria

Erythropoietic protoporphyria is a relatively common and mild form of porphyria, transmitted as an autosomal dominant trait and characterized by the
early onset of mild cutaneous photosensitivity and increased erythrocyte protoporphyrin levels. Erythrocyte protoporphyrin diffuses out of RBC into the
plasma. Photosensitivity is due to the presence of plasma protoporphyrins circulating in the skin. The skin lesions are variable and may be latent.

The primary enzymatic abnormality appears to be a decrease in
ferochelatase activity in immature RBC and in the liver cells. Excessive protoporphyrin accumulates in both sites and the condition is therefore also known
as *erythrohepatic protoporphyria*. Occasional complications are severe progressive liver disease and formation of gallstones containing protoporphyrin. The
lack of anemia is considered to be due to secondary regulating mechanisms that
lead to adequate heme formation.

### LABORATORY FINDINGS

Increased RBC protoporphyrin—characteristic finding

Increased fecal and plasma protoporphyrin

Fluorescence of marrow normoblasts, reticulocytes, and some circulating RBC

### HEPATIC PORPHYRIAS

## Acute Intermittent Porphyria

Acute intermittent porphyria, a common form of hepatic porphyria, is characterized by hepatic overproduction of the porphyrin precursors δ-aminolevulinic
acid (ALA) and porphobilinogen (PBG). It is inherited as an autosomal dominant trait. There are intermittent episodes of acute abdominal pain, hypertension, and various neurologic and psychiatric dysfunctions. The symptoms may
be precipitated by drugs, infections, estrogens or other steroids, alcohol consumption, or starvation.

The fundamental defect in this disease is a decrease in uroporphyrinogen I
synthetase (PBG deaminase) activity in the liver; this leads to an increase of ALA
synthetase activity and overproduction of ALA and PBG. The precipitating
factors indicated above are thought to induce increased ALA synthetase formation.

The neurologic symptoms result from of nerve damage by accumulated
porphyrin precursors, ALA, and PBG. Central neuropathy causes hypothalamic
dysfunction and a variety of psychiatric disorders. Peripheral neuropathy involving mesenteric nerves may cause intestinal spasm and severe abdominal
pain.

## LABORATORY FINDINGS

Increased urine PBG—characteristic finding, even during remission

If the qualitative test is negative, one should quantitatively test a properly preserved 24-hr urine specimen.

Decreased RBC PBG deaminase—characteristic finding

Urine may be of normal color when fresh and become brown, red, or black on standing because of conversion of colorless PBG to colored uroporphyrins.

Impaired glucose tolerance—similar to that in steroid-induced diabetes

Hypercholesterolemia (250 mg/dl–400 mg/dl)

Increased thyroxine ($T_4$), free $T_4$, or triiodothyronine ($T_3$) without clinical evidence of hyperthyroidism

Decreased serum sodium due to hypothalamic involvement, producing inappropriate antidiuretic hormone (ADH) secretion. Renal and GI sodium loss may also contribute to hyponatremia.

## *Variegate Porphyria*

Variegate porphyria is a relatively uncommon hepatic porphyria that is transmitted as an autosomal dominant trait. The disease may present cutaneous manifestations of photosensitivity, abdominal pain and neurologic features, or both. Clinical manifestations are variable. The acute abdominal and neurologic attacks are usually precipitated by drugs or hormones. This is probably due to ferrochelatase deficiency.

## LABORATORY FINDINGS

Increased fecal protoporphyrin and coproporphyrin—characteristic finding even during remission; higher levels occur during acute attacks

Increased urinary ALA and PBG during acute attacks

Increased urinary coproporphyrin and uroporphyrin

Plasma may fluoresce owing to increased coproporphyrin during acute photosensitivity attacks.

Increased serum cholesterol

## *Hereditary Coproporphyria*

Hereditary coproporphyria is a rare hepatic porphyria transmitted as an autosomal dominant trait; it clinically resembles acute intermittent porphyria. Acute attacks are frequently precipitated by certain drugs. Photosensitivity may occur. Hepatic ALA synthetase rises markedly during an acute attack but may be normal at other times. This suggests that the enzyme abnormality is a partial hepatic deficiency of coproporphyrinogen oxidase.

## LABORATORY FINDINGS

Increased fecal coproporphyrin III—characteristic finding, even in remission

Increased urinary ALA, PBG, and coproporphyrin—only during acute attacks

### Porphyria Cutanea Tarda

Porphyria cutanea tarda is characterized by excessive hepatic synthesis and urinary excretion of uroporphyrin I and by skin lesions. This is probably one of the most frequently occurring forms of porphyria. It is considered to be an autosomal dominant inherited disorder which becomes manifested *only* following certain precipitating factors. These factors include ingestion of drugs such as alcohol, hormonal effects, estrogens, infections, and starvation. Many consider this to be an acquired rather than an inherited disorder. Acute attacks of abdominal pain, neurologic disease, and increased urinary excretion of ALA and PBG, characteristic of the other forms of hepatic porphyria, do *not* occur in this disease.

In this disease there are increased skin fragility and acute cutaneous photosensitivity reactions. There is increased intestinal absorption of iron; this may be related to alcohol intake or to chronic liver disease. Alcoholic liver disease and hepatic iron accumulation are commonly associated with this disorder.

Porphyria cutanea tarda is probably caused by subnormal activity of hepatic and erythrocytic uroporphyrinogen decarboxylase.[7]

### LABORATORY FINDINGS

Increased urine uroporphyrin I and urine coproporphyrin; the former exceeds the latter—characteristic finding

Decreased RBC uroporphyrinogen decarboxylase

Increased serum iron—reflects increased intestinal absorption of iron

Increased hepatic porphyrins and iron

## AMYLOIDOSIS

*Amyloidosis* refers to accumulation in the tissues of a fibrillar protein in amounts sufficient to cause impaired function.[4] The term *amyloid* means starchlike or celluloselike.

Amyloidosis is not a single disease entity, but rather a variety of different disease processes resulting in the deposition of twisted fibrils formed from various proteins by several different mechanisms. This disease complex occurs not only in association with acute recurrent and chronic infections but also in association with a variety of immunologic disorders and with certain tumors. It is also commonly seen in aging.

Primary amyloidosis, which is associated with multiple myeloma or which occurs independent of any other disease, is the most common form of amyloidosis encountered in this country. The amyloid substance in the primary form of the disorder appears to be derived from the variable region of the light-chain molecule and from Bence Jones proteins in various plasma-cell diseases. It is designated *amyloid light chain.* Amyloidosis occurs in approximately 6% to 15% of cases of multiple myeloma.

Secondary amyloidosis is associated with various chronic infections and chronic inflammatory diseases. This form is now less common than the primary form of the disease. The protein of secondary amyloid is biochemically distinct from amyloid light chain and is designated as the *AA protein*. This is considered to be derived from a normal nonimmunoglobulin serum protein termed *SAA* (serum amyloid A related). Secondary amyloidosis is asssociated with rheumatoid arthritis in approximately 5% to 11% of cases. It also occurs with tuberculosis, syphilis, osteomyelitis, Hodgkin's disease, and cancer of the kidney.

Amyloid may be deposited in the heart, lungs, skin, tongue, thyroid gland, adrenal glands, lymph nodes, liver, spleen, kidneys, and blood vessels. Clinical features and laboratory findings are nonspecific and reflect the organ or system affected. Most patients with primary amyloidosis die as a consequence of cardiac involvement. Secondary systemic amyloidosis usually presents as nephrotic syndrome with accompanying enlargement of the liver and spleen. Renal failure is a common cause of death in secondary amyloidosis.

## LABORATORY FINDINGS

Tissue biopsy indicates the presence of amyloid deposits, which may be seen with special stains—essential for diagnosis

Laboratory findings of the primary disease, such as rheumatoid arthritis or multiple myeloma

Increased serum globulin and decreased serum albumin reflect chronic disease

Increased sedimentation rate

Normochromic, normocytic anemia reflects chronic disease

Leukocytosis ($>$12,000/$\mu$l)

**Laboratory Findings Associated With the Organ or System Involved**

Liver—increased alkaline phosphatase

Kidney—see Nephrotic Syndrome, Chapter 5

GI system—see Impaired Intestinal Absorption, Chapter 3

Endocrine system—see Addison's Disease, Chapter 6

Hematologic system—see Multiple Myeloma, Chapter 8

## *DISORDERS OF BILIRUBIN EXCRETION*

There is a group of metabolic disorders that affects bilirubin excretion at different stages of the excretory process. Interference with the normal process of conjugation of bilirubin to glucuronide in the liver results in increased blood levels of unconjugated bilirubin. Gilbert's syndrome and Crigler-Najjar syndrome are examples of this type of disorder.

Interference with the secretion, not conjugation, of bilirubin results in increased blood levels of conjugated bilirubin. Dubin-Johnson syndrome and Rotor's syndrome are examples of this type of disorder.

## UNCONJUGATED HYPERBILIRUBINEMIAS

### Gilbert's Syndrome

Gilbert's syndrome is a common disorder in which there is a mild chronic intermittent unconjugated hyperbilirubinemia. Serum bilirubin levels rise markedly during fasting, acute infections, severe physical exertion, congestive heart failure, thyrotoxicosis, or other metabolic stress. There is no evidence of other hepatic impairment, hemolysis, or ineffective erythropoiesis.

The physiologic defect exists at the sinusoidal membrane, or space of Disse. The bilirubin—albumin complex freely penetrates Disse's spaces and the unconjugated bilirubin is dissociated from albumin. There is, however, impaired transfer of bilirubin from sinusoidal blood into the hepatic cells. This impaired hepatic-cell uptake results in plasma retention of a large proportion of unconjugated bilirubin. There is also a greater than 50% decrease in conjugation. The hepatic defect is, therefore, in both the uptake and conjugation of bilirubin.

### LABORATORY FINDINGS

Increased unconjugated (indirect) serum bilirubin

Normal urine urobilinogen

Absent urine bilirubin

Normal fecal urobilinogen

### Crigler-Najjar Syndrome

Crigler-Najjar syndrome is a rare familial disease due to a marked congenital deficiency or lack of glucuronyl transferase. This enzyme is necessary for the conjugation of bilirubin to glucuronide in liver cells. From birth, affected patients have a rapid rise of unconjugated bilirubin in the serum. Bilirubin deposits in and stains adipose tissues and basal ganglia in the brain. The latter occurrence is known as *kernicterus*.

### LABORATORY FINDINGS

Increased unconjugated (indirect) serum bilirubin

Normal urine urobilinogen

Absent urine bilirubin

Normal fecal urobilinogen

## CONJUGATED HYPERBILIRUBINEMIAS

### Dubin-Johnson Syndrome

Dubin-Johnson syndrome is a hereditary disorder in which there is impaired secretion of conjugated bilirubin into the bile canaliculus. There is a chronic, fluctuating jaundice of moderate degree, retention of indocyanine green

(Cardio-Green) and gallbladder dye, and an accumulation of a brownish black pigment in the liver cells.

## LABORATORY FINDINGS

Increased conjugated (direct) serum bilirubin

Increased urine bilirubin and urobilinogen

Impaired Cardio-Green excretion

Other liver function tests are normal.

Liver biopsy shows brownish black pigment in liver cells.

### Rotor's Syndrome

Rotor's syndrome is a rare hereditary disorder in which there are impaired hepatic uptake of bilirubin and an impaired ability to store bilirubin in the liver cells. The reduced storage capacity results in reflux of conjugated bilirubin into the bloodstream. There is only minimal impairment of bilirubin secretion and no impairment of conjugation. No abnormal pigment occurs in the liver cells.

## LABORATORY FINDINGS

Increased conjugated (direct) serum bilirubin

Increased urine bilirubin and urobilinogen

Impaired Cardio-Green excretion

Other liver function tests are normal.

## REFERENCES

1. Boss GR, Seegmiller JE: Hyperuricemia and gout. N Engl J Med 300:1459–1468, 1979
2. Buehler BA: Inherited disorders of amino acid transport in relation to the kidney. Ann Clin Lab Sci 11:274–278, 1981
3. Civin WH, Epstein E: Enzyme defects in hereditary porphyria. Ann Clin Lab Sci 10:395–401, 1980
4. Glenner GG: Amyloid deposits and amyloidosis. N Engl J Med 302:1283–1292, 1333–1343, 1980
5. Goldring SR, Krane SM: Metabolic bone disease: Osteoporosis and osteomalacia. DM 27:1–103, 1981
6. Halpern SL: Quick Reference to Clinical Nutrition, p 5–7. Philadelphia, JB Lippincott, 1979
7. Kushner JP: The enzymatic defect in porphyria cutanea tarda. N Engl J Med 306:799–800, 1982
8. Nordin BEC, Peacock M, Aaron J et al: Osteoporosis and osteomalacia. Clin Endocrinol Metab 9:177–205, 1980
9. Whayne TF Jr: The hyperlipoproteinemias. J Fam Pract 11:789–799, 1980

## BIBLIOGRAPHY

Bondy PK, Rosenberg LE (eds): Metabolic Control and Disease, 8th ed. Philadelphia, WB Saunders, 1980

Rifkind BM, Levy RI: Hyperlipidemia: Diagnosis and Therapy. New York, Grune & Stratton, 1977

Stanbury JB, Wyngaarden JB, Fredrickson JS: The Metabolic Basis of Inherited Disease, 4th ed. New York, McGraw-Hill, 1978

# 11

# *INFECTIOUS DISEASES**

Amebiasis
Ascariasis
Chickenpox
Cytomegalovirus Infections
Enterobiasis
Giardiasis
Gonorrhea
  Infection in Men
  Infection in Women
  Disseminated Infection
  Neonatal Infection
Herpes Simplex Infections
Hookworm Disease

Infectious Mononucleosis
Measles
Mumps
Nongonococcal Urethritis
Rubella
Syphilis
  Primary Syphilis
  Secondary Syphilis
  Latent Syphilis
  Late Syphilis
  Congenital (Prenatal) Syphilis
Toxoplasmosis
Trichuriasis

## AMEBIASIS

Amebiasis is due to ingestion of cysts of the protozoan parasite *Entamoeba histolytica* in contaminated food or water. When intestinal mucosal resistance becomes lowered, trophozoites of the parasite invade the colonic mucosa, usually in the cecum or rectum. Ameboid movement and amebic enzymes facilitate mucosal penetration by the organisms. Invading trophozoites generally do not penetrate muscular layers of the colon but rather spread laterally in the submucosa, undermining the mucosa. As a consequence, the blood supply to the overlying mucosa is gradually destroyed, resulting in focal mucosal ulceration. This results in bloody diarrhea, which is also known as amebic dysentery.

Amebae may penetrate colonic capillaries and lymphatics and gain access to the liver through the portal vein. Only few of the amebae that reach the liver survive. Surviving amebae form hepatic abscesses. Rupture of a liver abscess may result in extension of the infestation to the lung, pleural cavity, or pericardium.

* This chapter includes only infections commonly encountered in the United States and those that have not been described in any of the previous chapters.

Humoral antibodies do not appear to confer immunity, except perhaps in the case of liver abscess. Thus, reinfections can occur in the presence of elevated antibody titers.

## LABORATORY FINDINGS

### Stool

Presence of *E. histolytica* cysts in stool, sigmoidoscopic aspirate, or rectal biopsy. If intestinal motility is rapid, trophozoites may be found in liquid stools.

Mucus and red blood cells (RBC) but very few leukocytes.

Mononuclear white blood cells (WBC) predominate over segmented WBC.

### Serologic Tests

Indirect hemagglutination test—fourfold rise in titer is diagnostic; >1 : 128 is clinically significant; >1 : 512 is suggestive of recent infection. The test becomes positive 2 weeks after infection and remains positive for 2 years after curative treatment. Titer does not correlate with the severity of the disease.

Serologic tests of approximately equal sensitivity are those using countercurrent electrophoresis and indirect fluorescent antibody techniques. All of these tests are more frequently positive in patients with amebic abscesses (>95% positive) than in patients with amebic dysentery. Patients with amebic dysentery have more positive serologic tests than are found in asymptomatic cyst carriers.

### Findings of Liver Abscess

Leukocytosis, increased sedimentation rate reflect active inflammation in presence of liver abscess

Identification of trophozoites of *E. histolytica* in the wall of a liver abscess and in necrotic abscess contents

## *ASCARIASIS*

Ascariasis is infection with the roundworm, *Ascaris lumbricoides*. Roundworms live in the small intestine, where the female lays approximately 200,000 eggs/day. Eggs passed in the feces are deposited in the soil, where they embryonate and develop into an infective stage. When embryonated eggs are ingested, they hatch in the duodenum, releasing larvae that penetrate the intestinal wall and enter the venules and lymphatics. Larvae pass from the portal circulation, through the liver and heart, into the lungs. They then migrate up the bronchioles to the pharynx, are swallowed, and eventually reach the small intestine. The complete migration cycle takes 2 to 3 months.

Most infections are clinically inapparent. Adult worms usually cause little or no damage to the intestine. Heavy infections may lead to appendicitis or intestinal twisting, kinking, telescoping, or obstruction, particularly in children. During the migration phase, heavy infections may provoke pulmonary inflammation with wheezing, difficult breathing, fever, and cough.

## LABORATORY FINDINGS

Stools contain *Ascaris lumbricoides* ova

Eosinophilia (30%–40%), especially during the migratory phase

## *CHICKENPOX*

Chickenpox (varicella) is a highly contagious viral disease caused by the varicella–zoster virus. The infection most commonly affects children and is generally a mild disease with few complications. In adults it is often associated with high fever, severe systemic symptoms, and pneumonia.

The virus is spread by respiratory secretions. It enters the respiratory tract, where it multiplies. The virus enters the bloodstream and is disseminated to the skin and internal organs. Viremia ceases 1 day to 4 days after onset of the rash and coincidentally with the appearance of measurable amounts of circulating antibody. Pathogenetic features of the infection are shown in Figure 11-1. Patients with impaired cellular immunity have prolonged and severe cutaneous eruptions.

Herpes zoster (shingles) is the recurrent form of chickenpox occurring predominantly in adults (see Chap. 7).

## LABORATORY FINDINGS

Scrapings of lesions or blister fluid contain large epithelial giant cells with intranuclear viral inclusions. The appearance of the cells is similar to that of those infected with herpes simplex virus.

Virus isolation from blister cells

Fourfold increase in complement fixing antibodies from acute-phase to convalescent-phase sera. Varicella cross-reacts with herpes simplex virus. Titers

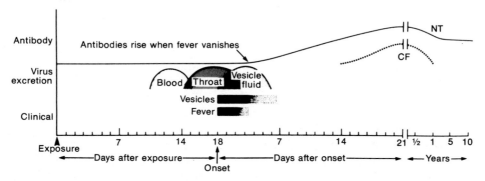

**Fig. 11-1.** Pathogenesis of chickenpox (varicella): Time course of clinical features, virus detection, and antibodies. (NT, neutralizing antibody; CF, complement-fixing antigen) (McLean DM: Virology in Health Care, p 218. Baltimore, Williams & Wilkins, 1980)

of complement-fixing antibodies decrease over a period of months; neutralizing, immune-adherence, and hemagglutinating antibodies, as well as antibodies to infected cell-membrane antigens, persist for many years.

Detection by fluorescence microscopy of antibody directed against membrane antigen—this is more sensitive and specific than the complement fixation test for determining susceptibility to varicella and for confirming the clinical diagnosis.

# CYTOMEGALOVIRUS INFECTIONS

Cytomegalovirus is a herpesvirus and is the most frequent known cause of perinatal infection.[6] Congenital infection may occur *in utero* or at the time of delivery. Most congenital infections are asymptomatic. However, cytomegalovirus is an important cause of fetal encephalitis and congenital deafness.

Most patients who acquire cytomegalovirus infection are usually asymptomatic during childhood or early adult years, or else have very mild, nonspecific clinical illnesses.[2] Transmission occurs by the oral or genital route, by blood transfusion, or following extracorporeal perfusion. The virus is thought to disseminate throughout the body in lymphocytes or mononuclear cells. Infected cells are most frequently seen in the lung, liver, and central nervous system (CNS).

The clinical picture resembles that of infectious mononucleosis, characterized by fever, malaise, and peripheral lymphocytosis. In contrast to mononucleosis, cytomegalovirus usually causes no sore throat or enlargement of lymph nodes, liver, or spleen. In a significant proportion of patients this infection is associated with the Guillain-Barré syndrome (see Chap. 7).

The host response to infection appears to vary with age, with the competency of the immune system, and with whether the infection is primary or recurrent. The high rate of asymptomatic infection suggests that host response may play an important role in development of clinical illness. The frequency and severity of infection are markedly increased in immune-suppressed patients and in those treated with cytotoxic drugs.

## LABORATORY FINDINGS

Lymphocytosis (>50% of WBC); >20% atypical lymphocytes

Negative heterophile antibody test and negative test for Epstein-Barr antibody

Increased alkaline phosphatase; normal serum glutamic-oxaloacetic transaminase (SGOT) (AST [aspartate aminotransferase])

Complement-fixing cytomegalovirus antibodies (IgG) show a fourfold increase from acute to chronic sera. Indirect fluorescent antibody and indirect hemagglutination tests appear to be more sensitive than the complement fixation method in detecting IgG antibody. These tests are not of diagnostic value before 6 months of age because maternal IgG crosses the placenta. Prior to that time, diagnosis requires identification of IgM antibodies, which may be demonstrated by indirect immunofluorescence. False-positive IgM reactions may occur with mononucleosis, varicella, or rheumatoid factor.

Detection of viral antigens in infected cells by direct immunofluorescence or immunoperoxidase techniques.

Urine sediment might show large intranuclear viral inclusions in renal tubular epithelial cells, especially in severely infected infants. Viral infected cells might also be found in bronchial and gastric washings.

Viral isolation from urine, saliva, or blood

Laboratory findings of an underlying condition—malignant lymphoma, leukemia, refractory anemia (see Chap. 8)

# ENTEROBIASIS

Enterobiasis is a common benign parasitic infection, occurring especially in school-age children. It is caused by the pinworm, *Enterobius vermicularis.* Infection occurs from ingestion of eggs of the parasite. The adult worms live in the cecum and ascending colon. The intestinal mucosa is not penetrated by this parasite. The gravid female worm migrates the length of the large intestine and deposits her eggs in the perianal folds. Perianal and perineal itching and scratching occur as a response to irritation of these areas from migration of the female and deposition of eggs. The eggs are fully embryonated and are infective within a few hours of the time they are deposited.

## LABORATORY FINDINGS

Scotch tape preparation of perianal area shows ova and, occasionally, adult worms. The specimen is best obtained when the patient first arises early in the morning.

# GIARDIASIS

Giardiasis is a protozoal small-intestine infection caused by *Giardia lamblia.* This organism is the most commonly identified pathogen in stool samples submitted for parasitologic examination.[8,10] An estimated 3% to 7% of American adults harbor the parasite. Following ingestion, cysts of *G. lamblia* pass into the duodenum, where trophozoites are released. Trophozoites attach superficially to the mucosa of the proximal small intestine. They persist in the small intestine for weeks to months and then move into the colon where they transform to the cyst stage for excretion in the stool. The entire cycle lasts for 6 to 15 days.

The parasites usually cause an asymptomatic infection, but may cause mild or moderately severe watery diarrhea. Severe infection, which is uncommon, may result in malabsorption. The exact mechanism of pathogenesis is not clearly understood. Repeated exposure results in some degree of humoral immunity.

## LABORATORY FINDINGS

Presence of cysts of *G. lamblia* in formed stool or trophozoites in watery stool

Presence of trophozoites in duodenal aspirates or obtained by string test[7]

Findings of impaired intestinal absorption in severe chronic infection (see Chap. 3)

## GONORRHEA

Gonorrhea is a genital infection transmitted by sexual contact and caused by *Neisseria gonorrhoeae.* The bacterium is a gram-negative diplococcus that has a cell wall covered by pili, which are hairlike structures. The pili enable the organisms to attach to the surface of epithelial cells. The bacteria reach the subepithelial tissues by penetrating between cells. Gonococci contain an endotoxin that contributes to their pathogenicity. Neutrophils are attracted to bacteria and engulf them, killing most of them. An inflammatory cellular response gives rise to the purulent urethral or cervical discharge characteristic of this disease. Repeated attacks of gonorrhea are common.

### INFECTION IN MEN

In heterosexual men, infection usually involves only the urethra. In homosexual men, infection may also involve the anal canal or pharynx. The usual incubation period of urethritis is 2 to 7 days. The disease is usually cured with treatment. Without treatment, symptoms of urethritis persist for an average of 8 weeks and are self-limited. In the chronic state, the infection may spread to involve the epididymis and prostate.

### INFECTION IN WOMEN

The most common site of infection in women is the cervix. Infection is usually mild and clinically inapparent. Other sites of infection are the urethra, anal canal, and pharynx. Cervical discharge presumably accounts for the occurrence of anorectal, urethral, and Bartholin's gland infections. Menstruation facilitates spread of the infection from the cervix upward into the endometrium and fallopian tubes. Tubal occlusion and sterility occur in about 20% of women with cervical gonorrhea. Infection may spread into the pelvic peritoneum, producing pelvic inflammatory disease.

### DISSEMINATED INFECTION

Some strains of gonococci tend to invade the bloodstream and are serum resistant.[4] Gonococcal septicemia has been detected in 1% of men and 3% of women with gonorrhea. Stages of disseminated infection include the bacteremic stage, characterized by positive blood cultures, dermatitis, and arthralgia. This is followed by the septic joint stage, characterized by positive synovial cultures and negative blood cultures. Other systemic manifestations include endocarditis, myopericarditis, and meningitis.

### NEONATAL INFECTION

Gonococcal infections of the newborn are contracted from the mother's infected birth canal. Infection may involve the conjunctivae, pharynx, respiratory tract, or anal canal. The risk of these infections increases with premature rupture of the fetal membranes during labor.

### LABORATORY FINDINGS

Urethral or endocervical smear shows gram-negative intracellular diplococci. Gram's stain is far more reliable in men than in women.

Positive endocervical culture in women; positive urethral culture in men. Possibly positive culture of pharynx and anal canal

Positive immunofluorescent stain of organisms on smear of suspected material

Blood culture may be positive in disseminated infection.

Synovial fluid culture may be positive in gonococcal arthritis (see Infectious Arthritis, Chap. 9).

Skin lesions may show the organism on smear or culture.

Conjunctivae of infected newborn may show the organism on smear or culture.

Findings of infective endocarditis may follow disseminated infection.

Findings of peritonitis may follow pelvic inflammatory disease.

Leukocytosis and increased sedimentation rate occur with inflammation of the fallopian tubes.

## *HERPES SIMPLEX INFECTIONS*

Herpes simplex viruses (HSV) consist of two antigenic types. HSV-1 is usually transmitted by oral and respiratory secretions. In adults and in children beyond the newborn age group, it involves nongenital sites, including the mouth, lips, skin above the waist, eyes, and brain. This type occurs with great frequency. Antibody is acquired in early childhood and may be found in 95% of people from 26 to 30 years of age. HSV-2 is most often transmitted sexually in adolescents and adults, usually causing infections of the genitalia and of the skin below the waist.[1,3] HSV-2 may also be transmitted from an infected mother's genitalia to the newborn as the infant passes through the infected vaginal canal.[11]

HSV infection of the fetus or newborn is a severe disease with high mortality and serious sequelae. In children 6 months to 4 years of age the major site of infection is the oral cavity. Up to the age of 14 years, herpes infections also involve the eyes and skin. During adolescence, genital herpetic infection is the predominant form. Older persons are more apt to experience recurrent herpetic infections at various sites, including the lips, corneas, skin, and genitalia. Herpetic encephalitis usually occurs after the age of 30 years (see Herpes Simplex Virus, Chap. 7).

The most striking characteristic of HSV infection is its propensity for persisting in a quiescent or latent state with recurrence of activity at irregular intervals. The initial infection occurs through a break in the mucous membranes or skin; local multiplication then ensues. From this focus, the virus spreads to regional lymph nodes, where it multiplies further. Viremia occurs only in immunologically compromised patients, including newborns, children who are malnourished or who have other associated infections, persons with skin disorders, and persons with congenital or acquired immunodeficiency. Bloodstream invasion results in widespread dissemination. During recovery, the virus clears from the blood. However, the virus persists as a latent infection, probably in a sensory ganglion adjacent to the major site of the primary disease. Viral survival occurs despite the presence of high antibody titer.

Genital HSV initially infects the genitalia but then ascends through nerves to the sacral ganglia, where it becomes latent and inaccessible to destruction by the host's immune mechanisms. It may remain latent lifelong. During reactivation, viral replication occurs within the ganglia. The reactivated virus then moves along the protected neural pathway, back to the skin or mucous membrane, causing recurrent genital infections. The factors influencing reactivation of genital HSV are poorly understood.[9] The virus may be shed while the patient is asymptomatic.

### LABORATORY FINDINGS

Scrapings of cells from blisters or ulcers or biopsies from skin or brain show characteristic multinucleated giant cells with prominent viral nuclear inclusions. (Cells are similar to those seen in varicella–zoster or cytomegalovirus infection.)

Isolation, using tissue culture, of HSV from lesions—this is the most definitive diagnostic laboratory test

Identification, using immunofluorescence or immunoperoxidase methods, of HSV-specific antigen in infected cells

Serologic findings are of limited diagnostic value, HSV-1 and HSV-2 produce similar antibodies; recurrent infection is usually *not* accompanied by a significant titer rise; HSV-1 antibodies are present in almost all adults. Primary acute infection might be documented by a fourfold rise in antibody titer 14–21 days after onset.

## HOOKWORM DISEASE

The adult *Necator americanus* (hookworm) lives in the small intestine. Eggs are passed in the feces; they then mature in the soil to rhabditiform and then filariform larvae. The latter penetrate the skin, enter the bloodstream, and are carried to the lungs. The pulmonary phase of the disease often evokes an inflammatory response producing pneumonia and small lung hemorrhages. The larvae migrate up the tracheobronchial tree, are swallowed, and reach the small intestine. The worms attach to the mucosa of the duodenum and jejunum to obtain blood for nourishment. The amount of blood consumed by the worms or lost in the stool and the intensity of the enteritis are proportional to the number of adult worms in the intestine.

### LABORATORY FINDINGS

Stools contain hookworm ova or rhabditiform larvae

Occult blood in stool

Hypochromic, microcytic anemia—iron deficiency type which is the result of chronic blood loss

Eosinophilia of 15%–30%

Normal WBC to slight leukocytosis

# INFECTIOUS MONONUCLEOSIS

Infectious mononucleosis is an acute disease caused by the Epstein-Barr virus (EBV). The virus infects only B-lymphocytes. The infection stimulates proliferation of T cells and leads to enlargement of lymph nodes, liver and spleen, and lymphocytosis. Viremia occurs, and the entire lymphoreticular system is involved. Following infection, EBV persists in lymphocytic tissues for years. Antibodies and lasting immunity occur.

The characteristic hematologic finding is the presence of "atypical" reactive lymphocytes in the peripheral blood. During the first week, these are predominantly immunoglobulin-secreting B-lymphocytes and lesser numbers of EBV-infected B-lymphocytes. After the second week, most of the atypical lymphocytes are activated T-lymphocytes, which have been shown *in vitro* to suppress or kill EBV-carrying cells.

The most frequent presenting symptoms are fever, sore throat, and enlarged cervical lymph nodes. Many patients have hepatic involvement with slightly elevated liver enzymes. Only about 5% are jaundiced. Thirty percent of patients have splenomegaly. Other, less common, clinical findings include hemolytic anemia, thrombocytopenia, splenic rupture, and Guillain-Barré syndrome.

## LABORATORY FINDINGS

### Hematologic Findings

Leukocytosis (10,000/$\mu$l–20,000/$\mu$l) after first week; >60% lymphocytes; 10%–20% of lymphocytes are atypical. Atypical lymphocytes appear 3 or 4 days after the onset of symptoms and reach a maximum by the 5th to 10th day. They usually decrease to normal by 3 weeks, but may persist for 3 months or more.

### Serologic Findings

Positive heterophile antibody test (>95% of adolescents and young adults with classical clinical features). Subsequent to EBV infection and lymphoid hyperplasia, IgM antibodies are produced that cross-react with antigens found in tissues of other animal species. They are therefore termed *heterophilic*. Differential absorption tests are used to differentiate heterophile from Forssman antibody. The heterophile antibody titer reaches diagnostically significant levels 1 week after symptoms appear. Highest heterophile titers occur in the 2nd or 3rd week of the illness and relatively high titers usually last for 2 to 8 weeks. The rise parallels atypical lymphocytosis and declines along with a decrease in lymphocytes. The titer is not related to clinical severity, but does parallel EBV-specific IgM antibody. A positive heterophile test is generally considered necessary to establish the diagnosis.

Heterophile-negative infectious mononucleosis is uncommon; it usually appears in young children. A rising titer of EBV antibody is required to establish the diagnosis of heterophile-negative infectious mononucleosis. This occurs in only 10%–20% of patients. EBV antibody may appear before, after, or coincidentally with the appearance of heterophile antibody. Heterophile-negative syndromes clinically resembling infectious mononucleosis are due to cytomegalovirus, adenovirus, rubella, or toxoplasmosis.

### Other Laboratory Findings

Increased lactate dehydrogenase (LDH), SGOT (AST) and serum glutamic-pyruvic transminase (SGPT) (ALT [alanine aminotransferase]) occur in 80%–100% of patients and remain elevated for 3–5 weeks.

Slight increase in bilirubin, usually <8 mg/dl

Positive cold agglutinin tests in 50% of patients, anti-i type

Markedly increased serum IgM early; moderately increased serum IgG later in the disease

## MEASLES

Measles is a highly contagious childhood viral disease characterized by fever and a rash. The upper respiratory tract or the conjunctiva are probably the primary portals of entry. This entry is followed by a period of viral replication in the mucosa and the regional lymph nodes. On the second or third day of illness, primary viremia disseminates the virus to lymphoid tissues throughout the body, where the virus multiplies. A more prolonged and extensive secondary viremia occurs after the sixth day and accounts for the fever. Blood, lymph nodes, spleen, kidneys, skin, and lungs are sites of viral replication. On or about the 14th day, the rash appears. From 24 to 48 hours later, coincidentally with the appearance of measurable amounts of circulating antibody, viremia ceases and symptoms begin to abate. Pathogenetic features are shown in Figure 11-2.

During the biphasic viremia, the measles virus seems to disseminate mainly within leukocytes. Viral multiplication within leukocytes is believed to account for the leukopenia and the increased incidence of chromosomal disruption that occur in measles.

The characteristic viremia in measles, in contrast to the more localized respiratory infections produced by influenza and parainfluenza viruses, probably contributes to the effective immunity conferred by the disease.

Skin lesions are caused by direct viral damage to the skin and blood vessels or result from a generalized, delayed hypersensitivity response to circulating virus–antibody complexes.

Evidence of measles pneumonia is present in 20% to 60% of patients. Secondary bacterial pneumonia, the leading cause of death in measles, is probably potentiated by the viral depression of pulmonary antibacterial activity. Bacterial middle-ear infection occurs in about 10% of patients with measles.

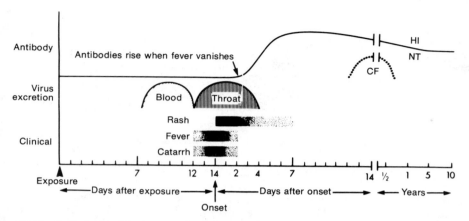

**Fig. 11-2.** Pathogenesis of measles: Time course of clinical features, virus detection, and antibodies. (CF, complement-fixing antigen; HI, hemagglutination inhibition; NT, neutralizing antibody) (McLean DM: Virology in Health Care, p 123. Baltimore, Williams & Wilkins, 1980)

### LABORATORY FINDINGS

Sputum, nasopharyngeal scrapings, and urine sediment may show multinucleated giant cells with intracellular viral inclusions.

Fluorescent antibody demonstration of measles antigen in nasopharyngeal scrapings and urine sediment cells

Virus can be isolated from blood, nasopharynx, or urine.

Positive serologic tests with fourfold rise in titer. Hemagglutination inhibition antibody first appears within 2–3 days after onset of the rash, attains peak titers after the 1st month, and gradually declines during the next 5 years. Persistence of antibodies correlates well with resistance to infection. Complement-fixation antibodies are first detected about 3 weeks after onset of the rash and usually become undetectable after 3–6 months.

Leukocytes—initially there is a slight increase; this later falls to 5000/$\mu$l with increased lymphocytes.

Mild thrombocytopenia, early

Cerebrospinal fluid (CSF)—<10% of patients show slightly increased protein and <500 mononuclear cells/$\mu$l.

## *MUMPS*

Mumps is an acute, contagious, generalized viral disease that usually causes painful enlargement of the salivary glands, most commonly the parotids. The virus is transmitted by saliva and respiratory secretions and its site of entry is the respiratory tract. Replication of the virus occurs in the upper-respiratory-tract epithelium and lymph nodes. This leads to primary viremia with dissemination to the salivary glands and other organs. A second viremia from these sites

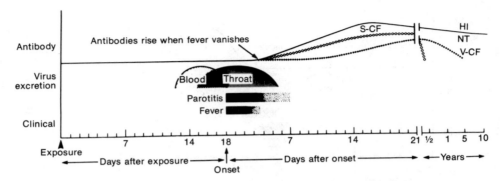

**Fig. 11-3.** Pathogenesis of mumps: Time course of clinical features, virus detection, and antibodies. (S-CF, soluble complement-fixing antigen; HI, hemagglutination inhibition; NT, neutralizing antibody; V-CF, viral complement-fixing antigen) (McLean DM: Virology in Health Care, p 110. Baltimore, Williams & Wilkins, 1980)

further extends the infection. Pathogenetic features are shown in Figure 11-3. Salivary-gland inflammation allows release of salivary amylase into the bloodstream. In postpubertal patients, complications include testicular or ovarian inflammation, pancreatitis, and (rarely) meningoencephalitis.

## LABORATORY FINDINGS

Increased serum and urine amylase during the first 10 days; these are of salivary gland origin.

Leukopenia

Increased cold agglutinins

Presence of IgM antibodies—maximum titer during the first 2 weeks; detectable for 6–9 months; indicates recent infection

Complement-fixation test for antibody is positive during the first week; this remains elevated for more than 6 weeks; convalescent sera show fourfold increase in titer when compared to acute-phase sera.

Isolation of virus from saliva up to 5 days after onset of salivary-gland symptoms

### Laboratory Findings of Complications

Testicular or ovarian inflammation—leukocytosis, increased sedimentation rate

Pancreatitis—leukocytosis, increased serum amylase and lipase, hyperglycemia

Meningitis—CSF usually contains fewer than 500 cells/$\mu$l; these are mononuclear cells; normal glucose; slightly elevated protein (20 mg/dl–125 mg/dl); isolation of virus from CSF within 1 day after onset of symptoms

## NONGONOCOCCAL URETHRITIS

*Chlamydia trachomatis* is the major cause of nongonococcal urethritis (NGU) in men. In women, asymptomatic cervicitis is the main genital infection caused by

*Chlamydia.* NGU is a sexually transmitted infection that is characterized by prolonged latency, a unique intracellular growth cycle, and development of incomplete host immunity.[5]

*Chlamydia* may be responsible for many cases of epididymitis, prostatitis, pelvic inflammatory disease, cystourethritis, Reiter's syndrome, and neonatal pneumonia, which may be contracted from an infected mother during birth.

## LABORATORY FINDINGS

Urethral discharge—≥5 neutrophils/oil immersion field (× 1000) in 5 fields

First morning urine—sediment of first portion of urine specimen contains ≥15 neutrophils/high dry field (× 400) in 1 or more of 5 high-power fields

Negative smear and culture for *N. gonorrhoeae*

Culture of *C. trachomatis* using tissue culture techniques

## *RUBELLA*

Rubella is a moderately contagious viral disease marked by an acute rash and enlargement of the lymph nodes in the back of the neck. Although rubella is typically a mild illness in children and young adults, when acquired in early pregnancy it may produce a severe general infection of the fetus, resulting in multiple congenital abnormalities.

The virus is spread by inhalation of infected droplet nuclei disseminated from the respiratory tract of an infected person. It is believed that initial viral replication occurs in the upper respiratory tract and in cervical lymph nodes. After multiplication in these sites, the virus spreads to other parts of the body through the bloodstream. Manifestations of viremia include arthritis, leukopenia, and occasional thrombocytopenia. Coincidentally with the development of the rash, or within 24 to 48 hours, neutralizing antibodies become detectable and circulating virus disappears from the blood. Pathogenetic features are shown in Figure 11-4. The rash may represent the inflammatory effect of an antibody–virus complex. Primary infection stimulates antibodies that confer immunity lifelong, including during pregnancy. Immunity may not protect the patient against a localized reinfection, which is of no danger to a fetus.

The pathogenesis of congenital rubella begins with maternal viremia. Infection is most dangerous for the fetus during the first 8 gestational weeks because of greater placental transmission of virus early in pregnancy. Fetal infection is present throughout gestation and after birth. Serious congenital defects or fetal death results from direct tissue damage or from retarded growth of primitive fetal cells during periods of rapid cellular differentiation and organ formation. Cataracts and cardiac malformations are the major fetal consequences.

## LABORATORY FINDINGS

### Postnatal Acquired Rubella

Fourfold increase in hemagglutination-inhibition antibody titer from acute-phase to convalescent-phase sera. Increased titer occurs within less than 1 week following the rash and rises rapidly for 1–2 weeks. Titers persist for many

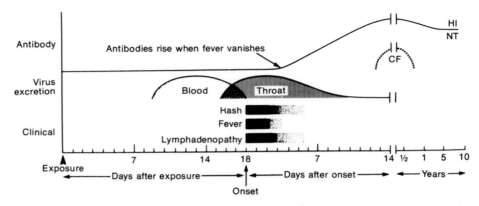

**Fig. 11-4.** Pathogenesis of rubella: Time course of clinical features, virus detection, and antibodies. (CF, complement-fixing antigen; HI, hemagglutination inhibition; NT, neutralizing antibody) (McLean DM: Virology in Health Care, p 140. Baltimore, Williams & Wilkins, 1980)

years but slowly decline. The height of the titer does not distinguish recent from remote infection. This technique measures both IgG and IgM antibodies.

Complement-fixation antibodies appear within 1 week after the rash. They last for 8 months to several years. This test is less sensitive than are other serologic procedures.

Passive hemagglutination tests detect antibody 4–5 weeks after onset of clinical disease. A positive test indicates that a patient has antibody and is immune to a repeat infection. This technique also detects both IgG and IgM antibodies.

Indirect immunofluorescence tests can be used to detect IgG and IgM antibodies. IgM antibody appears with the onset of the rash, peaks approximately 10 days after appearance of the rash, and disappears within 50 days. This appears *only* following a primary infection. IgG antibody appears and peaks similarly to IgM antibody, but remains elevated indefinitely. IgG antibody appears after a primary infection or reinfection.

Isolation of virus from nasopharynx and blood

Leukocytes are variably decreased before the rash. This reflects viral replication in lymphocytes. Lymphocytes are increased during the rash; atypical lymphocytes are frequently seen.

Decreased platelet count occurs within 1 week of the rash.

### Congenital Rubella

Presence of IgM antibodies in the first 6 months. Maternal infections early in pregnancy result in a greater incidence of infants with IgM antibody than do maternal infections occurring later in pregnancy.

Persistence of hemagglutination-inhibition antibody after 6 months. Prior to 6 months, the infant's antibody titer is not diagnostic because it represents the composite of passively acquired maternal IgG antibody and fetal IgM antibody formed in response to the congenital infection.

Infant's antibody titer level usually parallels that of the mother.

Isolation of rubella virus from amniotic fluid or infant's throat, urine, or CSF. Virus excretion in the throat or urine may persist for several months after birth, and rubella virus may be detected in CSF for 1 year or longer.

### Laboratory Findings of Systemic Disease

Thrombocytopenia (see Chap. 8)

Hemolytic anemia (see Chap. 8)

Hepatitis (see Chap. 4)

Encephalitis (see Chap. 7)

## SYPHILIS*

Syphilis is caused by *Treponema pallidum* and is usually transmitted by sexual contact. The spirochetal organisms enter the body through minute breaks in the skin or by penetrating intact mucous membranes. They reach the lymphatic system within 30 minutes of penetration and bloodstream dissemination follows. Systemic spread occurs long before appearance of the primary syphilitic lesion, the chancre.

### PRIMARY SYPHILIS

After an incubation period of about 3 to 4 weeks, a chancre develops at the site of entry of the treponemal organisms. Enlargement of lymph nodes in the groin usually occurs. The chancre heals within 3 to 6 weeks.

### SECONDARY SYPHILIS

The secondary stage becomes manifest about 4 to 8 weeks after the appearance of the chancre. Although secondary syphilis involves many organs of the body, it is usually most evident on the skin and mucous membranes. These lesions contain large number of spirochetes and are highly infectious. Symptoms of systemic illness are often present. These manifestations disappear spontaneously after several weeks or up to 1 year.

### LATENT SYPHILIS

In the latent stage of the disease, the patient is asymptomatic but the serologic tests remain positive. This stage occurs between the secondary and late stages. In the first 4 years of this stage, the disease is considered to be infectious. After 4 years the disease is considered noninfectious except in the case of a pregnant woman, who may transmit the disease to her fetus. The latent stage may continue throughout life except in those patients who develop the serious manifestations of late syphilis.

* See also Chapter 1 and Chapter 7.

## LATE SYPHILIS

*Late syphilis* is also called *tertiary syphilis* and it includes late benign syphilis, cardiovascular syphilis, and neurosyphilis. In this stage there are very few organisms but there are extensive tissue damage and scar formation.

The gumma is the characteristic lesion of late benign syphilis. This develops in approximately 15% of untreated syphilitics 1 to 10 years after the initial infection. Gummas are found mainly in the skin and bones, but visceral lesions involving the liver, cardiovascular system, or CNS may occur. Cardiovascular involvement occurs in approximately 10% of late untreated syphilitics. This occurs 10 or more years following the initial infection. The basic vascular lesion is an obliterative endarteritis of the vessels nourishing the arch of the aorta. This results in destruction of the elastic fibers of the aorta with calcification, aortic-valve insufficiency, or aneurysm formation (see Chap. 1). Neurosyphilis develops in approximately 8% of cases of untreated syphilis. Although treponemal invasion of the CNS occurs during the early stages of syphilis, symptoms do not generally appear until 5 to 35 years after infection. (see Neurosyphilis, Chap. 7)

## CONGENITAL (PRENATAL) SYPHILIS

Infection is transmitted from a pregnant woman across the placenta, usually after the 16th week of pregnancy. This may reflect the onset of fetal immunologic responsiveness. Approximately 50% of infected infants die before or shortly after birth. Of those who survive infancy, 40% develop findings of acute symptomatic syphilis characterized by massive treponemal invasion of nearly all body tissues.

## LABORATORY FINDINGS

Treponemal tests are more specific than are nontreponemal tests, and the antibody detected is usually related only to treponemal infection. These tests are, therefore, helpful in confirming the diagnosis of syphilis and in identifying persons with false-positive nontreponemal tests. The fluorescent treponemal antibody absorption (FTA-ABS) test has evolved as the standard treponemal test used today. The FTA-ABS test is more sensitive than are nontreponemal tests for primary, latent, and late syphilis. Once reactive, all treponemal tests tend to remain so for many years. None of the treponemal tests distinguishes between syphilis and other treponemal diseases.

Nontreponemal tests are available as screening tests and for evaluating treatment responses, because they fall quickly after therapy. The Veneral Disease Research Laboratory (VDRL) test is the most widely used nontreponemal test.

### Primary Syphilis

Demonstration of *T. pallidum* in darkfield examination of a chancre

Reactive nontreponemal test (76% of patients)

Reactive FTA-ABS test (90% of patients)—this is more sensitive and specific than the nontreponemal tests.

The serologic tests become reactive 1 week to 3 weeks after the chancre appears.

### Secondary Syphilis

Demonstration of *T. pallidum* in darkfield examination of skin or mucous membrane lesions

Reactive treponemal and nontreponemal serologic tests (100% of patients); high titers

### Latent Syphilis

FTA-ABS test is more frequently reactive (97%) than are the nontreponemal tests (72%).

Negative serologic test of CSF

### Late Syphilis

FTA-ABS test is more frequently reactive (95%) than are the nontreponemal tests (77%).

### Congenital Syphilis

Demonstration of *T. pallidum* in darkfield examination of skin or mucous-membrane lesions or umbilical cord

Reactive VDRL test is high titer; rising infant's titer or infant's titer higher than mother's titer establishes the diagnosis.

One must establish that the infant's reactive serum is not reflecting passively transmitted maternal antibody.

### Neurosyphilis

See Chapter 7.

## TOXOPLASMOSIS

Toxoplasmosis is a common infection caused by an intracellular protozoon, *Toxoplasma gondii*. The parasite infects most animals, but the definitive hosts are cats. The incidence in normal adults ranges from 20% to 70%, depending on age and geographic location. Because most infections are not clinically evident, the incidence is based on positive serologic tests.

The two major routes of transmission to humans are oral and congenital. Uncooked infected beef, lamb, pork, or poultry is probably the major source of human infection. Women acquiring acute infections during pregnancy expose their fetuses to the risk of transplacental infection. As pregnancy nears term, the risk of transmission to the fetus increases greatly. Congenital toxoplasmosis is a very serious disease, involving predominantly the brain and eyes.

The recognition of a parasite cycle in domestic cats has led to their being considered a major reservoir and source of infection for humans and other animals. The importance of this source of infection in any given area remains to be determined. Most epidemiologic studies have been unable to demonstrate an association of household cats with positive serologic tests for *T. gondii*.

After multiplication at the site of entry, trophozoites disseminate through the blood and lymphatics. Proliferation of trophozoites usually results in destruction of the invaded cells. However, development of humoral and cellular immunity resolves the acute infection and most of the parasites are destroyed. Those organisms that form cysts in tissue survive. Parasitic cysts may be found in every organ, but the brain, skeletal muscle, and cardiac muscle appear to be the most common sites. The cyst form of the infection is asymptomatic and is referred to as *chronic* or *latent toxoplasmosis*. Patients with this form of disease have positive serologic tests.

## LABORATORY TESTS

Identification of organisms in CSF sediment or in a biopsy of lymph node or muscle

CSF—increased protein (<2000 mg/dl); WBC 50/$\mu$l–500/$\mu$l, chiefly monocytes

### Serologic Tests

Sabin-Feldman dye test and indirect fluorescent antibody test—these detect IgG antibodies, which appear 1–2 weeks after an acute infection, peak at 6–8 weeks, and persist at low levels for life. The titer does not correlate with the severity of illness. A rising titer of antibodies is present in sera obtained 2–3 weeks following an acute infection.

Indirect hemagglutination test—antibodies appear 2–4 weeks after an acute infection, peak at 8–16 weeks, and persist for life. This is a screening test.

IgM fluorescent antibody test—IgM antibodies appear 5 days to 2 weeks after an acute infection, peak at 3–4 weeks, and usually disappear by 3–4 months. This test is useful in the diagnosis of acute toxoplasmosis.

## TRICHURIASIS

Trichuriasis is infection with the whipworm, *Trichuris trichiura*. Infection is acquired by ingestion of ova in contaminated food or water. Adult worms live in the cecum and ascending colon. Although the anterior two thirds of the adult *T. trichiura* is embedded in the colonic mucosa, the hemorrhagic lesions that result are considered less important than is the mechanical irritation caused by large masses of worms. When infection is heavy, hemorrhagic colitis may develop and lead to sloughing of the mucosa.

### LABORATORY FINDINGS

Stool contains ova of *T. trichiura* or, possibly, occult blood.

Mild eosinophilia (10%–15%)—result of heavy infection

Possible hypochromic, microcytic anemia due to chronic blood loss from heavy infection

## REFERENCES

1. Alexander H: Herpes simplex virus: A cause for concern. Am J Med Tech 48:241–245, 1982
2. Betts RF: Syndromes of cytomegalovirus infection. Adv Intern Med 26:447–466, 1980

3. Editorial: Herpes simplex, changing patterns. Lancet 2:1025–1026, 1981
4. Eisenstein BI, Masi AT: Disseminated gonococcal infection and gonococcal arthritis. Semin Arth Rheum 10:155–172, 1981
5. Felman YM, Nikitas JA: Nongonococcal urethritis: A clinical review. JAMA 245:381–386, 1981
6. Panjvani ZFK, Hanshaw JB: Cytomegalovirus in the perinatal period. Am J Dis Child 135:56–60, 1981
7. Rosenthal P, Liebman WM: Comparative study of stool examinations, duodenal aspiration and pediatric Entero-Test for giardiasis in children. J Ped 96:278–279, 1980
8. Strausbaugh LJ, Rogers WA: Giardiasis: An update on our most common parasite. Mo Med 77:393–397, 1980
9. Tummon IS, Dudley DKL, Walters JH: Genital herpes simplex. Canad Med Assoc J 125:23–29, 1981
10. Visvesvara GS: Giardia lamblia: America's No. 1 intestinal parasite. Diagn Med 4:25–28, 1981
11. Whitley RJ, Nahmias A, Visintine A et al: The natural history of herpes simplex virus infection of mother and newborn. Pediatrics 66:489–494, 1980

## *BIBLIOGRAPHY*

**Davis BD, Dulbecco R, Eisen HN et al (eds):** Microbiology, 3rd ed. Hagerstown, Harper & Row, 1980
**Hoeprich PD (ed):** Infectious Diseases, 2nd ed. Hagerstown, Harper & Row, 1977
**McLean DM:** Virology in Health Care. Baltimore, Williams & Wilkins, 1980
**Rose NR, Friedman F:** Manual of Clinical Immunology, 2nd ed. Washington, Am Soc Microbiol, 1980
**Wehrle PF, Top FH (eds):** Communicable and Infectious Diseases, 9th ed. St Louis, CV Mosby, 1981

# *INDEX*

The letter *f* following a page number indicates a figure; the letter *t* represents tabular material.